DEDICATION

We dedicate this work on medication safety to the countless healthcare professionals worldwide who work tirelessly to prevent medication errors and ensure patient safety. Your daily vigilance, commitment to continuous improvement, and unwavering dedication to patient care inspire us all. To the patients and families who have been affected by medication errors—your experiences drive our determination to improve healthcare systems and prevent future harm. To our students, who represent the future of pharmacy practice and medication safety—may this work guide you in creating safer healthcare environments for all

FUNDAMENTALS OF MEDICATION SAFETY MONITORING

Dr. Rajkiran Kolakota
Mr. Sri Venkatesh Uriti
Mr. Manoj Kumar Gembali
Mrs. Manjulatha Kornu

ISBN: 9788197973147

Scan to view online

Editors

Dr. Rajkiran Kolakota

Mr. Sri Venkatesh Uriti

Mr. Manoj Kumar Gembali

Mrs. Manjulatha Kornu

First Edition: 2025
ISBN: 9788197973147

Maximum Retail Price: Rs. 1000/- (Inclusive of all taxes)

Published by ThinkPlus Pharma Publications,
9-15/1, Indrapalem, Kakinada, AP-533006, India.
Website: www.books.jopir.in

Cover Page Illustration: Kiran Priyam Kumar Sarella

Printed at Tarangini Printing Works, Subhadra Arcade, Bhanugudi, Kakinada, AP-533003, India.

CONTENTS

ACKNOWLEDGMENTS

The creation of this textbook has been a great journey that would not have been possible without the support and contributions of many individuals and organizations. First and foremost, we express our profound gratitude to the management of Sri Sivani College of Pharmacy for their unwavering support, encouragement, and provision of resources that made this academic endeavor possible.

We extend our heartfelt thanks to our esteemed colleagues who generously shared their expertise, provided valuable feedback, and offered constructive suggestions throughout the development of this work.

We are deeply indebted to the reviewers who meticulously reviewed our manuscript and provided invaluable insights that significantly enhanced the quality and accuracy of the content.

To our families, we express our deepest gratitude for their patience, understanding, and unwavering support during the countless hours devoted to researching and writing this book. Your sacrifices have not gone unnoticed.

Finally, we thank our readers—healthcare professionals, students, administrators, and safety advocates—for your commitment to advancing medication safety. We hope this work serves as a valuable resource in your important mission

CHAPTER 1

INTRODUCTION TO MEDICATION SAFETY

Abstract

Medication safety has evolved from reactive responses to preventable tragedies toward systematic prevention approaches, catalyzed by sentinel events like the 1995 death of Betsy Lehman from chemotherapy overdose. This foundational healthcare domain encompasses processes designed to prevent patient harm throughout the medication use continuum, addressing both actual errors and potential risks. The medication use process involves multiple interdependent stages from prescribing through monitoring, with vulnerability at each transition point. The main concepts include medication error definitions, near-miss events, high-alert medications, and safety culture affecting organizational behaviors. Healthcare facilities increasingly recognize medication safety as a strategic priority requiring leadership commitment, resource allocation, and system-level interventions beyond individual vigilance. Global challenges persist through communication barriers, resource disparities, technological infrastructure variations, and inconsistent regulatory systems across different healthcare settings, necessitating context-appropriate adaptation of safety principles.

Keywords: *Medication use, Harm prevention, Safety culture, Sentinel events, Healthcare systems*

Learning Objectives

After completion of the chapter, the learners should be able to:

- Remember the key historical events that shaped modern medication safety practices.
- Understand the fundamental terminology and concepts in medication safety.
- Apply medication safety principles to identify vulnerabilities in the medication use process.
- Analyze how medication errors can occur at different stages of the medication use process.
- Evaluate the impact of safety culture on medication error prevention within healthcare organizations.
- Create strategies to address global medication safety challenges in diverse healthcare settings

HISTORY

The evolution of medication safety as a distinct discipline within healthcare has roots that extend back several centuries, though its formal recognition as a critical component of patient care is relatively recent. In early medical practice, little distinction existed between the roles of physician and apothecary, with limited standardization of medications and their preparation. The 19th century marked a significant turning point with the emergence of modern pharmaceutical manufacturing, creating a need for greater oversight of medication quality and safety.

The thalidomide tragedy of the late 1950s and early 1960s represents a watershed moment in medication safety history. This sedative, prescribed to pregnant women for morning sickness, caused thousands of severe birth defects globally before being withdrawn from market.

Table 1.1: Historical Events in Medication Safety

Year	Event	Impact on Medication Safety
1937	Sulfanilamide Disaster	100+ deaths from diethylene glycol led to the 1938 Federal Food, Drug, and Cosmetic Act requiring safety testing before marketing
1962	Thalidomide Tragedy	Birth defects from thalidomide led to Kefauver-Harris Drug Amendments requiring proof of efficacy and stricter reporting
1975	First hospital-based medication error reporting program	Establishment of systematic error detection and monitoring in hospitals
1995	Creation of United States Pharmacopeia (USP) Medication Errors Reporting Program	Formalized national voluntary reporting system for medication errors
1999	"To Err is Human" IOM Report	Estimated 7,000 deaths annually from medication errors; catalyzed national focus on medication safety
2004	WHO launched World Alliance for Patient Safety	Beginning of coordinated global effort including medication safety initiatives
2010	Affordable Care Act (US)	Introduction of financial incentives tied to medication safety outcomes

Year	Event	Impact on Medication Safety
2017	WHO Global Patient Safety Challenge: Medication Without Harm	International commitment to reduce severe, avoidable medication-related harm by 50% in 5 years
2020	COVID-19 Pandemic	Highlighted vulnerabilities in medication supply chains and accelerated telehealth medication management

This catastrophe catalyzed the development of more rigorous drug approval processes and post-marketing surveillance systems in many countries, most notably leading to the Kefauver-Harris Amendments to the Federal Food, Drug, and Cosmetic Act in the United States in 1962.

By the late 20th century, medication safety had evolved from a primarily regulatory concern to a systems-based approach. The publication of the Institute of Medicine's landmark report "To Err is Human" in 1999 represented another pivotal moment, revealing that between 44,000 and 98,000 patients died annually in American hospitals due to preventable medical errors, with medication errors comprising a significant portion. This report shifted the paradigm from individual blame to recognizing system failures, establishing medication safety as a critical priority in healthcare delivery systems worldwide.

The 21st century has seen medication safety mature into a multidisciplinary science, incorporating principles from human factors engineering, informatics, and quality improvement methodologies. The development of medication safety organizations, dedicated research centers, and specialized professionals reflects the field's growing sophistication and importance in contemporary healthcare.

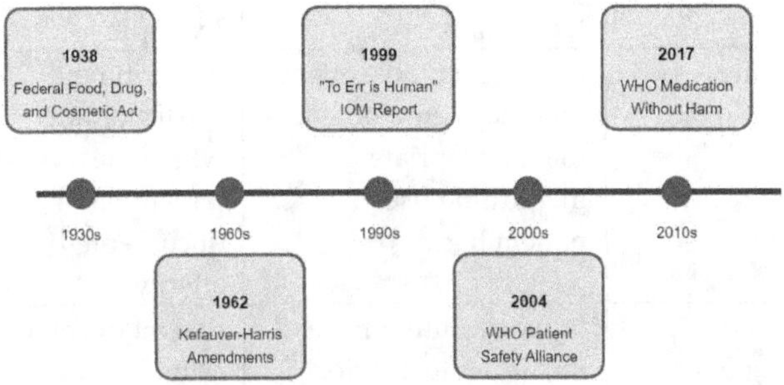

Figure 1.1 Major Milestones in Medication Safety

BASIC CONCEPTS AND TERMINOLOGY

Understanding medication safety requires familiarity with a standardized lexicon that facilitates clear communication among healthcare stakeholders. Medication safety, broadly defined, encompasses the activities and processes designed to prevent, minimize, or mitigate harm associated with medication use. This includes interventions across the medication use process: prescribing, transcribing, dispensing, administration, and monitoring.

A medication error refers to any preventable event that may cause or lead to inappropriate medication use or patient harm while the medication is in the control of the healthcare professional, patient, or consumer. Such errors may occur at any point in the medication use process and may or may not result in harm. The concept of near miss—an error that has the potential to cause harm but is intercepted before reaching the patient—is equally important in proactive safety management.

Adverse drug events (ADEs) describe injuries resulting from medication use.

Table 1.2: Medication Safety Terminology

Term	Definition	Example
Medication Error	Any preventable event that may cause or lead to inappropriate medication use or patient harm	Prescribing a medication to which the patient has a documented allergy
Adverse Drug Event (ADE)	Injury resulting from medical intervention related to a drug	Patient develops acute kidney injury after receiving contrast media
Adverse Drug Reaction (ADR)	Noxious and unintended response to a medicinal product occurring at normal doses	Rash developing after antibiotic use without any error in prescribing
Near Miss	An error that could have caused harm but did not reach the patient due to chance or intervention	Wrong dose caught by pharmacist before dispensing
Medication Reconciliation	Process of creating an accurate list of all medications a patient is taking and comparing against new orders	Comparing pre-hospital medications with admission orders
High-Alert Medications	Drugs with heightened risk of causing significant patient harm when used in error	Insulin, anticoagulants, chemotherapy agents
Safety Culture	Shared values and beliefs about the importance of safety in an organization	Environment where reporting concerns is encouraged and valued

These events can be categorized as preventable (resulting from medication errors) or non-preventable (adverse drug reactions occurring despite proper medication use). Adverse drug reactions (ADRs) specifically refer to harmful, unintended responses to medications at normal doses used for prophylaxis, diagnosis, or treatment.

High-alert medications warrant special attention, as they carry heightened risks of causing significant patient harm when used in error. Examples include anticoagulants, insulin, opioids, and concentrated electrolyte solutions. The concept of a medication use system describes the interdependent processes comprising medication selection, procurement, prescribing, order processing, dispensing, administration, and monitoring, emphasizing the interconnected nature of medication safety.

Just culture represents an organizational approach that balances accountability with a non-punitive response to errors, encouraging error reporting while maintaining professional accountability. This concept underpins modern approaches to medication safety improvement.

IMPORTANCE IN HEALTHCARE DELIVERY

Medication safety constitutes a cornerstone of healthcare quality, affecting virtually every aspect of patient care. Medications represent the most common healthcare intervention, with nearly all patients encountering pharmaceutical therapy during their healthcare journey. The economic impact of medication errors is substantial—estimated annual costs exceed $40 billion globally, with preventable ADEs adding significant length to hospital stays and increasing healthcare expenditures.

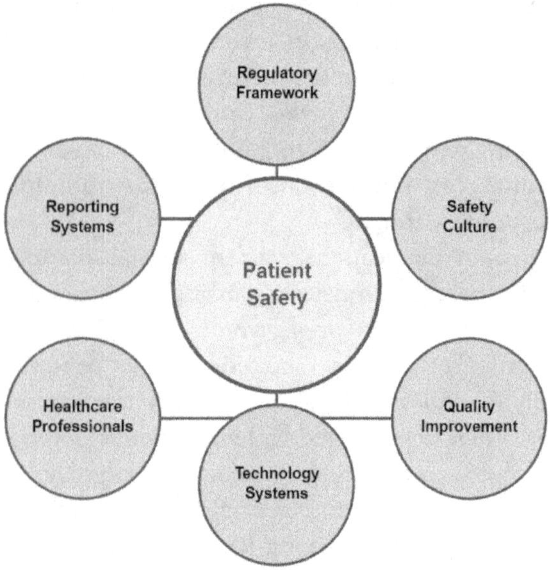

Figure 1.2 Medication Safety Systems

Beyond economic considerations, medication safety directly impacts clinical outcomes and patient experience. Preventable ADEs cause unnecessary suffering, diminish patient trust in healthcare systems, and in severe cases, result in permanent disability or death. Healthcare providers experience significant psychological distress when involved in serious medication errors, contributing to burnout and decreased job satisfaction.

Medication safety also plays a crucial role in healthcare resource allocation. Resources devoted to managing preventable medication-related harm could otherwise support positive healthcare initiatives. As healthcare systems globally face increasing financial pressures, medication safety improvements represent a significant opportunity for enhancing efficiency while improving care quality.

Table 1.3: Economic Impact of Medication Safety

Impact Domain	Statistics	Source/Year
Mortality	7,000-9,000 deaths annually from medication errors in the US	Institute of Medicine, 1999
	Estimated 1.3 million people injured annually from medication errors globally	WHO, 2017
Morbidity	1 in 10 hospital patients experience an adverse drug event	Agency for Healthcare Research and Quality, 2018
	28% of adverse drug events are preventable	Systematic review by Kanjanarat et al., 2003
Economic Cost	$40 billion in annual costs worldwide from medication errors	WHO, 2017
	$528,000 average annual cost of ADEs for a 700-bed teaching hospital	Bates et al., 1997
	$5,857 average additional hospital cost per preventable ADE	Bates et al., 1997
Healthcare Utilization	1 in 5 ADEs in ambulatory settings lead to emergency department visits	Sarkar et al., 2011
	700,000 emergency department visits annually in the US due to ADEs	CDC, 2018
	120,000 hospitalizations annually resulting from medication-related events	CDC, 2018

The intersection of medication safety with other healthcare domains underscores its systemic importance. Patient transitions between care settings—hospital admission, transfer between units, and discharge—represent particular vulnerability points for medication errors. Coordinated medication safety practices across these transitions directly affect readmission rates, patient satisfaction, and overall care continuity. In ambulatory care, medication adherence and proper administration significantly influence chronic disease management outcomes.

GLOBAL MEDICATION SAFETY

Despite advancements in healthcare delivery, medication safety remains a global challenge with significant variations across geographic, economic, and cultural contexts. The World Health Organization has designated medication safety as a global patient safety challenge, recognizing that medication-related harm represents a leading cause of preventable injury worldwide.

In high-income countries, complex healthcare systems, polypharmacy, and fragmented care present significant challenges. The aging population—often managing multiple chronic conditions with numerous medications—faces heightened risks of adverse drug interactions and medication errors. Healthcare specialization, while advancing medical knowledge, can result in communication gaps between providers regarding medication regimens. Additionally, the rapid implementation of health information technology, while offering potential safety benefits, introduces new error types when poorly designed or implemented.

Low- and middle-income countries face fundamentally different challenges. Limited regulatory infrastructure may result in substandard or falsified medications entering supply chains. Healthcare workforce shortages, particularly of pharmacists and specialized nursing staff, compromise medication safety monitoring capabilities. Limited access to electronic health records and decision support tools impedes systematic error prevention. Furthermore, patient literacy regarding medication use may be lower, complicating proper administration and adherence.

Globally shared challenges include standardization of medication naming, labeling, and packaging to prevent confusion; development of systematic approaches to medication reconciliation across care transitions; implementation of effective pharmacovigilance systems; and creation of robust error reporting cultures that encourage transparency without blame. The internationalization of pharmaceutical manufacturing and distribution adds complexity to regulatory oversight and quality assurance.

Addressing these challenges requires coordinated efforts across international bodies, national governments, healthcare organizations, professional societies, and educational institutions. Emerging approaches emphasize knowledge sharing across borders, adaptation of successful interventions to diverse contexts, patient engagement as active partners in medication safety, and leveraging technology while mitigating its risks.

Table 1.4: Global Medication Safety Challenges by Region

Region	Primary Challenges	Notable Initiatives
North America	High cost of medications Fragmented healthcare systems Complex electronic health record systems Prescription drug misuse	High-reliability organization systems Comprehensive state reporting systems FDA Sentinel Initiative Prescription drug monitoring programs
Europe	Cross-border pharmaceutical regulation Varying healthcare systems across countries Aging population with polypharmacy Multilingual medication information	European Medicines Agency pharmacovigilance European Network for Patient Safety Cross-border electronic prescriptions Falsified Medicines Directive
Asia-Pacific	Variability in regulatory systems Counterfeit medications Limited healthcare resources in some areas Rapid adoption of new technologies	Asia Pacific Economic Cooperation Regulatory Harmonization PharmacoVigilance Africa (PAVIA) WHO Western Pacific medication safety networks
Latin America	Inconsistent medication access Variable regulatory enforcement Self-medication practices Limited pharmacovigilance	Pan American Network for Drug Regulatory Harmonization PAHO Strategic Fund Regional

Region	Primary Challenges	Notable Initiatives
	infrastructure	pharmacovigilance networks
Africa	Limited healthcare infrastructure Counterfeit medication prevalence Medication shortages Limited trained personnel	African Medicines Regulatory Harmonization African Vaccine Regulatory Forum WHO essential medicines programs
Middle East	Variable regulatory systems Medication storage in extreme heat Language barriers in multinational workforces Varying levels of healthcare technology	Gulf Cooperation Council centralized drug registration Middle East & North Africa Pharmacovigilance Congress National pharmacovigilance centers

Things to Remember

- ☑ Medication safety has evolved from reactive responses to preventable tragedies toward systematic prevention following sentinel events like the 1995 death of Betsy Lehman.
- ☑ The medication use process involves multiple interdependent stages (prescribing, transcribing, dispensing, administering, and monitoring) with vulnerability at each transition point.
- ☑ Medication errors can occur without patient harm (near misses), while adverse drug events may occur even with correct medication use.
- ☑ Safety culture significantly influences medication safety through shared beliefs, values, and behaviors regarding error reporting and

prevention.

☑ System-based approaches recognize that errors typically result from multiple system failures rather than individual negligence.

☑ Global medication safety challenges include communication barriers, resource disparities, infrastructure limitations, and varied regulatory systems requiring context-appropriate solutions.

Multiple Choice Questions

1. Which sentinel event in 1995 is often cited as a catalyst for modern medication safety initiatives?
   a) The Elixir Sulfanilamide disaster
   b) The death of Betsy Lehman from chemotherapy overdose
   c) The thalidomide tragedy
   d) The heparin contamination crisis
2. The medication use process includes which of the following stages? (Select all that apply)
   a) Prescribing
   b) Marketing
   c) Dispensing
   d) Administering
   e) Manufacturing
3. Which of the following best defines a "near miss" in medication safety?
   a) A medication error that causes patient harm
   b) A medication error that is intercepted before reaching the patient
   c) An adverse drug reaction from correct medication use

d) A manufacturing defect in a pharmaceutical product

4. According to systems thinking in medication safety, errors most commonly result from:
   a) Individual incompetence or negligence
   b) Patient non-compliance with medication regimens
   c) Multiple system failures rather than individual factors
   d) Inadequate regulatory oversight of pharmaceutical products
5. Which of the following is NOT considered a high-alert medication category?
   a) Anticoagulants
   b) Insulin
   c) Antibiotics
   d) Chemotherapy agents
6. What concept describes an organization's shared beliefs, values, and behaviors regarding error reporting and prevention?
   a) Regulatory compliance
   b) Safety culture
   c) Quality assurance
   d) Clinical governance
7. The "Five Rights" of medication administration include all of the following EXCEPT:
   a) Right patient
   b) Right dose
   c) Right manufacturer
   d) Right time
8. Which of the following represents a transition point in the medication use process that

presents vulnerability for errors?
a) From prescribing to transcribing
b) From manufacturing to marketing
c) From research to development
d) From patenting to licensing

9. Global medication safety challenges include all of the following EXCEPT:
a) Communication barriers between healthcare providers
b) Resource disparities between healthcare systems
c) Uniform regulatory systems across all countries
d) Variable technological infrastructure

10. Which approach to medication safety focuses on preventing errors through system design rather than individual vigilance?
a) Punitive approach
b) Education-based approach
c) Systems-based approach
d) Regulatory approach

Self-Assessment Questions

1. Describe the historical evolution of medication safety as a discipline, highlighting key events and their impact on modern healthcare practices.
2. Explain the fundamental concepts and terminology in medication safety, including definitions of medication errors, adverse drug events, and near misses.
3. Critically analyze the importance of medication safety in healthcare delivery systems and its impact on patient outcomes and healthcare costs.
4. Compare and contrast global approaches to medication safety, including initiatives by major organizations such as WHO and differences between high and low-resource countries.
5. Evaluate how the patient safety movement has influenced the development of medication safety practices over the past three decades.
6. Discuss the relationship between medication safety and healthcare quality, explaining how they are interconnected within healthcare delivery systems.
7. Analyze the economic impact of medication errors and the cost-effectiveness of medication safety programs.
8. Examine the role of organizational culture in promoting medication safety and strategies for cultivating a culture of safety.

9. Explain the concept of a "just culture" and its importance in medication safety reporting and improvement.
10. Discuss how medication safety metrics are defined, measured, and used to improve safety practices globally.

Bibliography

1. Bates DW, Cullen DJ, Laird N, Petersen LA, Small SD, Servi D, et al. Incidence of adverse drug events and potential adverse drug events. Implications for prevention. ADE Prevention Study Group. JAMA. 1995;274(1):29-34.
2. Kohn LT, Corrigan JM, Donaldson MS, editors. To Err Is Human: Building a Safer Health System. Washington, DC: National Academies Press; 2000.
3. Leape LL, Brennan TA, Laird N, Lawthers AG, Localio AR, Barnes BA, et al. The nature of adverse events in hospitalized patients. Results of the Harvard Medical Practice Study II. N Engl J Med. 1991;324(6):377-84.
4. Aspden P, Wolcott J, Bootman JL, Cronenwett LR, editors. Preventing Medication Errors: Quality Chasm Series. Washington, DC: National Academies Press; 2007.
5. Phillips J, Beam S, Brinker A, Holquist C, Honig P, Lee LY, et al. Retrospective analysis of mortalities associated with medication errors. Am J Health Syst Pharm. 2001;58(19):1835-41.
6. Leape LL, Bates DW, Cullen DJ, Cooper J, Demonaco HJ, Gallivan T, et al. Systems analysis of adverse drug events. ADE Prevention Study Group. JAMA. 1995;274(1):35-43.
7. WHO. Medication Without Harm - Global Patient Safety Challenge on Medication Safety. Geneva: World Health Organization; 2017.
8. Cohen MR, editor. Medication Errors. 2nd ed. Washington, DC: American Pharmacists Association; 2010.
9. Reason J. Human error: models and management. BMJ. 2000;320(7237):768-70.
10. Wachter RM. Understanding Patient Safety. 3rd ed. New York: McGraw-Hill Education; 2018.

CHAPTER 2

REGULATORY STANDARDS

Abstract

Regulatory standards provide essential structure for medication safety through multilayered oversight addressing different aspects of pharmaceutical use. International bodies including WHO and ICH establish baseline standards, harmonize approaches across borders, and facilitate global collaboration through programs like Medication Without Harm. National regulatory authorities such as FDA, EMA, and MHRA enforce country-specific requirements through approval processes, post-marketing surveillance, and enforcement mechanisms with varying approaches to safety oversight. Professional organizations including ISMP, JCI, and discipline-specific associations provide specialized guidance through accreditation programs, practice standards, and evidence-based recommendations complementing governmental regulation. Healthcare facilities must navigate complex compliance requirements involving documentation standards, mandatory reporting obligations, staff credentialing verification, technology validation processes, and ongoing quality assessment activities, often requiring dedicated resources for monitoring evolving requirements and maintaining regulatory adherence across diverse operational areas.

Keywords: *Regulatory oversight, Compliance verification, Standards harmonization, Accreditation, Safety legislation*

Learning Objectives

After completion of the chapter, the learners should be able to:

- Remember the key international and national regulatory bodies governing medication safety.
- Understand how different levels of regulation complement each other in the medication safety framework.
- Apply regulatory requirements to develop compliant medication safety practices in healthcare settings.
- Analyze the relationship between professional standards and governmental regulations in medication safety.
- Evaluate the effectiveness of specific regulatory approaches in preventing medication errors.
- Create a compliance monitoring system addressing multiple regulatory requirements in a healthcare setting

INTERNATIONAL REGULATIONS

International regulations establish fundamental principles for medication safety while accommodating regional variations in healthcare delivery. The World Health Organization (WHO) serves as the primary global coordinator for medication safety initiatives through its Essential Medicines Programme and pharmacovigilance activities. The WHO's International Drug Monitoring Programme, established in 1968, now encompasses over 170 countries in a collaborative network for adverse drug reaction monitoring, with the Uppsala Monitoring Centre in Sweden serving as its operational headquarters.

The International Council for Harmonisation of Technical Requirements for Pharmaceuticals for Human Use (ICH) represents a pivotal organization in global medication regulation. Formed in 1990, the ICH brings together regulatory authorities and pharmaceutical industry representatives to harmonize guidelines for drug development and registration. Its guidelines on Good Clinical Practice (GCP), Good Manufacturing Practice (GMP), and pharmacovigilance have been widely adopted internationally, establishing consistent standards for medication safety across jurisdictions.

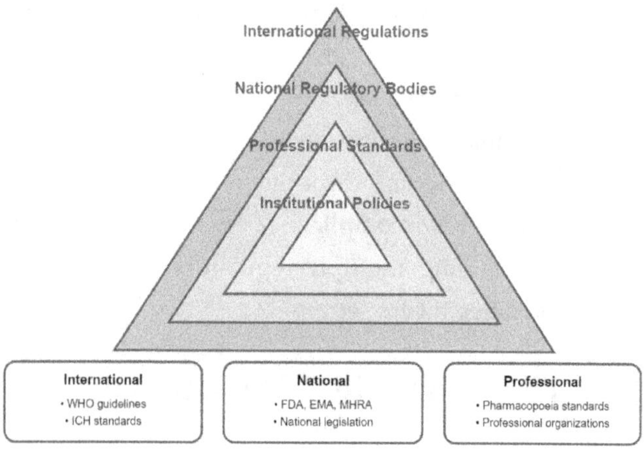

Figure 2.1 Hierarchy of Medication Safety Regulatory Bodies

The International Organization for Standardization (ISO) contributes to medication safety through standards development in areas including medical device safety, quality management systems, and risk management in pharmaceutical manufacturing. ISO 9001 certification has become a recognized benchmark for quality management in pharmaceutical organizations worldwide.

International conventions governing narcotic drugs and psychotropic substances provide systems for controlling medications with abuse potential while ensuring appropriate medical access.

Table 2.1: International Regulatory Bodies and Their Roles in Medication Safety

Organization	Medication Safety Functions	Initiatives
World Health Organization (WHO)	Sets international standards Coordinates global safety initiatives Promotes medication safety research Monitors global trends	Global Patient Safety Challenge: Medication Without Harm International Drug Monitoring Programme Essential Medicines List Prequalification of medicines
International Council for Harmonisation (ICH)	Harmonizes technical requirements Develops quality, safety, and efficacy guidelines Standardizes pharmacovigilance practices	Common Technical Document format Good Clinical Practice standards MedDRA standardized medical terminology E2B electronic transmission of ADR reports
International Organization for Standardization (ISO)	Develops technical standards Creates medication safety-related standards	ISO 9001 Quality Management Systems ISO 13485 Medical Devices Quality

Organization	Medication Safety Functions	Initiatives
	Establishes quality management systems	Management ISO/TS 22224 Medication Management ISO 31000 Risk Management
European Medicines Agency (EMA)	Centralizes drug approvals Monitors medication safety Coordinates pharmacovigilance activities Issues safety alerts	EudraVigilance database European Risk Management Strategy Falsified Medicines Directive Good Pharmacovigilance Practices (GVP)
Pan American Health Organization (PAHO)	Regional medication safety coordination Strengthens regulatory systems Promotes access to safe medicines	Strategic Fund for essential medicines Pan American Network for Drug Regulatory Harmonization Regional Platform on Access and Innovation
Asia-Pacific Economic Cooperation (APEC)	Promotes regulatory convergence Facilitates information sharing Strengthens supply chain integrity	APEC Regulatory Harmonization Steering Committee Supply Chain Security Toolkit Roadmap for Medical Product Regulatory Convergence

The Single Convention on Narcotic Drugs (1961), Convention on Psychotropic Substances (1971), and Convention Against Illicit Traffic in Narcotic Drugs and Psychotropic Substances (1988) establish reporting requirements, import/export controls, and manufacturing limitations that profoundly influence medication safety practices for controlled substances.

Harmonization efforts continue to face challenges, particularly in balancing regulatory stringency with practical implementation across varied economic contexts. The WHO's prequalification programme for medications represents a pragmatic approach, providing quality assurance for essential medicines in regions with limited regulatory capacity, thereby addressing medication safety beyond traditional regulatory systems.

NATIONAL REGULATORY BODIES

National regulatory agencies serve as primary authorities for ensuring medication safety within their jurisdictions, with substantial variation in scope, authority, and resources. The United States Food and Drug Administration (FDA) represents one of the most influential regulatory bodies, with comprehensive authority over drug approval, manufacturing standards, post-marketing surveillance, and product recalls. The FDA's Adverse Event Reporting System (FAERS) collects voluntary reports of adverse drug reactions and medication errors, generating signals for potential safety concerns requiring investigation.

Table 2.2: National Regulatory Authorities and Their Medication Safety Oversight

Country	Regulatory Authority	Primary Medication Safety Functions	Main Programs
United States	Food and Drug Administration (FDA)	Pre-market approval Post-market surveillance Safety communications Regulatory enforcement	MedWatch reporting system Sentinel Initiative Risk Evaluation and Mitigation Strategies (REMS) Safety labeling changes
United Kingdom	Medicines and Healthcare products Regulatory Agency (MHRA)	Marketing authorizations Post-market surveillance Medication alerts Device regulation	Yellow Card Scheme Drug Safety Update Good Pharmacovigilance Practice Falsified Medicines Directive implementation
Japan	Pharmaceuticals and Medical Devices Agency (PMDA)	Drug approvals Safety monitoring Quality standards Relief services for health	Japanese Adverse Drug Event Report database Relief System for Adverse Drug Reactions Early

Country	Regulatory Authority	Primary Medication Safety Functions	Main Programs
		damage	Postmarketing Phase Vigilance Medical Information for Risk Assessment Initiative
Australia	Therapeutic Goods Administration (TGA)	Product registration Safety monitoring Compliance activities Adverse event reporting	Database of Adverse Event Notifications Black Triangle Scheme Pharmacovigilance Inspection Program Medicine Shortages Information Initiative
Canada	Health Canada	Drug authorization Post-market surveillance Compliance and enforcement Risk communication	Canada Vigilance Program Protecting Canadians from Unsafe Drugs Act Risk Management Plans Summary Safety Review program
India	Central Drugs	Drug approval Standards	Pharmacovigilance

Country	Regulatory Authority	Primary Medication Safety Functions	Main Programs
	Standard Control Organization (CDSCO)	setting Import licensing Post-marketing surveillance	Programme of India Indian Pharmacopoeia Schedule H1 to control antimicrobial resistance New Drugs and Clinical Trials Rules
Brazil	Brazilian Health Regulatory Agency (ANVISA)	Marketing authorization Pharmacovigilance Inspection and enforcement Quality control	National Pharmacovigilance System Drug Safety Alerts Post-registration Monitoring Antimicrobial Control Program

The European Medicines Agency (EMA) operates with a different organizational model, coordinating the European Union's decentralized network of national regulatory authorities. The EMA's centralized approval procedure enables simultaneous medication authorization across all EU member states, while its EudraVigilance system aggregates adverse event reports throughout Europe. Following the United Kingdom's exit from the European Union, the Medicines and Healthcare products Regulatory Agency (MHRA) has resumed independent regulatory functions with continued reciprocal recognition arrangements.

Japan's Pharmaceuticals and Medical Devices Agency (PMDA) exercises regulatory oversight through a system that incorporates unique ethnopharmacological considerations reflecting genetic variations in Japanese populations. China's National Medical Products Administration (NMPA) has undergone significant reform to enhance regulatory capacity commensurate with the country's expanding pharmaceutical sector.

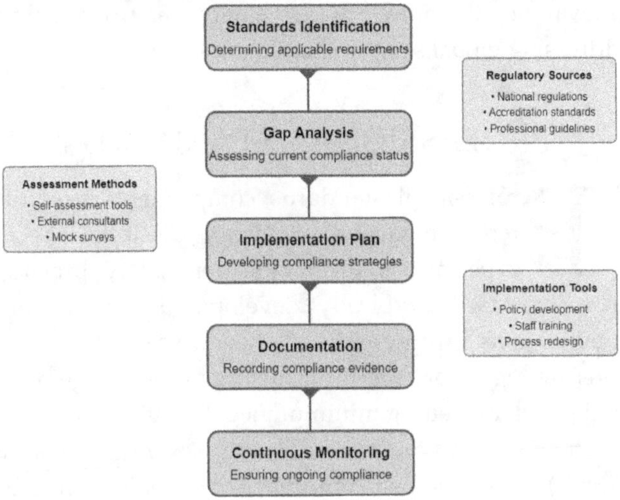

Figure 2.2 Process of Medication Safety Regulatory Compliance

In emerging economies, regulatory capacity varies substantially. Brazil's Agência Nacional de Vigilância Sanitária (ANVISA) and India's Central Drugs Standard Control Organization (CDSCO) have developed increasingly sophisticated regulatory systems, though implementation challenges persist. The South African Health Products Regulatory Authority (SAHPRA) exemplifies evolving regulatory structures in Africa, with increasing capacity for both pre-market evaluation and post-marketing surveillance.

Regardless of variations in structure and resources, national regulatory authorities typically share core functions essential to medication safety: pre-market evaluation of safety and efficacy, manufacturing oversight, pharmacovigilance, labeling and packaging requirements, and enforcement actions for non-compliance. Contemporary challenges include regulating digital health technologies, balancing timely access to innovative therapies with safety assurance, and addressing global supply chain complexity.

PROFESSIONAL STANDARDS

Professional standards complement regulatory requirements by establishing discipline-specific expectations for medication safety practices. These standards, typically developed by professional organizations representing healthcare disciplines, translate regulatory requirements into practical guidance while often exceeding minimum legal requirements.

The American Society of Health-System Pharmacists (ASHP) has developed comprehensive medication safety standards addressing medication use processes across healthcare settings. These standards provide detailed guidance on high-alert medications, technology implementation, and safety monitoring systems. Similarly, the International Pharmaceutical Federation (FIP) establishes global standards for pharmaceutical practice that incorporate medication safety principles adaptable to diverse practice environments.

Nursing standards, such as those developed by the American Nurses Association and International Council of Nurses, delineate medication administration safety practices, documentation requirements, and patient education responsibilities. These standards emphasize the nurse's role in medication reconciliation, independent verification of high-risk medications, and vigilant monitoring for adverse effects.

Medical professional organizations, including the American Medical Association and Royal Colleges of Physicians, have established prescribing standards addressing legibility, completeness, and documentation of medication orders. Increasingly, these standards incorporate guidance on electronic prescribing practices and communication during care transitions to prevent medication errors.

Table 2.3: Professional Standards Organizations and Their Medication Safety Guidelines

Organization	Medication Safety Standards	Implementation Resources
Institute for Safe Medication Practices (ISMP)	High-alert medication lists Error-prone abbreviations Medication storage guidelines Best practices for medication safety	Self-assessment tools Focused safety assessments Error reporting programs Targeted medication safety best practices
The Joint Commission (TJC)	National Patient Safety Goals Medication management standards Reconciliation requirements High-alert medication standards	Implementation guides Tracers methodology Sentinel Event Alert publications Center for Transforming Healthcare resources
American Society of Health-System Pharmacists (ASHP)	Practice standards for acute and ambulatory care Guidelines for preventing medication errors	Policy positions Practice advancement initiatives Best practice tools Professional guidelines

Organization	Medication Safety Standards	Implementation Resources
	Sterile product preparation standards Controlled substance guidelines	
European Association of Hospital Pharmacists (EAHP)	European Statements of Hospital Pharmacy Standards for clinical pharmacy services Guidelines for medication preparation Automation utilization standards	Implementation toolkit Common training framework Self-assessment tools Position papers
International Pharmaceutical Federation (FIP)	Good Pharmacy Practice standards Patient safety systems Medication use competencies Guidelines for pharmacist interventions	Practice transformation toolkits Continuing education programs Global pharmacy standards Policy statements
Society of Hospital Pharmacists of Australia (SHPA)	Standards of Practice Medication safety position statements Guidelines for high-risk medications Pharmacist intervention documentation	Practice guidelines Don't Rush to Crush handbook Pharmacy residency framework Medication Safety Position Statements

Accreditation standards represent a particularly influential category of professional standards with direct implications for organizational practices. The Joint Commission's medication management standards in the United States and similar requirements from Accreditation Canada and the Australian Council on Healthcare Standards establish comprehensive organizational expectations that significantly exceed regulatory minimums. These standards address medication storage, preparation, administration, documentation, and ongoing quality improvement activities.

A contemporary development in professional standards involves increased interprofessional collaboration in standard development. Organizations such as the Institute for Safe Medication Practices (ISMP) have pioneered multidisciplinary approaches to developing medication safety guidelines that transcend traditional professional boundaries, reflecting the systemic nature of medication safety challenges.

COMPLIANCE REQUIREMENTS

Compliance with medication safety regulations and standards involves systematic organizational processes for implementation, documentation, and verification. Healthcare organizations must establish robust medication safety programs that integrate regulatory requirements, accreditation standards, and professional guidelines into operational practices while demonstrating measurable adherence.

Documentation requirements constitute a fundamental aspect of compliance, encompassing medication administration records, adverse event reports, quality improvement activities, and staff competency verification. Contemporary electronic health record systems incorporate structured documentation tools designed to ensure regulatory compliance while supporting clinical workflows, though implementation quality varies substantially.

Mandatory reporting systems represent significant compliance obligations in many jurisdictions. In the

United States, the FDA's MedWatch program requires reporting of serious adverse events and product quality issues for approved medications. Similar requirements exist through the EMA's EudraVigilance system in Europe and the Yellow Card Scheme in the United Kingdom. Healthcare organizations must establish internal processes to identify reportable events, submit required information within specified timeframes, and maintain records of submissions.

Risk Evaluation and Mitigation Strategies (REMS) in the United States and Risk Management Plans (RMPs) in Europe represent structured programs required for certain medications with significant safety concerns. These programs may mandate restricted distribution systems, special certification for prescribers or dispensers, patient registries, or enhanced monitoring protocols. Healthcare organizations must integrate these requirements into medication use processes to maintain compliance and access to these medications.

Controlled substance regulations impose particularly stringent compliance requirements. These include secure storage systems, perpetual inventory maintenance, documentation of each dose, regular reconciliation procedures, and reporting of discrepancies. Electronic systems for controlled substance management have improved compliance efficiency while preserving necessary controls.

Compliance verification occurs through internal audit processes and external inspections. Organizations typically implement tiered audit approaches, with routine operational audits complemented by periodic comprehensive evaluations against regulatory standards. External verification may include regulatory inspections, accreditation surveys, or third-party certifications, each evaluating different aspects of medication safety compliance.

Penalties for non-compliance range from improvement plans to financial sanctions, operational restrictions, or in extreme cases, facility closure. The compliance function increasingly emphasizes proactive risk identification and mitigation rather than reactive responses to identified deficiencies, reflecting evolving perspectives on regulatory effectiveness in complex healthcare systems

Table 2.4: Regulatory Compliance Requirements for Healthcare Organizations

Domain	Typical Requirements	Monitoring and Enforcement
Medication Management Systems	Written medication management policies Clear lines of responsibility Medication administration standards Storage and security controls	Internal audits External regulatory surveys Quality measure reporting Incident review processes
Staff Competency and Training	Demonstrated competencies Initial and ongoing education Specialty training for high-risk areas Documentation of training	Competency assessments Direct observation Knowledge testing Peer review processes
Error Reporting and Analysis	Error reporting system Near-miss reporting	Reporting rates tracking Types of events reported

	Root cause analysis for serious events Performance improvement processes	Implementation of improvements External mandatory reporting
Medication Reconciliation	Process at all transitions of care Defined responsibilities Documentation requirements Quality monitoring	Compliance rate monitoring Discrepancy tracking Patient outcome measures Documentation audits
High-Alert Medications	Identification of high-alert medications Special handling procedures Documentation requirements Additional safety controls	Compliance observations Targeted audits Event analysis Outcome measures
Technology Implementation	Technology safety assessments User training requirements Downtime procedures Maintenance standards	Technology utilization rates Override monitoring Workaround tracking Alert fatigue assessment

Things to Remember

- ☑ International regulations provide baseline standards through WHO's Medication Without Harm initiative and ICH guidelines harmonizing requirements across regions.
- ☑ National regulatory bodies including FDA, EMA, and MHRA oversee medication approval, surveillance, and safety communication with varying approaches to oversight.
- ☑ Professional standards complement governmental regulations through organizations like ISMP, JCI, and discipline-specific associations providing specialized guidance.
- ☑ Compliance requirements include documentation standards, mandatory reporting obligations, staff credentialing verification, technology validation, and ongoing quality assessment.
- ☑ Regulatory expectations continuously evolve, requiring dedicated resources for monitoring requirements and maintaining adherence.
- ☑ Effective compliance balances technical requirement satisfaction with meaningful safety improvement rather than purely administrative focus.

Multiple Choice Questions

1. Which international organization launched the "Medication Without Harm" global patient safety challenge?

   a) International Pharmaceutical Federation (FIP)

   b) World Health Organization (WHO)

   c) International Council of Nurses (ICN)

d) International Society for Pharmacovigilance (ISOP)

2. The International Council for Harmonisation (ICH) primarily focuses on:
   a) Setting standards for pharmacist education globally
   b) Harmonizing pharmaceutical regulations across different regions
   c) Developing nursing practice guidelines for medication administration
   d) Establishing hospital accreditation standards worldwide
3. Which national regulatory body is responsible for medication approval and safety monitoring in the United States?
   a) European Medicines Agency (EMA)
   b) Medicines and Healthcare products Regulatory Agency (MHRA)
   c) Food and Drug Administration (FDA)
   d) Therapeutic Goods Administration (TGA)
4. Professional standards for medication safety differ from governmental regulations in that they typically:
   a) Have stronger legal enforcement mechanisms
   b) Focus more on specialized practice areas and clinical considerations
   c) Are developed without input from practicing clinicians
   d) Change less frequently than governmental regulations
5. Which organization provides specialized medication safety guidelines through its

International Medication Safety Self-Assessment tool?
a) Joint Commission International (JCI)
b) Institute for Safe Medication Practices (ISMP)
c) Agency for Healthcare Research and Quality (AHRQ)
d) International Organization for Standardization (ISO)

6. Hospital accreditation standards addressing medication safety:
a) Replace the need for compliance with national regulatory requirements
b) Focus exclusively on documentation practices
c) Typically require interdisciplinary approaches to medication management
d) Are identical across all countries and healthcare settings

7. Compliance with medication safety regulations requires:
a) Focus solely on documentation practices
b) Annual review of requirements by a single designated individual
c) Dedicated resources for ongoing monitoring of evolving requirements
d) Prioritizing governmental regulations over professional standards

8. Which of the following is NOT typically included in regulatory compliance requirements for medication safety?
a) Staff credentialing verification
b) Technology validation processes

c) Marketing strategies for pharmaceutical products

d) Mandatory error reporting obligations

9. The primary goal of medication safety regulations should be:

   a) Creating administrative documentation

   b) Preventing patient harm through safe practices

   c) Limiting liability for healthcare organizations

   d) Streamlining the medication use process

10. Regulatory oversight of medication safety can be described as:

    a) Static, with infrequent changes to requirements

    b) Focused exclusively on pharmaceutical manufacturers

    c) Multilayered, with international, national, and professional components

    d) Consistent across all countries and healthcare settings

Self-Assessment Questions

1. Compare and contrast the medication safety regulatory approaches of three major international organizations (e.g., WHO, ICH, EMA), highlighting their unique contributions.
2. Critically analyze how the FDA's regulatory framework for medication safety has evolved over time and its impact on healthcare delivery in the United States.
3. Evaluate the effectiveness of professional standards from organizations like ISMP, ASHP, and JCI in promoting medication safety globally.
4. Discuss the challenges healthcare organizations face in maintaining compliance with multiple regulatory requirements and strategies to address these challenges.
5. Analyze the impact of regulatory harmonization efforts on global medication safety practices and patient outcomes.
6. Explain how regulatory bodies enforce medication safety standards and the consequences of non-compliance for healthcare organizations.
7. Evaluate the role of accreditation processes in promoting medication safety and their relationship with regulatory requirements.
8. Compare the approaches to medication safety regulation in at least three different countries, analyzing strengths and weaknesses of each system.

9. Discuss how medication safety regulations address emerging technologies and practices, including the challenges of regulating novel pharmaceutical products and delivery systems.
10. Critically analyze the balance between regulatory oversight and innovation in medication safety practices, with examples of how this balance affects healthcare delivery

Bibliography

1. World Health Organization. The third WHO Global Patient Safety Challenge: Medication Without Harm. Geneva: World Health Organization; 2017.
2. International Council for Harmonisation of Technical Requirements for Pharmaceuticals for Human Use (ICH). Quality Guidelines. Geneva: ICH; 2020.
3. Ndomondo-Sigonda M, Miot J, Naidoo S, Dodoo A, Kaale E. Medicines regulation in Africa: current state and opportunities. Pharmaceut Med. 2017;31(6):383-97.
4. Lexchin J. Health Canada's use of its priority review process for new drugs: a cohort study. BMJ Open. 2015;5(5):e006816.
5. Hamburg MA, Sharfstein JM. The FDA as a public health agency. N Engl J Med. 2009;360(24):2493-5.
6. European Medicines Agency. Guideline on good pharmacovigilance practices (GVP). London: European Medicines Agency; 2017.
7. Therapeutic Goods Administration. Pharmacovigilance responsibilities of medicine sponsors: Australian recommendations and requirements. Canberra: Australian Government Department of Health; 2018.
8. U.S. Food and Drug Administration. Strategic Plan for Preventing and Mitigating Drug Shortages. Silver Spring, MD: FDA; 2013.
9. Medicines and Healthcare products Regulatory Agency. Good pharmacovigilance practice guide. London: MHRA; 2009.
10. The Joint Commission. Comprehensive Accreditation Manual for Hospitals: The Patient Safety Systems Chapter. Oakbrook Terrace, IL: The Joint Commission; 2020.

CHAPTER 3

MEDICATION ERRORS AND PREVENTION

Abstract

Medication errors encompass various types including prescribing inaccuracies, transcription omissions, dispensing mistakes, administration failures, and monitoring oversights, with classification systems addressing both error characteristics and harm outcomes. Root cause analysis methodologies identify systemic factors contributing to errors, distinguishing between active failures at the point of care and latent conditions within organizational systems through structured investigation techniques. Prevention strategies incorporate high-reliability principles through technological safeguards like computerized order entry and barcode scanning, standardized processes reducing unnecessary variation, human factors engineering addressing cognitive limitations, and redundant verification systems providing multiple error detection opportunities. Reporting systems enable systematic learning from errors through confidential mechanisms that separate occurrence identification from punitive consequences while supporting aggregate analysis for pattern recognition, priority setting, and intervention effectiveness evaluation driving continuous improvement.

Keywords: *Error classification, Root cause analysis, Prevention measures, Reporting systems, Systems thinking*

Learning Objectives

After completion of the chapter, the learners should be able to:

- Remember the different types and classifications of medication errors.
- Understand how root cause analysis methodologies identify underlying factors contributing to medication errors.
- Apply the hierarchy of effectiveness principles to select optimal error prevention strategies.
- Analyze how both active failures and latent conditions contribute to medication error occurrence.
- Evaluate the effectiveness of different error prevention approaches based on evidence and theoretical systems.
- Create a comprehensive error reporting and analysis system that supports learning while maintaining appropriate accountability.

TYPES OF MEDICATION ERRORS

Medication errors encompass a diverse spectrum of events occurring throughout the medication use process, each with distinct characteristics, contributing factors, and preventive approaches. Understanding the taxonomy of medication errors provides a foundation for targeted prevention strategies and systematic improvement efforts.

Prescribing errors represent the most frequent type of medication error, occurring when a medication order is written incorrectly or inappropriately. These errors include inappropriate drug selection for the patient's condition, incorrect dosage calculations, failure to account for patient-specific factors such as renal impairment or allergies, contraindicated drug combinations, and incomplete or illegible orders. Computerized prescriber order entry systems have reduced traditional illegibility issues but introduced new error mechanisms such as selection of incorrect items from dropdown menus and alert fatigue from excessive warnings.

Transcription errors occur when medication orders are incorrectly transferred from their original form to another documentation system. Although increasingly rare in electronic health record environments, these errors persist in hybrid paper-electronic systems and during system downtime procedures. Common transcription errors include misinterpretation of abbreviations, decimal point misplacement, and omission of essential order components such as route or frequency.

Dispensing errors occur during the medication preparation and distribution process, typically within pharmacy departments. These include selection of incorrect medications (particularly those with look-alike packaging or sound-alike names), compounding errors involving incorrect calculations or ingredients, inappropriate packaging or labeling, and failure to identify contraindications or interactions during verification processes. Environmental factors such as lighting, interruptions, and workspace design significantly influence dispensing error rates.

Administration errors occur when medications are incorrectly provided to patients. These include wrong patient errors (failure to verify patient identity), wrong time errors (medications given outside acceptable timeframes), wrong dose errors (including incorrect measurement of liquid medications), wrong route errors (such as oral solutions administered intravenously), and omission errors (failure to administer ordered medications). Administration errors represent the final opportunity for error interception before reaching the patient, making their prevention particularly critical.

Table 3.1: Types of Medication Errors by Process Stage

Process Stage	Error Types	Common Causes
Prescribing	Wrong drug Wrong dose/frequency Wrong route Omission errors Inappropriate medication Therapeutic duplication Incomplete orders Illegible handwriting	Knowledge deficits Calculation errors Inadequate patient information Look-alike/sound-alike drugs Distractions Alert fatigue
Transcribing	Misinterpretation of orders Incorrect entry into systems Dropped or added information Unit conversion errors	Illegible handwriting Sound-alike medications Abbreviation misinterpretation Distractions Communication barriers
Dispensing	Wrong drug Wrong dose/quantity Wrong formulation Wrong patient Labeling errors Compounding errors	Look-alike packaging Similar medication names Workload pressures Storage problems

Process Stage	Error Types	Common Causes
Administration	Wrong patient Wrong time Wrong dose Wrong route Omitted doses Extra doses Technique errors	Failure to verify identity Interruptions Documentation errors Poor communication Workflow issues Lack of standardization
Monitoring	Failure to monitor Failure to intervene Inadequate follow-up Missed laboratory tests Failure to recognize adverse effects	Lack of assigned responsibility Communication breakdowns Inadequate monitoring parameters Knowledge deficits Fragmented care

Monitoring errors involve failures to appropriately assess patient responses to medications, recognize adverse effects, or make necessary adjustments to therapy. These include inadequate laboratory monitoring for medications requiring serum level or organ function assessment, failure to recognize or respond to signs of adverse drug reactions, and inappropriate continuation of medications despite changing patient conditions. Monitoring errors frequently involve communication failures across care transitions or between healthcare team members.

Each error type exhibits characteristic patterns influenced by medication complexity, patient factors, environmental conditions, and system design. High-alert medications such as anticoagulants, insulin, opioids, and electrolyte solutions present disproportionate risks, with errors involving these agents more likely to cause serious harm. Understanding the specific mechanisms of different error types enables development of targeted prevention strategies addressing their unique contributing factors.

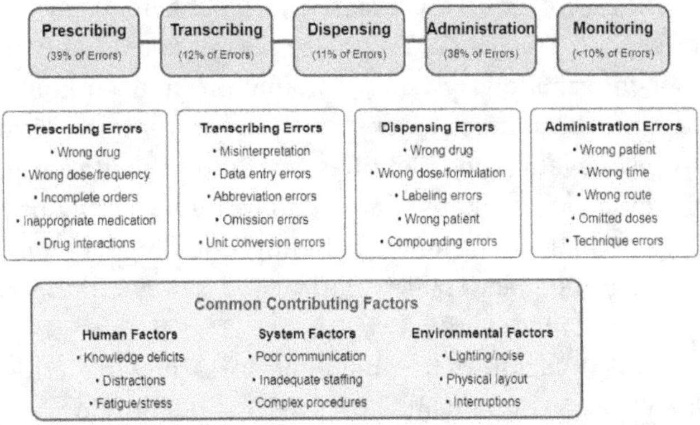

Figure 3.1 Types of Medication Errors by Process

ROOT CAUSE ANALYSIS

Root cause analysis (RCA) represents a structured methodology for investigating medication errors to identify underlying system vulnerabilities rather than focusing on individual performance. This approach recognizes that serious medication errors typically result from multiple system failures rather than isolated human mistakes, aligning with James Reason's "Swiss cheese model" of accident causation in complex systems.

The RCA process typically begins with comprehensive event description, establishing what occurred without attribution of blame or responsibility. This phase involves detailed timeline construction, identification of involved personnel and their roles, examination of documentation, and assessment of actual or potential patient impact. Multiple information sources are triangulated to develop a comprehensive understanding of the event sequence.

Investigation then progresses to identification of contributing factors across several domains. Human factors analysis determines how environmental conditions, cognitive processes, and behavioral patterns influenced the event. Technology assessment evaluates how information systems, automation, and equipment design contributed to or failed to prevent the error. Process evaluation identifies workflow inefficiencies, communication gaps, and procedural ambiguities. Organizational factors including staffing patterns, training adequacy, policy clarity, and safety culture are systematically identified.

Causal factor determination represents the critical analytical component of RCA, identifying the relationships between contributing factors and distinguishing proximate causes from underlying systemic vulnerabilities.

Table 3.2: Root Cause Analysis Components for Medication Errors

Root Cause Category	**Investigation Methods**	**Sample Questions**
Human Factors	Interviews with involved staff Workload analysis Performance observation Clinical knowledge assessment Simulation of event	What was the workload at the time? Were there distractions or interruptions? Did staff have necessary knowledge? How were handoffs conducted? Were cognitive biases present?
Environmental Factors	Physical environment assessment	How was the physical layout designed? Did environment

Root Cause Category	Investigation Methods	Sample Questions
	Ergonomic evaluation Noise/light measurements Workflow mapping Staffing analysis	contribute to the error? Was staffing appropriate? Where were medications stored? Were there competing priorities?
System/Process Factors	Policy review Process mapping Failure mode and effects analysis System testing Documentation review	Were processes designed optimally? Did policies exist and were they followed? Were there adequate safety checks? Did technology help or hinder? Were there previous similar events?
Organizational Factors	Culture surveys Leadership interviews Budget/resource analysis Organizational structure review Incentive analysis	How does leadership respond to errors? Are resources adequate for safety? Is there a culture of safety? Are there competing priorities? What are the accountability systems?
External Factors	Regulatory review Market analysis Literature review Community needs assessment Patient	Did external regulations affect the process? Were there economic constraints? Did patient factors contribute? Did external standards influence decisions?

Techniques such as the "5 Whys" method and fishbone diagrams facilitate progressive exploration beyond superficial explanations. For example, an investigation of a dosing error might progress from initial identification of a calculation mistake (what happened) to recognition of contributing factors including confusing medication packaging, interruption-prone work environments, and inadequate dosing references, ultimately identifying systemic issues in staff training and reference material accessibility.

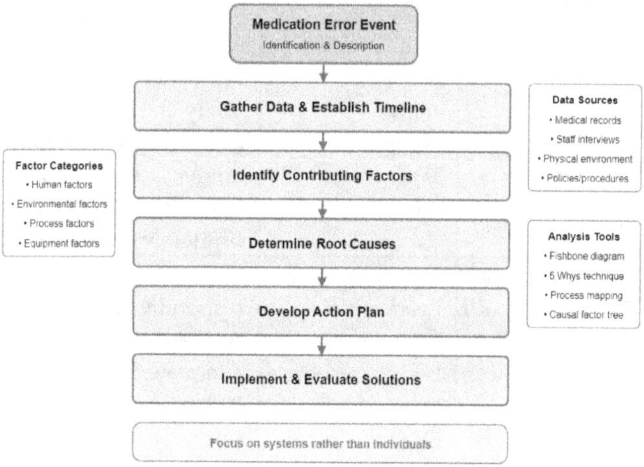

Figure 3.2 Medication Errors by Process

RCA culminates in development of corrective action plans designed to address identified system vulnerabilities. Effective corrective actions typically incorporate multiple interventions targeting different system components, prioritized based on feasibility, resource requirements, and potential impact. Implementation timelines with designated responsibility assignments and measurement strategies ensure accountability for improvement actions.

Healthcare organizations increasingly employ more

sophisticated RCA variants, including apparent cause analysis for less severe events and aggregate RCA for identifying patterns across multiple similar incidents. Contemporary approaches emphasize the importance of strong vs. weak actions—favoring system redesign and forcing functions over additional warnings or educational initiatives with limited sustained impact. Patient inclusion in the RCA process, when appropriate, provides valuable perspectives and reinforces organizational commitment to transparency.

Despite its widespread adoption, traditional RCA approaches face criticism regarding limited effectiveness in preventing error recurrence. Contemporary methodologies increasingly incorporate resilience engineering principles, focusing on understanding how systems succeed under varying conditions rather than exclusively examining failure modes. This perspective shift supports development of more robust systems capable of adapting to changing circumstances rather than optimizing for specific known error types.

PREVENTION MEASURES

Medication error prevention requires multifaceted approaches addressing vulnerabilities throughout the medication use process. Contemporary prevention strategies integrate technological solutions, process standardization, human factors engineering, and cultural interventions to create comprehensive safety systems with redundant safeguards.

Table 3.3: Medication Error Prevention Strategies by System Level

System Level	Preventive Measures	Implementation
Individual Level	Education and training Competency validation Cognitive aids Error awareness training Personal practices (e.g., double-checking, SBAR communication)	Requires reinforcement Must be role-specific Limited impact without system changes May create false sense of safety
Team Level	Standardized communication tools Team training Briefings and debriefings Peer coaching Collaborative medication reviews Defined team roles	Requires team stability Needs leadership support Cultural adaptation required Needs interprofessional commitment
Clinical Unit/Department Level	Standardized processes Medication safety zones Environmental redesign Unit-based pharmacists Local error reporting Safety huddles	Requires local champions Resource-intensive Must fit specific workflow Needs ongoing reinforcement
Organizational Level	Technology implementation Medication safety programs High-alert medication protocols Standard order sets Formulary management Just culture	Significant resource investment Requires leadership commitment Needs system-wide coordination Long implementation time

System Level	Preventive Measures	Implementation
Healthcare System Level	Medication naming/packaging standards Electronic health record interoperability Regulatory requirements Pay-for-performance metrics Regional error sharing Population health approaches	Multiple stakeholders required Political considerations Difficult to implement quickly May have unintended consequences
National /International Level	Labeling standards Manufacturing requirements Regulatory systems Look-alike/sound-alike precautions International safety alerts Medication naming conventions	Slow implementation Industry resistance National differences in practices Regulatory jurisdiction issues

Standardization represents a fundamental prevention strategy, reducing unnecessary variation that creates error opportunities. Standardized order sets, medication concentrations, administration times, and documentation formats establish consistent expectations that simplify cognitive processing and facilitate pattern recognition. Implementation of tall-man lettering for look-alike drug names (e.g., hydrOXYzine/hydrALAzine) and standardized terminology for medication instructions exemplify targeted standardization interventions addressing specific error mechanisms.

Technology solutions play increasingly prominent roles in medication error prevention. Computerized provider order entry (CPOE) with integrated clinical decision support eliminates illegibility issues while providing real-time alerts for potential overdoses, allergies, and drug interactions. Barcode medication administration systems verify patient identity and medication accuracy at the point of care. Automated dispensing cabinets with built-in safety features reduce selection errors through guided retrieval processes. Smart infusion pumps with drug libraries and dose-checking capabilities prevent intravenous medication administration errors.

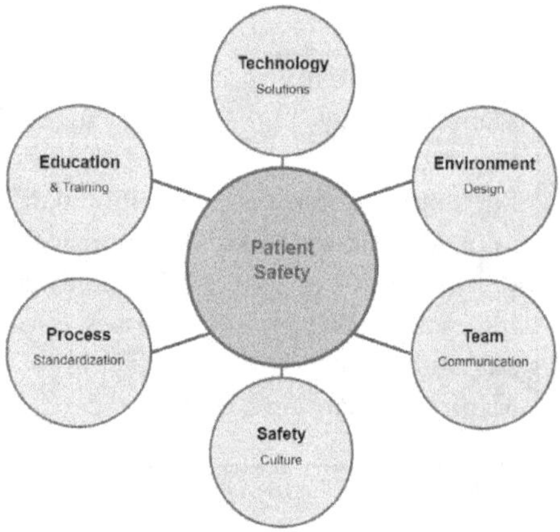

Figure 3.3: Medication Error Prevention

Environmental design modifications address physical and cognitive factors contributing to medication errors. Dedicated medication preparation areas with minimal interruptions, adequate lighting, and ergonomic design reduce dispensing and preparation errors. Visual cues such as colored labeling for high-alert medications enhance situational awareness. Noise reduction strategies in medication administration areas minimize distractions during critical safety checks.

Independent double-checks represent a procedural

intervention for high-risk medications and processes. These checks, when properly implemented, involve two clinicians separately verifying critical medication parameters rather than simultaneously reviewing the same information. Effective double-check procedures specify which elements require verification, establish clear responsibility boundaries, and avoid over-implementation that could lead to diminished effectiveness through normalization.

Patient engagement strategies recognize patients and families as valuable partners in error prevention. Medication education programs that encourage patients to question unfamiliar medications, maintain accurate medication lists, and report adverse effects create an additional safety layer. Some organizations implement patient-accessible medication administration records to facilitate participation in the verification process.

Simulation training provides healthcare professionals with opportunities to practice error prevention strategies in realistic but consequence-free environments. Particularly effective for high-risk procedures and emergency situations, simulation enables teams to develop communication skills, practice safety protocols, and identify system vulnerabilities before encountering similar scenarios in clinical practice.

Just culture implementation addresses the organizational context for error prevention by balancing accountability with psychological safety. This approach distinguishes between normal human error, at-risk behavior, and reckless conduct, applying appropriate responses to each. Healthcare organizations with established just cultures typically demonstrate higher error reporting rates, more proactive identification of system vulnerabilities, and more effective implementation of prevention strategies.

Effectiveness evaluation represents an essential component of prevention programs, with organizations increasingly employing outcome measures (actual error rates and harm events), process measures (compliance with safety practices), and structural measures (implementation of safety systems) to assess comprehensive program performance. Trigger tool methodologies and global trigger tools provide standardized approaches for detecting adverse events that might indicate medication errors, supplementing voluntary reporting systems with more objective measurement techniques.

ERROR REPORTING SYSTEMS

Error reporting systems provide structured mechanisms for collecting, analyzing, and learning from medication errors and near-miss events. These systems serve multiple purposes: identifying emerging safety concerns, evaluating prevention strategy effectiveness, sharing lessons across departments or organizations, and demonstrating organizational commitment to continuous improvement.

Internal reporting systems operate within healthcare organizations, collecting information about medication errors and near-misses occurring in local practice settings. Effective internal systems emphasize accessibility through multiple reporting modalities (electronic, paper, telephone), clear inclusion criteria, and streamlined processes that minimize reporting burden. Contemporary systems increasingly incorporate mobile reporting capabilities and integration with electronic health records to facilitate real-time error documentation.

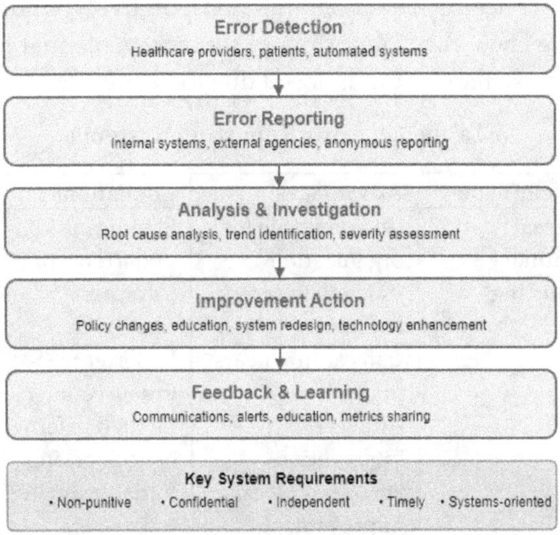

Figure 3.4 Components of Medication Error Reporting System

Anonymous reporting options within internal systems address fear of punitive responses, particularly in organizations transitioning toward just culture principles. While anonymity may limit follow-up investigation capacity, it often captures events that would otherwise remain unreported. Some organizations implement confidential rather than anonymous reporting, maintaining reporter privacy while enabling targeted follow-up when necessary.

External reporting systems aggregate medication error information across multiple organizations, providing broader perspective on error patterns and facilitating widespread dissemination of prevention strategies. The Institute for Safe Medication Practices (ISMP) Medication Error Reporting Program represents a pioneering voluntary external system, collecting reports from healthcare professionals and patients to identify emerging safety concerns. The program's non-punitive, confidential nature encourages reporting of serious events that might otherwise remain undisclosed due to liability concerns.

Table 3.4: Error Reporting Systems

System Type	Advantages	Limitations
Internal Voluntary Reporting	Customizable to organization Immediate access to data Can capture near-misses Allows rapid intervention Focuses on local improvement	Significant underreporting (captures ~5% of errors) Reporter bias Resource-intensive Limited external benchmarking Variable quality of reports
External Voluntary Reporting	Aggregates data across institutions Identifies rare events Provides comparative analysis May include expert recommendations Supports organizational learning	Distance from local context Delayed feedback Limited details No denominator data Selected reporting
Mandatory Reporting	Captures serious events Ensures minimum reporting Enables system-wide monitoring May drive policy changes Accountability	Focus on harmful outcomes Compliance-oriented Minimal learning focus May discourage transparency

Automated Trigger Detection	Identifies events missed by reporting More consistent detection Not dependent on reporting culture Can identify patterns May enable earlier intervention	Technology-dependent False positives/negatives Limited to available data May miss contextual factors Implementation complexity
Patient/Family Reporting	Captures patient perspective Identifies gaps in care coordination Reveals communication issues Identifies unreported events Engages patients in safety	Variable quality/reliability Different definition of error Limited clinical knowledge May focus on service issues Requires interpretation

Mandatory reporting requirements exist in many jurisdictions for errors resulting in serious harm or death. These systems, typically operated by governmental agencies or accrediting bodies, ensure systematic collection of serious event information. In the United States, The Joint Commission requires reporting of sentinel events, including medication errors resulting in death or permanent harm, through its Sentinel Event Alert system. Similar requirements exist internationally, though definitions and thresholds for mandatory reporting vary substantially across jurisdictions.

Analysis methodologies for reported errors have evolved from simple categorization to sophisticated pattern detection approaches. Contemporary systems employ both quantitative and qualitative analysis techniques. Statistical process control methods identify significant changes in error rates or patterns. Natural language processing applied to narrative descriptions identifies emerging themes across multiple reports. Machine learning algorithms increasingly supplement human analysis by detecting subtle patterns across large datasets that might escape manual review.

Feedback mechanisms represent a critical component of effective reporting systems. Organizations with mature systems provide both individual feedback to reporters (acknowledging submissions and describing actions taken) and systemic feedback to the broader organization (aggregated data on error patterns, improvement initiatives, and outcome measures). Transparency regarding actions taken in response to reports reinforces the value of reporting and sustains participation.

Information sharing across organizational boundaries enhances the learning potential from reported errors. Patient Safety Organizations (PSOs) in the United States facilitate confidential sharing of error information with federal legal protections. International collaboratives such as the Global Patient Safety Alert system enable cross-border learning from serious medication errors. These mechanisms extend the impact of individual reports beyond their originating organizations, multiplying their preventive potential.

Despite their importance, reporting systems face significant challenges. Underreporting remains pervasive, with research suggesting that voluntary systems capture only 5-20% of actual medication errors. Reporting bias skews toward certain error types, particularly those with observable consequences, potentially distorting organizational understanding of safety vulnerabilities. Resource limitations for analysis and response can create reporting fatigue when participants perceive limited organizational response to submitted reports. Contemporary approaches address these challenges through simplified reporting processes, emphasis on high-value reports rather than capturing all errors, and clear communication about improvement actions resulting from reported events.

Things to Remember

- ☑ Medication errors include prescribing inaccuracies, transcription omissions, dispensing mistakes, administration failures, and monitoring oversights with varying harm potential.
- ☑ Classification systems address both error characteristics (type, stage, severity) and outcomes (NCC MERP categories from no error to death).
- ☑ Root cause analysis investigates system factors beyond individual performance, distinguishing between active failures at the point of care and latent conditions within organizational systems.
- ☑ Prevention strategies employ high-reliability principles through technological safeguards, standardized processes, human factors engineering, and redundant verification.
- ☑ The hierarchy of effectiveness ranks safety interventions from most effective (forcing functions, automation) to least (policies, education).
- ☑ Reporting systems require non-punitive cultures separating error identification from blame, while maintaining accountability for reckless behavior.

Multiple Choice Questions

1. Which of the following is NOT a common type of medication error?
   a) Prescribing errors
   b) Transcription errors
   c) Marketing errors
   d) Administration errors
2. Root cause analysis in medication safety:
   a) Focuses primarily on identifying individual responsible for errors
   b) Is only necessary for errors resulting in serious patient harm
   c) Identifies both active failures and latent conditions contributing to errors
   d) Should be conducted exclusively by quality improvement departments without clinical input
3. According to the hierarchy of effectiveness, which intervention would likely be MOST effective in preventing medication errors?
   a) Additional staff education about error-prone medications
   b) New policies requiring double-checking high-alert medications
   c) Forcing functions preventing dangerous medication combinations
   d) Warning labels on high-alert medications
4. Active failures in medication error occurrence include:
   a) Inadequate staffing levels
   b) Poor lighting in medication preparation areas
   c) Administering medication to the wrong

patient
d) Lack of standardized protocols

5. A just culture in medication error reporting:
a) Focuses on punishing individuals responsible for errors
b) Balances accountability for reckless behavior with non-punitive approach to unintentional errors
c) Eliminates all personal accountability for medication errors
d) Prioritizes organizational reputation over transparency
6. The NCC MERP index categorizes medication errors by:
a) The type of medication involved
b) The healthcare professional responsible
c) The harm outcome, from no error to death
d) The setting where the error occurred
7. Which of the following is an example of a latent condition that could contribute to medication errors?
a) A nurse administering medication without checking patient identification
b) A pharmacist selecting the wrong medication from a shelf
c) Sound-alike medications stored alphabetically next to each other
d) A physician writing an illegible prescription
8. Error reporting systems are most effective when they:
a) Focus exclusively on errors causing serious harm

b) Require detailed information about who was responsible
c) Separate error identification from punitive consequences
d) Are managed exclusively by regulatory agencies

9. Which approach to error prevention addresses the cognitive limitations of healthcare providers?
a) Regulatory compliance
b) Human factors engineering
c) Staff disciplinary procedures
d) Increased documentation requirements

10. Standardization in medication processes reduces errors by:
a) Eliminating the need for clinical judgment
b) Reducing unnecessary variation in routine tasks
c) Increasing individual accountability
d) Focusing exclusively on high-alert medications

Self-Assessment Questions

1. Describe the different types of medication errors using a comprehensive classification system, providing examples and explaining the potential consequences of each type.
2. Explain the methodology of root cause analysis in investigating medication errors, with a detailed example demonstrating how this approach identifies system failures.
3. Critically evaluate the effectiveness of various prevention measures for medication errors across the medication use process.
4. Compare and contrast voluntary and mandatory error reporting systems, analyzing their respective strengths, limitations, and impact on safety improvement.
5. Analyze how human factors engineering principles can be applied to medication safety to reduce errors and improve safety systems.
6. Evaluate the concept of "high-reliability organizations" and how their principles can be applied to prevent medication errors in healthcare settings.
7. Discuss the psychological impact of medication errors on healthcare professionals and strategies to support "second victims" while maintaining safety.
8. Analyze the role of patients and families in preventing medication errors and strategies to effectively engage them as partners in medication safety.

9. Evaluate how technological solutions have changed the landscape of medication error prevention, including both benefits and unintended consequences.
10. Discuss how medication error data should be collected, analyzed, and utilized to drive continuous quality improvement within a healthcare organization

Bibliography

1. Aronson JK. Medication errors: definitions and classification. Br J Clin Pharmacol. 2009;67(6):599-604.
2. Bates DW, Spell N, Cullen DJ, Burdick E, Laird N, Petersen LA, et al. The costs of adverse drug events in hospitalized patients. JAMA. 1997;277(4):307-11.
3. National Coordinating Council for Medication Error Reporting and Prevention. NCC MERP Index for Categorizing Medication Errors. Rockville, MD: NCC MERP; 2001.
4. Flynn EA, Barker KN, Pepper GA, Bates DW, Mikeal RL. Comparison of methods for detecting medication errors in 36 hospitals and skilled-nursing facilities. Am J Health Syst Pharm. 2002;59(5):436-46.
5. Reason J. Human error: models and management. BMJ. 2000;320(7237):768-70.
6. Wu AW, Lipshutz AK, Pronovost PJ. Effectiveness and efficiency of root cause analysis in medicine. JAMA. 2008;299(6):685-7.
7. Pham JC, Kim GR, Natterman JP, Cover RM, Goeschel CA, Wu AW, et al. ReCASTing the RCA: an improved model for performing root cause analyses. Am J Med Qual. 2010;25(3):186-91.
8. ISMP. ISMP List of High-Alert Medications in Acute Care Settings. Horsham, PA: Institute for Safe Medication Practices; 2018.
9. Leape LL, Berwick DM, Bates DW. What practices will most improve safety? Evidence-based medicine meets patient safety. JAMA. 2002;288(4):501-7.
10. Nuckols TK, Smith-Spangler C, Morton SC, Asch SM, Patel VM, Anderson LJ, et al. The effectiveness of computerized order entry at reducing preventable adverse drug events and medication errors in hospital settings: a systematic review and meta-analysis. Syst Rev. 2014;3:56.

CHAPTER 4

RISK MANAGEMENT IN MEDICATION SAFETY

Abstract

Risk management provides structured approaches to medication safety through systematic hazard identification and mitigation before patient harm occurs. Proactive assessment methodologies include FMEA identifying potential process failures, prospective risk assessment examining planned changes before implementation, and socio-technical probabilistic analyses quantifying risk likelihood and severity. Comprehensive mitigation strategies employ hierarchy of effectiveness principles prioritizing system redesign and forcing functions over education and policies, with tailored interventions addressing specific identified vulnerabilities. Implementation typically involves defined responsibility assignment, resource allocation matched to risk magnitude, and structured evaluation confirming effectiveness. Documentation systems maintain records of assessment findings, intervention decisions, implementation actions, and evaluation results supporting both operational accountability and regulatory compliance. Quality indicators measure risk management effectiveness through outcome metrics tracking actual harm events, process measures assessing mitigation implementation, and structural indicators evaluating program components, creating balanced evaluation supporting continuous improvement beyond incident-driven response.

Keywords: *Proactive assessment, Mitigation hierarchy, Risk quantification, Intervention effectiveness, Safety metrics*

Learning Objectives

After completion of the chapter, the learners should be able to:

- Remember the key risk assessment methodologies used in medication safety.
- Understand how the hierarchy of effectiveness guides risk mitigation strategy selection.
- Apply appropriate risk assessment techniques to identify medication safety vulnerabilities.
- Analyze documentation systems for capturing risk assessment findings and mitigation activities.
- Evaluate the effectiveness of risk mitigation strategies using appropriate quality indicators.
- Create a comprehensive risk management program addressing medication safety in a healthcare setting

RISK ASSESSMENT METHODS

Risk assessment in medication safety employs structured methodologies to identify, analyze, and evaluate potential sources of medication-related harm before adverse events occur. This proactive approach contrasts with reactive analyses of errors that have already occurred, enabling prevention through systematic examination of medication systems and processes.

Failure Mode and Effects Analysis (FMEA) represents a cornerstone methodology in medication safety risk assessment. This team-based, systematic technique studies processes to identify potential failure points, their potential effects, and their relative priority for intervention. The FMEA process begins with process mapping to establish a shared understanding of workflow and system components. Teams then systematically identify potential failure modes at each process step, estimating severity, probability, and detectability of each potential failure. These estimates generate Risk Priority Numbers (RPNs) that guide prioritization of improvement efforts. In medication safety applications, FMEA has proven particularly valuable for evaluating high-risk processes such as chemotherapy ordering and preparation, anticoagulation management, and patient-controlled analgesia implementation.

Probabilistic Risk Assessment (PRA) applies quantitative methods to estimate the likelihood and consequences of adverse medication events. This approach, adapted from high-reliability industries such as aviation and nuclear power, construct's fault trees and event trees representing the potential pathways to medication errors. PRA enables sophisticated modeling of complex systems with multiple failure points and interdependencies. While more resource-intensive than qualitative methods, PRA provides detailed risk quantification that supports cost-benefit analysis of potential interventions. Healthcare organizations increasingly employ simplified PRA variants that maintain methodological rigor while requiring less specialized expertise.

Sociotechnical Probabilistic Risk Assessment (ST-PRA) extends traditional PRA by incorporating human and organizational factors more explicitly. This methodology recognizes that medication errors frequently occur at the intersection of technical systems and human behavior, with organizational context significantly influencing both.

ST-PRA help us to know how technology design, workflow, organizational policies, and cultural factors interact to create or mitigate risk. This approach has proven particularly valuable for evaluating health information technology implementations where technical functionality alone does not determine safety outcomes.

Hazard Analysis and Critical Control Points (HACCP), originally developed for food safety, has been successfully adapted to medication safety applications, particularly in compounding and preparation processes. This method identifies critical points in processes where monitoring or intervention can prevent hazards from reaching harmful levels. HACCP emphasizes establishing measurable control parameters at these critical points, with defined actions when monitoring indicates deviation from safe ranges. In sterile compounding applications, HACCP principles guide identification of contamination risks and establishment of appropriate environmental monitoring programs.

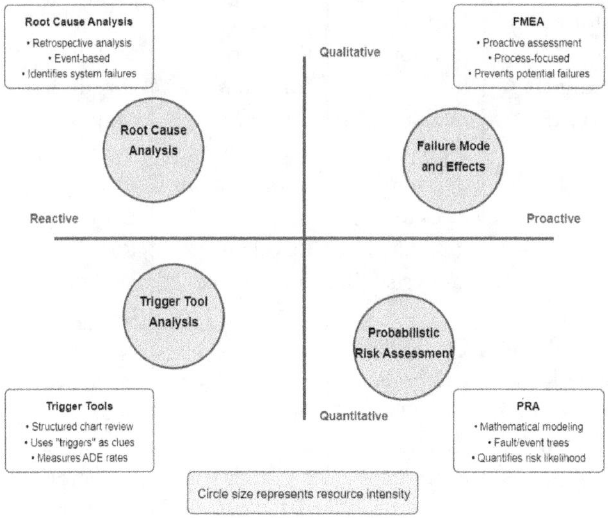

Figure 4.1 Methods for Medication Safety Risk Assessment

Table 4.1: Comparison of Risk Assessment Methods for Medication Safety

Method	Description	Applications	Limitations
Failure Mode and Effects Analysis (FMEA)	Systematic, proactive approach to identify process failure points and their potential effects before they occur	Before implementing new processes Prior to technology implementation High-risk medication systems After serious errors to prevent recurrence	Resource-intensive Relies on team knowledge Subjective risk scoring May miss rare combinations of failures
Healthcare Failure Mode and Effect Analysis (HFMEA)	Streamlined version of FMEA developed for healthcare with decision trees for hazard analysis	Complex clinical processes Resource-constrained settings Team-based improvement projects Regulatory compliance	Less comprehensive than FMEA Still time-consuming May oversimplify complex failures Requires facilitator training
Probabilistic Risk Assessment (PRA)	Quantitative approach using fault trees and event trees to determine probability	High-consequence processes When quantitative risk data needed Complex	Requires extensive data Mathematically complex Time and resource intensive

Method	Description	Applications	Limitations
	of specific failure sequences	system interactions Regulatory requirements	Requires specialized expertise
Root Cause Analysis (RCA)	Retrospective structured investigation to identify underlying causes of specific incidents	After serious events Recurrent problems Regulatory requirements Complex, multifactorial errors	Reactive rather than proactive Hindsight bias Single incident focus Implementation challenges
Structured What-If Technique (SWIFT)	Facilitated team-based approach using "what-if" questions to identify risks	Rapid assessment needs Limited resources Preliminary risk screening Team engagement	Less structured than FMEA Depends on team imagination May miss systematic risks Variable depth of analysis
Bow-Tie Analysis	Visual method showing pathways from hazards to consequences, with preventive and mitigating controls	Complex risk visualization Multiple control evaluation Communication of risk strategies Barrier analysis	Simplified representation Limited quantification Focuses on single events Dependency challenges

Healthcare Failure Mode and Effect Analysis (HFMEA) represents a modification of traditional FMEA developed by the Veterans Health Administration to address healthcare-specific needs. This methodology incorporates decision trees to focus analysis on the most critical failure modes and includes more explicit consideration of human factors. HFMEA typically employs multidisciplinary teams including frontline staff, safety specialists, and subject matter experts to ensure comprehensive risk identification. The structured nature of HFMEA makes it particularly suitable for organizations beginning formalized risk assessment programs.

Ethnographic approaches complement structured methodologies by directly observing medication processes in their natural settings. These approaches employ trained observers who document workflow patterns, workarounds, interruptions, and environmental factors influencing medication safety. Ethnographic assessment often reveals discrepancies between official procedures and actual practice, identifying informal adaptations that may either enhance safety through resilience or create vulnerabilities through procedural deviation. The rich contextual understanding provided by ethnographic methods helps explain why similarly designed medication systems may perform differently across different organizational settings.

Risk assessment timing significantly influences effectiveness, with proactive assessment before implementation of new medications, technologies, or processes yielding the greatest preventive benefit. Periodic reassessment at defined intervals captures emerging risks from changes in patient populations, staff composition, or connected systems. Event-triggered assessments following significant medication errors or near-misses enable targeted examination of specific vulnerabilities identified through actual events.

RISK MITIGATION

Risk mitigation in medication safety encompasses interventions designed to eliminate, reduce, or control identified risks through systematic application of safety principles. Effective mitigation strategies address risks at multiple system levels, creating redundant safeguards that maintain safety despite individual component failures.

The hierarchy of controls framework, adapted from occupational safety, provides a structured approach to medication safety interventions. This framework ranks interventions from most to least effective: elimination (removing the hazardous process or medication), substitution (replacing high-risk medications or processes with safer alternatives), engineering controls (designing systems to prevent errors), administrative controls (policies, procedures, and training), and personal protection (individual vigilance and double-checks). This hierarchy guides organizations toward higher-leverage interventions with greater reliability and less dependence on perfect human performance.

Engineering controls represent particularly robust interventions, designing safety into medication systems rather than relying on procedural compliance. Physical constraints that prevent misconnections between incompatible medication delivery systems exemplify this approach. Forcing functions in electronic health records that require confirmation of unusual doses or contraindicated medications create technical barriers to potential errors. Smart infusion pumps with hard limits on medication concentrations physically prevent administration of potentially lethal doses. These technological safeguards function regardless of operator knowledge, attention, or intention.

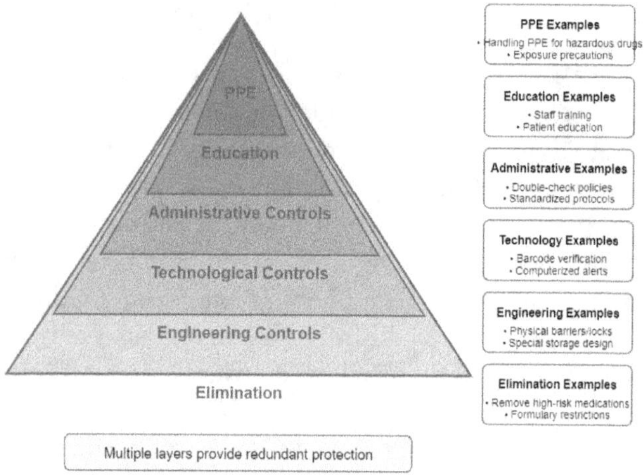

Figure 4.2 Medication Safety Risk Mitigation

Risk mitigation for high-alert medications requires particularly comprehensive approaches given their potential to cause severe harm. Strategies include distinctive packaging and labeling to enhance recognition, restricted storage to prevent inadvertent access, standardized ordering processes to eliminate ambiguity, independent double-checks at critical points, and enhanced monitoring requirements. Organizations increasingly implement medication-specific protocols addressing the unique risk profiles of agents such as insulin, anticoagulants, opioids, and chemotherapeutic agents.

Differentiating strategies address risks from look-alike/sound-alike medications that can be confused during ordering, dispensing, or administration. Beyond tall-man lettering conventions, effective approaches include physical separation in storage areas, distinctive auxiliary labels, barcode verification requirements, and inclusion in high-alert medication protocols. Some organizations implement annual reviews of look-alike/sound-alike medication pairs to systematically identify and address confusion potential.

Environmental modifications mitigate risks associated with workspace design and workflow patterns. Dedicated, well-lit medication preparation areas minimize distractions during critical tasks. Visual cues such as color-coded zones for different risk levels create situational awareness. Noise reduction strategies in medication administration areas support concentration during safety-critical activities. Adequate workspace and appropriate equipment placement reduce workarounds that often introduce unintended risks.

Standardization represents a fundamental risk mitigation strategy, reducing unnecessary variation that creates error opportunities. Standardized order sets, medication concentrations, administration times, and dosing protocols establish consistent expectations that simplify cognitive processing and facilitate error detection when deviations occur. This approach proves particularly valuable for complex or high-risk medications where calculation errors present significant hazards.

Redundancy and independent verification provide protection against single-point failures in medication processes. Critical steps with high error potential warrant redundant safeguards through both technical and human verification. The Swiss cheese model of accident causation illustrates how multiple safeguards create cumulative protection, requiring simultaneous failure of multiple safety layers for errors to reach patients. Implementation of redundant safeguards requires careful design to ensure true independence rather than superficial verification that may perpetuate initial errors.

Table 4.2: Risk Mitigation Strategies for Common Medication Safety Hazards

Hazard Category	Example Hazards	Preventive Measures
High-Alert Medications	Insulin Anticoagulants Opioids Neuromuscular blockers Concentrated electrolytes	Standardized concentrations Restricted access Tall-man lettering Order sets Dose range limits
Look-Alike/Sound-Alike Medications	Hydroxyzine/hydralazine Vinblastine/vincristine Morphine/hydromorphone Metoprolol/metronidazole Prednisolone/prednisone	Tall-man lettering Separated storage Alert prompts Barcode verification Distinct labeling
Medication Administration Errors	Wrong patient Wrong time Wrong route Wrong technique Omission errors	Barcode verification Independent checks Standardized procedures Distraction-free zones Patient involvement
Calculation Errors	Decimal point errors Unit conversions Weight-based dosing Infusion rate errors Compounding errors	Standardized worksheets Electronic calculators Independent calculations Dose range limits

Communication Failures	Handoff errors Unclear orders Abbreviation misinterpretation Verbal order errors Documentation gaps	SBAR communication Prohibited abbreviation lists Read-back protocols Standardized documentation Electronic orders
Medication Reconciliation Failures	Omitted medications Duplicate therapy Wrong dose/frequency Contraindicated medicines Wrong formulations	Structured reconciliation tools Patient involvement Multiple information sources Pharmacist review High-risk patient identification

Technology implementation represents increasingly important risk mitigation, though requiring careful design and implementation. Computerized provider order entry with clinical decision support addresses risks in the prescribing phase. Barcode medication administration systems mitigate patient identification and medication selection errors. Automated dispensing cabinets with security features and guided selection reduce dispensing errors. Effective implementation requires attention to potential new risks introduced by technology, including alert fatigue, workflow disruption, and over-reliance on technological safeguards.

Implementation science principles guide effective risk mitigation deployment, recognizing that intervention design alone does not ensure safety improvement. Consideration of local context, stakeholder engagement, appropriate training, and sustainability planning significantly influence intervention effectiveness. Pilot testing with subsequent refinement enables adaptation to specific organizational environments before full-scale implementation. Post-implementation monitoring with defined success metrics ensures intended risk reduction without unintended consequences.

DOCUMENTATION AND MONITORING

Documentation and monitoring systems provide the information infrastructure necessary for ongoing medication safety risk management, enabling both proactive surveillance for emerging risks and evaluation of mitigation effectiveness. Comprehensive approaches integrate documentation across the medication use process, establishing continuity from prescribing through administration and monitoring.

Medication ordering documentation has evolved substantially with electronic health record implementation, incorporating structured fields that eliminate illegibility issues while enabling clinical decision support. Contemporary systems capture not only basic order parameters but also clinical indications, relevant laboratory values, patient-specific factors influencing medication selection, and prescriber rationales for overriding safety alerts. This enriched documentation supports both individual patient safety and aggregate analysis of prescribing patterns to identify potential improvement opportunities.

Dispensing documentation addresses both individual medication preparation and system-level inventory management. For individual preparations, particularly compounded sterile products, documentation includes preparation environment conditions, component lot numbers, preparer and verifier identities, and beyond-use dating calculations. Automated compounding devices generate detailed records of ingredients and volumes, creating verification opportunities before patient administration. At the system level, inventory management documentation enables tracking of medication movement throughout organizations, supporting both diversion monitoring and recall management.

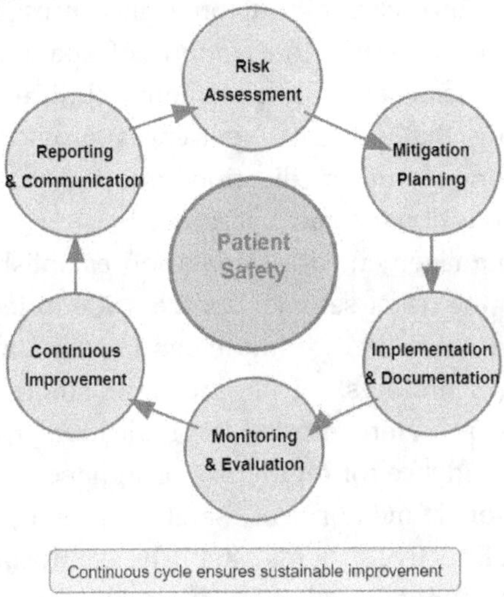

Figure 4.2 Medication Safety and Monitoring Cycle

Administration documentation serves multiple safety functions beyond basic legal requirements. Contemporary medication administration records (MARs) incorporate verification protocols, administration timing, patient response observations, and reasons for any omitted or delayed doses. Barcode medication administration systems generate detailed transaction logs capturing the timing and sequence of verification steps. Smart infusion pump documentation records not only basic infusion parameters but also pump programming changes, alarm responses, and overrides of safety limits, enabling identification of potential unsafe practices requiring intervention.

Patient monitoring documentation integrates medication-specific parameters with broader clinical assessment, creating a comprehensive view of medication effects. Structured documentation supports tracking of therapeutic drug monitoring results, adverse effect screening, and clinical outcome measures related to medication therapy. Integration of patient-reported outcomes increasingly complements clinical measures, recognizing that patient experiences provide valuable information about medication effects not captured through traditional clinical parameters.

Risk management documentation establishes formal records of the risk assessment process, identified hazards, mitigation decisions, implementation status, and evaluation findings. This documentation supports continuity in safety efforts across leadership changes, provides evidence for regulatory compliance, and creates organizational memory of safety investigations and decisions. Effective systems establish clear documentation standards while avoiding excessive administrative burden that could divert resources from actual safety improvement.

Surveillance monitoring represents a proactive approach to identifying medication safety risks before serious harm occurs. Trigger tool methodologies systematically scan clinical documentation for indicators of potential adverse drug events, such as abnormal laboratory values, antidote administration, or unexpected clinical deterioration. More sophisticated systems employ machine learning algorithms to identify subtle patterns suggesting emerging medication safety concerns not detectable through traditional monitoring approaches.

Compliance monitoring assesses adherence to established safety protocols and best practices. This includes both direct observation of medication processes and retrospective record review to identify deviations from expected practice. Effective compliance monitoring differentiates between procedural variations representing appropriate clinical judgment and those indicating safety risks requiring intervention. Sampling strategies balance comprehensive surveillance with resource efficiency, often employing risk-stratified approaches that focus greater attention on high-risk medications and processes.

Outcome monitoring estimates the actual safety performance of medication systems through tracking of medication errors, adverse drug events, and near-misses. Contemporary approaches recognize the limitations of voluntary reporting and supplement this data with more objective measures such as trigger tool reviews, focused chart audits, and direct observation studies. Organizations increasingly track both actual harm events and "good catches" representing successfully intercepted errors, recognizing that the latter provide valuable information about both system vulnerabilities and effective safeguards.

Integration of monitoring data across sources creates comprehensive medication safety dashboards that support both operational management and strategic improvement. Effective dashboards present information at appropriate levels of aggregation for different audiences, providing executive-level summary metrics while enabling drill-down capabilities for detailed analysis. Visual representation through statistical process control charts enables distinction between normal variation and significant changes requiring investigation. Regular review cadences ensure that monitoring data translates into improvement action rather than merely documenting existing conditions.

Table 4.3: Documentation and Monitoring Elements for Medication Safety Risk Management

Documentation Element	Components	Frequency	Primary Responsibility
Risk Register	Identified medication risks Risk scores and prioritization Mitigation strategies Timelines and responsibilities Current status	Initial comprehensive assessment Quarterly review Annual comprehensive update After significant incidents	Medication Safety Officer Pharmacy Leadership Risk Management Department Quality Committee
Safety Action Plans	Specific improvement initiatives Implementation timelines Required resources Responsible individuals Success measures	Monthly progress updates Quarterly comprehensive review Project-specific milestones Annual strategic review	Project leaders Department managers Quality improvement teams Executive sponsors
Medication Safety Dashboards	Key performance indicators Trend analyses	Monthly data collection Quarterly comprehensi	Data analysts Quality department Pharmacy

Documentation Element	Components	Frequency	Primary Responsibility
	Benchmark comparisons High-alert medication metrics Process compliance measures	ve analysis Annual strategic review Real-time critical indicators	leadership IT support Clinical leadership
Incident Investigation Reports	Event description Contributing factors Root causes Recommended actions Implementation plans Effectiveness measures	Within 30-45 days of serious events Monthly aggregate review Quarterly trend analysis Annual comprehensive review	Investigation teams Quality/risk departments Medication safety committee Department leadership Executive leadership
Safety Assessments and Audits	Proactive risk assessments Compliance with best practices High-risk process evaluations Technology safety evaluations Environmental assessments	Annual comprehensive audits Quarterly focused assessments Post-implementation reviews Event-triggered assessments	Medication safety team Department managers External consultants Regulatory specialists Inter-professional committees

QUALITY INDICATORS

Quality indicators provide standardized metrics for assessing medication safety performance, enabling objective evaluation of improvement initiatives, comparison across organizations, and identification of priority areas for intervention. Effective indicator systems balance comprehensiveness with feasibility, focusing measurement resources on aspects of medication safety with greatest impact on patient outcomes.

Structure indicators assess the fundamental components and resources of medication safety systems. These include implementation of recommended technologies (computerized provider order entry, barcode medication administration, smart infusion pumps), staffing patterns (pharmacist-to-patient ratios, nursing workload measures), physical environment characteristics (dedicated medication rooms, appropriate lighting), and governance structures (medication safety committees, designated medication safety officers). While structure indicators do not directly measure safety outcomes, they provide essential information about organizational capacity for safe medication management.

Process indicators measure adherence to evidence-based safety practices throughout the medication use system. Common process measures include compliance rates with independent double-checks for high-alert medications, barcode scanning rates during medication administration, appropriate venous thromboembolism prophylaxis ordering, and timely administration of time-critical medications. These indicators typically employ random sampling methodologies with standardized definitions and exclusion criteria to ensure measurement validity. Organizations increasingly implement electronic data capture for process measures, reducing manual audit burden while increasing sample size and measurement frequency.

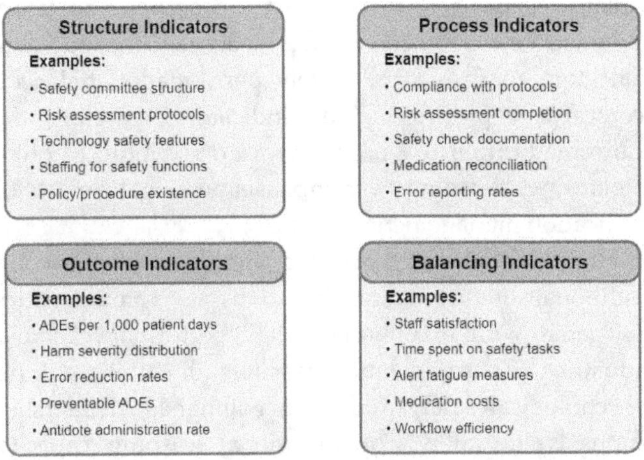

Figure 4.4 Quality Indicators for Medication Safety Risk Management

Outcome indicators directly assess the results of medication safety efforts through measures of actual or potential patient harm. Traditional outcome measures include medication error rates by type and severity, preventable adverse drug event incidence, and triggers suggesting medication misadventures (antidote administration, abrupt medication discontinuation). More sophisticated outcome measurement incorporates patient-reported outcomes regarding medication experiences, recognizing that patients often detect adverse effects not documented in clinical records. Risk-adjusted outcome measures account for variation in patient populations when comparing performance across organizations or units.

Balanced scorecard approaches integrate structure, process, and outcome indicators to provide comprehensive medication safety assessment. This methodology recognizes the complementary nature of different measurement types—structure indicators explain capacity for safety, process indicators demonstrate reliability of safety practices, and outcome indicators confirm actual safety performance. Balanced scorecards typically include indicators spanning the entire medication use process from prescribing through monitoring, avoiding overemphasis on single aspects of medication management.

High-reliability organization metrics extend beyond traditional quality indicators to assess characteristics associated with exceptional safety performance across industries. These include measures of safety culture (psychological safety, reporting willingness, leadership emphasis on safety), organizational learning capacity (error investigation thoroughness, implementation of identified improvements), and resilience (ability to maintain safety during disruptions, effectiveness of contingency responses). While less standardized than traditional medication indicators, these measures provide valuable context for understanding variation in safety performance among organizations with similar technical capabilities.

Composite indicators aggregate multiple individual measures into summary metrics designed to provide overall assessment of medication safety performance. The Medication Safety Thermometer exemplifies this approach, combining measures across multiple safety domains into a single metric for executive-level monitoring. While valuable for high-level oversight, composite indicators require careful construction to ensure appropriate weighting of component measures and clear operational definitions to support improvement efforts when deficiencies are identified.

Table 4.4: Quality Indicators for Medication Safety Risk Management

Indicator Category	Example Indicators	Measurement Methodology	Use in Improvement
Outcome Measures	Adverse drug events per 1,000 patient days Percentage of patients with ADEs Severity-adjusted medication harm index Preventable ADEs per 100 admissions ADE-related readmissions	Chart review Trigger tool methodology Voluntary reporting Administrative data analysis Patient interviews Claims data analysis	Strategic priority setting Board-level monitoring External reporting Public transparency Pay-for-performance metrics
Process Measures	Compliance with medication reconciliation Barcode medication administration scanning rate High-alert medication independent verification Override rates for dose warnings Medication order review	Electronic system reports Direct observation Documentation audits Workflow analysis Process compliance audits	Process improvement Staff feedback Unit-level performance Technology optimization Workflow redesign

Indicator Category	Example Indicators	Measurement Methodology	Use in Improvement
	by pharmacists		
Structural Measures	Medication safety committee activity Staff trained in safety practices High-alert medication protocols implemented Technology safety features enabled Safety resources allocation	Program documentation review Policy analysis Resource allocation tracking Technology configuration audits Training records review	Program development Resource allocation Strategic planning Accreditation preparation Infrastructure investment
Balancing Measures	Time spent on medication administration Alert fatigue measures Staff satisfaction with safety systems Time to medication availability Medication cost per patient day	Time-motion studies Staff surveys Workload analysis Financial data analysis Patient satisfaction surveys	Workflow optimization Alert refinement Staff engagement Efficiency improvement Cost-effectiveness analysis

Indicator Category	Example Indicators	Measurement Methodology	Use in Improvement
Patient-Reported Measures	Patient knowledge of medications Patient-reported medication problems Patient satisfaction with medication information Patient engagement in medication safety Patient-reported administration discrepancies	Patient surveys Post-discharge interviews Teach-back assessments Patient reporting systems Focus groups	Patient education Communication improvement Discharge planning Patient engagement Experience enhancement
High-Reliability Measures	Safety culture survey scores Near-miss reporting rates Proactive risk assessment completion Learning from errors implementation Safety suggestion implementation rate	Culture surveys Reporting system analysis Risk assessment tracking Implementation monitoring Staff feedback systems	Culture development Leadership engagement Organizational learning Innovation promotion Staff empowerment

Benchmarking employs quality indicators to compare performance across organizations, units, or time periods, identifying opportunities for improvement through comparison with best practices. External benchmarking programs such as the Leapfrog Hospital Safety Grade and Centers for Medicare and Medicaid Services (CMS) quality reporting initiatives publish comparative medication safety metrics. Internal benchmarking within healthcare systems compares performance across similar units to identify both successful practices for dissemination and underperforming areas requiring intervention. Effective benchmarking requires standardized definitions, risk adjustment methods, and appropriate peer groupings to ensure valid comparisons.

Indicator selection and implementation involve careful consideration of measurement properties, resource requirements, and strategic alignment. Validity assessment determines whether indicators genuinely measure intended safety aspects rather than documentation artifacts or surrogate processes. Reliability testing ensures consistent measurement across different observers, time periods, and clinical contexts. Implementation feasibility considers data accessibility, collection burden, and sustainability within operational workflows. Strategic alignment ensures that measured aspects of medication safety reflect organizational priorities and known safety challenges rather than simply convenient measurement opportunities.

Contemporary approaches increasingly emphasize parsimony in indicator selection, focusing on high-value measures with demonstrated links to patient outcomes rather than comprehensive measurement of all possible safety aspects. Regular review and refinement of indicator sets ensure continued relevance as medication practices, technologies, and known safety risks evolve. Integration of indicator monitoring into routine operational oversight rather than separate quality initiatives supports sustained attention to medication safety performance beyond specific improvement projects or regulatory requirements.

Things to Remember

- ☑ Risk assessment methods include FMEA for process failure analysis, prospective assessment for planned changes, and socio-technical probabilistic approaches quantifying risk likelihood and severity.
- ☑ Effective mitigation follows hierarchy of effectiveness principles, prioritizing system redesign and forcing functions over education and policies.
- ☑ Implementation requires defined responsibility assignment, resource allocation matched to risk magnitude, and structured evaluation confirming effectiveness.
- ☑ Documentation maintains comprehensive records of assessment findings, intervention decisions, implementation actions, and evaluation results.
- ☑ Quality indicators include outcome metrics tracking harm events, process measures assessing mitigation implementation, and structural indicators evaluating program components.
- ☑ Risk management transforms safety from reactive event response to proactive vulnerability identification and systematic mitigation.

Multiple Choice Questions

1. Which risk assessment methodology proactively examines potential failure modes, effects, and their criticality?
   a) Root cause analysis (RCA)
   b) Failure mode and effects analysis (FMEA)
   c) Tracer methodology
   d) Retrospective chart review
2. According to the hierarchy of effectiveness, which risk mitigation strategy would be LEAST effective?
   a) Forcing functions preventing dangerous medication combinations
   b) Automated dose calculators reducing mathematical errors
   c) Standardized order sets for complex medications
   d) Educational reminders about high-alert medications
3. Socio-technical probabilistic risk assessment involves:
   a) Exclusive focus on technology failures without human factors
   b) Qualitative analysis without quantitative components
   c) Quantifying risk likelihood and severity through mathematical modeling
   d) Retrospective analysis of errors that have already occurred
4. Effective documentation of risk management activities should include:
   a) Only successful mitigation strategies without failed attempts

b) Assessment findings, intervention decisions, implementation actions, and evaluation results
c) Technical details without contextual information about implementation
d) Exclusively incidents resulting in patient harm

5. Structural indicators in medication safety quality measurement assess:
a) Actual harm events occurring within the organization
b) Staff compliance with established safety protocols
c) Program components and resource allocation
d) Patient satisfaction with medication education

6. Prospective risk assessment differs from reactive approaches by:
a) Examining planned changes before implementation
b) Focusing exclusively on technology-related risks
c) Requiring less interdisciplinary involvement
d) Producing findings that are only relevant for regulatory reporting

7. Which of the following best describes risk mitigation implementation?
a) One-time activities completed at project initiation
b) Defined responsibility assignment, resource allocation, and structured evaluation

c) Focusing primarily on documentation rather than actual practice changes
d) Responsibility assigned exclusively to quality departments without clinical involvement

8. Quality indicators measuring risk management effectiveness should include:
a) Exclusively outcome measures tracking harm events
b) Primarily financial metrics related to liability reduction
c) A balanced approach including outcome, process, and structural measures
d) Focus only on regulatory compliance requirements

9. Effective risk management transforms medication safety from:
a) Clinical practice to administrative functions
b) Individual responsibility to regulatory compliance
c) Reactive event response to proactive vulnerability identification
d) Evidence-based practice to consensus-based guidelines

10. Resource allocation in risk management should be:
a) Equal across all identified risks regardless of severity
b) Matched to risk magnitude with higher resources for greater risks
c) Focused exclusively on risks with regulatory implications

Self-Assessment Questions

1. Compare and contrast different risk assessment methodologies used in medication safety, including FMEA, HFMEA, and PRA, analyzing the strengths and limitations of each.
2. Explain the comprehensive process of medication risk mitigation, from identification to implementation of safety measures, using a specific high-risk medication as an example.
3. Critically evaluate the role of risk management documentation in medication safety and how it contributes to organizational learning and safety culture.
4. Analyze how quality indicators for medication safety should be selected, validated, and implemented to effectively monitor risk management strategies.
5. Discuss the relationship between risk management and patient harm, including approaches to prioritizing risks and allocating resources to prevention efforts.
6. Evaluate the impact of proactive versus reactive risk management approaches in medication safety, providing examples of each and their outcomes.
7. Analyze how risk management strategies differ across various healthcare settings (acute care, ambulatory care, long-term care) and the rationale for these differences.
8. Discuss the role of risk perception in medication safety decision-making among

healthcare professionals and its influence on safety practices.

9. Evaluate the integration of medication risk management within the broader organizational risk management framework, including governance structures and reporting mechanisms.
10. Analyze the ethical considerations in medication risk management, including resource allocation, transparency, and disclosure of risks to patients

Bibliography

1. Marx DA, Slonim AD. Assessing patient safety risk before the injury occurs: an introduction to sociotechnical probabilistic risk modelling in health care. Qual Saf Health Care. 2003;12 Suppl 2:ii33-8.
2. Card AJ, Ward JR, Clarkson PJ. Beyond FMEA: the structured what-if technique (SWIFT). J Healthc Risk Manag. 2012;31(4):23-9.
3. DeRosier J, Stalhandske E, Bagian JP, Nudell T. Using health care Failure Mode and Effect Analysis: the VA National Center for Patient Safety's prospective risk analysis system. Jt Comm J Qual Improv. 2002;28(5):248-67.
4. ECRI Institute. Risk Management, Quality Improvement, and Patient Safety. Healthcare Risk Control. Plymouth Meeting, PA: ECRI Institute; 2016.
5. Bonnabry P, Cingria L, Sadeghipour F, Ing H, Fonzo-Christe C, Pfister RE. Use of a systematic risk analysis method to improve safety in the production of paediatric parenteral nutrition solutions. Qual Saf Health Care. 2005;14(2):93-8.
6. Carayon P, Wetterneck TB, Rivera-Rodriguez AJ, Hundt AS, Hoonakker P, Holden R, et al. Human factors systems approach to healthcare quality and patient safety. Appl Ergon. 2014;45(1):14-25.
7. Aronson JK. Risk assessment in clinical pharmacology and clinical pharmacy: a systematic approach. Clin Pharmacol Ther. 2014;95(3):239-40.
8. Shebl NA, Franklin BD, Barber N. Failure mode and effects analysis outputs: are they valid? BMC Health Serv Res. 2012;12:150.
9. Duwe B, Fuchs BD, Hansen-Flaschen J. Failure mode and effects analysis application to critical care medicine. Crit Care Clin. 2005;21(1):21-30.
10. Vincent C, Taylor-Adams S, Chapman EJ, Hewett D, Prior S, Strange P, et al. How to investigate and analyse clinical incidents: clinical risk unit and association of litigation and risk management protocol. BMJ. 2000;320(7237):777-81

CHAPTER 5

PHARMACOVIGILANCE SYSTEMS

Abstract

Pharmacovigilance systems provide techniques to medication safety surveillance beyond pre-approval clinical trials, detecting and analyzing adverse effects throughout product lifecycles. Adverse drug reaction monitoring employs multiple methods including spontaneous reporting from healthcare providers and patients, active surveillance through established patient cohorts, and database studies analyzing large-scale health records for signal detection. Signal detection methodologies employ statistical algorithms identifying potential safety concerns through disproportionality analysis, sequence pattern recognition, and multivariate techniques detecting subtle associations. Reporting mechanisms include national systems like FDA MedWatch and Yellow Card Scheme, manufacturer reporting requirements, and international networks coordinated through WHO's Uppsala Monitoring Centre, with standardized case definitions enhancing data quality. Analysis and interpretation involve causality assessment distinguishing true adverse reactions from coincidental events, risk characterization establishing clinical significance, regulatory impact determination driving potential interventions, and communication for appropriate awareness while preventing unwarranted medication abandonment, ultimately supporting benefit-risk balance optimization throughout medication use.

Keywords: *Post-marketing surveillance, Signal detection algorithms, Causality assessment, Reporting, Benefit-risk evaluation*

Learning Objectives

After completion of the chapter, the learners should be able to:

- Remember the key methods used in adverse drug reaction monitoring.
- Understand how signal detection methodologies identify potential medication safety concerns.
- Apply appropriate reporting mechanisms for identified adverse drug reactions.
- Analyze pharmacovigilance data to determine causality and clinical significance.
- Evaluate the effectiveness of different pharmacovigilance approaches in various healthcare contexts.
- Create a comprehensive pharmacovigilance monitoring plan for a healthcare organization.

ADVERSE DRUG REACTION MONITORING

Adverse drug reaction (ADR) monitoring constitutes the cornerstone of pharmacovigilance systems, providing systematic approaches to identifying, documenting, and evaluating unintended and harmful responses to medications. These monitoring systems operate across multiple levels, from individual patient assessment to global surveillance networks, creating a comprehensive safety net for detecting medication-related harm.

At the patient level, clinical monitoring establishes baseline parameters before medication initiation and tracks relevant physiological markers throughout therapy. This monitoring ranges from routine vital sign assessment to sophisticated laboratory evaluation of organ function, drug levels, or biomarkers indicative of adverse effects. Evidence-based monitoring protocols define appropriate parameters, frequency, and threshold values for specific medications based on their known safety profiles. For example, clozapine monitoring requirements include regular white blood cell counts to detect agranulocytosis, while lithium therapy necessitates serum concentration monitoring alongside thyroid and renal function assessment.

Active surveillance programs represent structured approaches to ADR detection for specific medications with significant safety concerns. These programs, often mandated by regulatory authorities as post-marketing requirements, employ more intensive monitoring strategies than standard clinical care. Pregnancy registries track outcomes in women exposed to medications during pregnancy, providing critical safety data for agents where pre-marketing pregnancy studies were unethical or impractical. Patient registries for high-risk therapies such as clozapine, isotretinoin, and certain biologics combine clinical monitoring data with demographic information and treatment outcomes, enabling detection of rare adverse effects that might not appear in clinical trials.

Targeted clinical reviews employ standardized assessment of specific adverse effects known to be associated with particular medications. Screening tools such as the Abnormal Involuntary Movement Scale (AIMS) for tardive dyskinesia, the Liverpool Adverse Drug Reaction Causality Assessment Tool, and the Naranjo Algorithm for causality assessment provide structured approaches to evaluating suspected ADRs. These instruments enhance detection consistency and documentation quality while supporting appropriate clinical decision-making regarding therapy continuation, dose adjustment, or discontinuation.

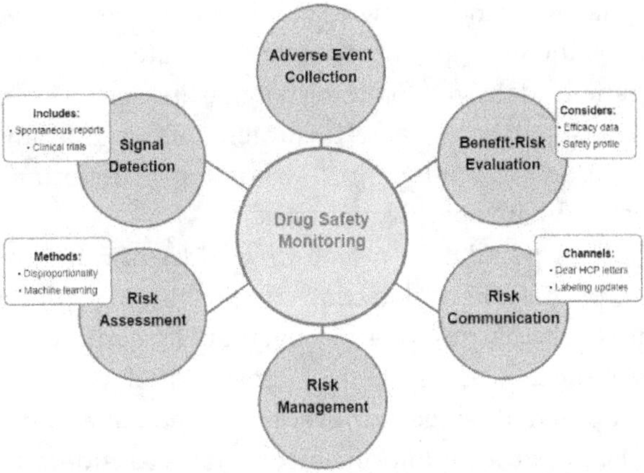

Figure 5.1: Components of Pharmacovigilance System

Hospital-based ADR monitoring programs employ both passive and active surveillance strategies within inpatient settings. Passive approaches rely on spontaneous reporting by healthcare professionals, while active surveillance involves dedicated personnel conducting systematic chart reviews, patient interviews, and targeted laboratory data screening. Hybrid models increasingly predominate, with computerized alert systems flagging potential ADRs for investigation by trained pharmacovigilance specialists. Such programs frequently prioritize high-risk patient populations, including geriatric patients, those with renal or hepatic impairment, and recipients of multiple potentially interacting medications.

Community-based ADR monitoring presents unique challenges due to less intensive patient contact and distributed care delivery. Strategies to enhance outpatient ADR detection include systematic post-dispensing follow-up contacts, patient-reported outcome measures incorporated into routine care, and integration of community pharmacy surveillance into broader pharmacovigilance networks. Electronic health record systems increasingly incorporate automated screening of outpatient data for patterns suggesting adverse drug reactions, such as new symptom reports following medication initiation or laboratory abnormalities associated with specific therapies.

Special population monitoring addresses the unique ADR profiles and detection challenges in vulnerable groups. Pediatric pharmacovigilance employs age-appropriate assessment tools and considers developmental stage in evaluating potential adverse effects. Geriatric monitoring incorporates consideration of altered pharmacokinetics, multiple comorbidities, and polypharmacy effects. Pharmacogenomic approaches increasingly inform individualized monitoring protocols based on genetic variants affecting drug metabolism or target receptor function, enabling precision pharmacovigilance that accounts for inter-individual variability in adverse effect susceptibility.

Integration of patient-reported outcomes into ADR monitoring represents a significant advancement in comprehensive pharmacovigilance. Structured assessment tools such as the Patient-Reported Outcomes version of the Common Terminology Criteria for Adverse Events (PRO-CTCAE) enable systematic collection of symptom information directly from patients. These approaches recognize that patients often detect adverse effects before they become clinically apparent to providers and may identify effects not routinely assessed in standard monitoring protocols, particularly those affecting quality of life or functional status.

Table 5.1: Global Pharmacovigilance Systems and Their Characteristics

System	Coordinating Organization	Features
WHO Programme for International Drug Monitoring	Uppsala Monitoring Centre (UMC)	VigiBase global database VigiLyze analysis tool Signal detection methodology International standards Capacity building
FDA Adverse Event Reporting System (FAERS)	U.S. Food and Drug Administration	MedWatch for voluntary reporting Electronic submission gateway Sentinel Initiative active surveillance Public dashboards Safety communications
EudraVigilance	European Medicines Agency	Centralized EU database Electronic reporting gateways Signal management processes PROTECT methodology Cross-border monitoring
Yellow Card Scheme	UK Medicines and Healthcare products Regulatory Agency	Patient reporting portal Mobile app reporting Signal detection

System	Coordinating Organization	Features
		algorithms Drug Safety Update bulletins AI-powered analysis
Canadian Vigilance Program	Health Canada	MedEffect Canada portal Consumer reporting Regional reporting centers Targeted surveillance Canadian Adverse Reaction Newsletter
Japanese Adverse Drug Event Report (JADER)	Pharmaceuticals and Medical Devices Agency	Direct healthcare provider reporting Early post-marketing vigilance Patient ADR reporting system Signal detection algorithms Relief system for health damage

SIGNAL DETECTION

Signal detection includes the methodologies used to identify potential associations between medications and adverse effects, particularly those not recognized during pre-marketing evaluation. These approaches range from evaluation of individual case reports to sophisticated statistical analyses of large healthcare databases, collectively enabling identification of safety signals that warrant further investigation or regulatory action.

Spontaneous reporting systems represent the traditional foundation of signal detection, collecting reports of suspected adverse drug reactions from healthcare professionals, manufacturers, and increasingly, patients themselves. Individual case evaluation assesses the temporal relationship between medication exposure and adverse effects, biological plausibility, presence of alternative explanations, response to dechallenge (medication discontinuation) or rechallenge (reintroduction), and consistency with known pharmacological properties. While individual cases rarely provide definitive evidence of causality, they often serve as initial signals prompting more rigorous investigation, particularly for rare or severe reactions.

Disproportionality analysis applies statistical methods to spontaneous reporting databases to identify medication-event combinations reported more frequently than expected based on background reporting patterns. Metrics such as the proportional reporting ratio (PRR), reporting odds ratio (ROR), and empirical Bayes geometric mean (EBGM) quantify the strength of association between specific medications and adverse events. These analyses control for reporting biases by comparing the proportion of specific adverse event reports for a medication of interest against the proportion for all other medications in the database. Signal thresholds typically combine statistical criteria (e.g., lower bound of the 95% confidence interval exceeding 1.0) with clinical criteria (minimum number of cases, seriousness of the reaction).

Sequential analysis methods enable continuous monitoring of accumulating safety data with formal statistical adjustment for multiple testing over time. These approaches, including sequential probability ratio tests and maximized sequential probability ratio tests, maintain appropriate statistical properties while allowing early signal detection when sufficient evidence accumulates. Implementation in major pharmacovigilance databases supports regular screening of new reports to identify emerging safety concerns requiring evaluation.

Pattern recognition techniques employ machine learning algorithms to identify complex relationships within pharmacovigilance data that might escape traditional analytical approaches. Natural language processing extracts structured information from narrative case descriptions, enabling analysis of clinical details not captured in coded fields. Neural networks and other advanced algorithms detect subtle patterns across multiple variables that may indicate previously unrecognized adverse effect associations. These techniques prove particularly valuable for identifying drug-drug interactions where conventional analysis focused on single medications may miss important safety signals.

Healthcare database studies utilize electronic health records, insurance claims data, and prescription databases for population-level signal detection. These data sources offer advantages including larger sample sizes, reduced reporting bias, availability of denominator data, and longitudinal patient information. Observational study designs employed for signal detection include cohort studies comparing event rates between exposed and unexposed populations, case-control studies examining medication exposure rates in patients with and without specific outcomes, self-controlled case series analyzing event rates during exposed and unexposed periods within the same patients, and prescription sequence symmetry analysis examining the sequence of medication initiation and event occurrence.

Table 5.2: Methods of Signal Detection in Pharmacovigilance

Signal Detection Method	Advantages	Limitations
Disproportionality Analysis	Requires minimal resources Can detect rare signals Allows automation Works with large databases No denominator needed	False positives common Confounding not addressed Reporting biases affect results Limited by data quality No causal assessment
Sequential Probability Ratio Test (SPRT)	Early signal detection Controls false positive rate Efficient for active surveillance Adjustable thresholds Works with limited data	Complex implementation Requires ongoing monitoring Needs accurate baseline Less effective for rare events Parameter specification
Multivariate Logistic Regression	Controls for confounding Quantifies variable relationships Can incorporate multiple factors Estimates adjusted risk	Requires large datasets Computationally intensive Model specification critical Needs complete data Complex interpretation

	Tests multiple hypotheses	
Case Series Analysis	Detailed clinical information Reveals temporal relationships Identifies unique presentations Detects rare/serious events Includes dechallenge/rechallenge	Labor intensive Small sample size Subjective assessment Limited generalizability Selection bias
Bayesian Neural Networks	Handles complex relationships Learning capabilities Detects novel patterns Improves with more data Automated signal identification	"Black box" results Requires extensive training Technical expertise needed Computational resources Validation challenges
Natural Language Processing (NLP)	Leverages unstructured data Processes large text volumes Detects novel terminology Extracts contextual information Supplements structured data	Language/terminology challenges Accuracy varies by context Requires validation Resource intensive Privacy considerations

Targeted surveillance studies prospectively collect data regarding specific safety concerns based on theoretical risks or preliminary signals. These studies employ standardized monitoring protocols focusing on predefined outcomes of interest, often employing enriched enrollment strategies to increase statistical power for detecting rare events. Event adjudication committees typically review potential cases using standardized criteria to ensure consistent outcome classification. Such studies frequently represent post-marketing requirements for medications approved with significant uncertainty regarding specific safety aspects.

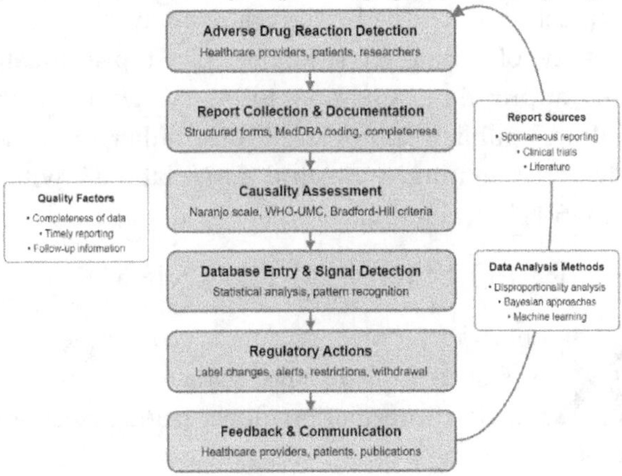

Figure 5.2: Adverse Drug Reaction (ADR) Processing

Signal strengthening involves triangulation of evidence across multiple data sources and methodologies to confirm initial signals before regulatory action or major clinical practice changes. This process evaluates signal consistency across different study designs, populations, and data sources; biological plausibility based on pharmacological properties and potential mechanisms; dose-response relationships supporting causal association; and confounding factors that might explain apparent associations. Signal strengthening recognizes that individual detection methods have specific limitations and biases, with convergent evidence across complementary approaches providing stronger support for true safety signals.

Signal prioritization systems guide resource allocation for further investigation based on signal characteristics. Priority factors typically include the seriousness of the potential adverse effect, strength of the evidence supporting the association, potential public health impact based on medication utilization patterns, availability of therapeutic alternatives, and whether the effect represents a previously unidentified risk or alteration in frequency or severity of a known risk. Structured prioritization ensures appropriate attention to signals with greatest clinical and public health significance rather than those merely representing statistical associations without meaningful clinical implications.

REPORTING MECHANISMS

Reporting mechanisms constitute the infrastructure through which adverse drug reaction information flows from detection to analysis, forming the backbone of effective pharmacovigilance systems. These mechanisms operate at individual, organizational, national, and international levels, incorporating both mandatory and voluntary components to create comprehensive safety monitoring networks.

Spontaneous reporting systems represent the most widespread pharmacovigilance reporting mechanism, collecting voluntary reports of suspected adverse drug reactions from healthcare professionals, patients, and manufacturers. Major national systems include the FDA Adverse Event Reporting System (FAERS) in the United

States, the Yellow Card Scheme in the United Kingdom, and the Canadian Vigilance Program. These systems typically employ standardized reporting forms capturing essential information including patient characteristics, suspected medications, adverse event descriptions, and outcome data. While historically paper-based, contemporary systems increasingly offer electronic submission options including web interfaces and mobile applications to reduce reporting barriers.

Table 5.3: Adverse Drug Reaction Reporting Systems

Stakeholder	Primary Reporting Methods	Information Typically Reported
Healthcare Professionals	Web-based forms Electronic health record integration Mobile applications Paper forms Telephone hotlines	Drug information Adverse event description Patient characteristics Treatment details Clinical outcomes Causality assessment
Patients/Consumers	Web portals Mobile applications Paper forms Call centers Through healthcare providers Patient organizations	Symptom descriptions Timing of events Impact on quality of life Treatment changes Medication details Personal experiences
Pharmaceutical Industry	Electronic gateways E2B formatted	Comprehensive case details Follow-up

Stakeholder	Primary Reporting Methods	Information Typically Reported
	submissions Database management systems Expedited reporting Periodic safety reports Literature monitoring	information Literature findings Clinical trial data Post-marketing surveillance Causality assessments Global safety data
Healthcare Organizations	Internal reporting systems Medication error systems Quality improvement databases Electronic health records External regulatory reporting	Event details Contributing factors System issues Patient outcomes Corrective actions Process deviations Local trends
Research Organizations	Clinical trial safety reporting Literature publications Research databases Safety monitoring boards Registry studies Collaborative networks	Trial-related adverse events Unexpected findings Statistical analyses Risk factor identification Comparative data Long-term outcomes

Mandatory reporting requirements establish legal

obligations for adverse event reporting by pharmaceutical manufacturers and sometimes healthcare organizations. In most jurisdictions, manufacturers must report serious, unexpected adverse reactions within strict timeframes (typically 15 days for serious, unexpected reactions) and submit periodic safety update reports summarizing cumulative safety experience. Some regulatory systems also mandate reporting of medication errors, quality defects, and emerging safety concerns not manifesting as specific adverse events. Compliance with these requirements typically undergoes regulatory inspection with potential penalties for systematic non-compliance.

Patient reporting mechanisms increasingly complement traditional healthcare professional reporting, recognizing that patients often detect adverse effects not documented in clinical records. Dedicated patient reporting portals offer structured forms adapted for lay terminology and direct experience description. Some systems incorporate validated patient-reported outcome measures to standardize symptom reporting. Research indicates that patient reports frequently contain more detailed descriptions of symptom experience and impact on quality of life, providing valuable perspective complementing clinical assessment.

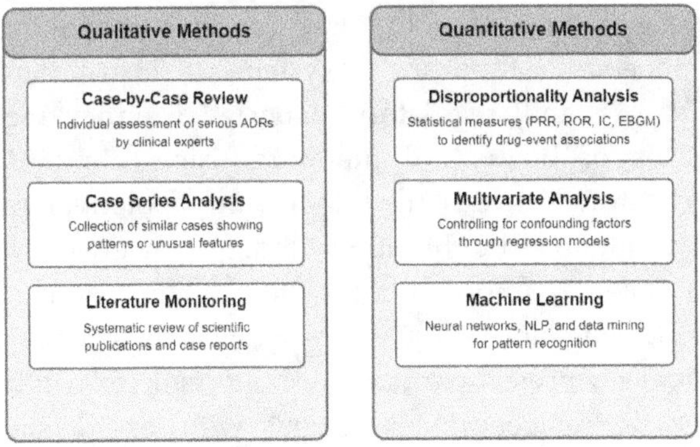

Figure 5.3: Signal Detection Methods

Hospital adverse drug reaction reporting systems operate within individual healthcare facilities, collecting information about medication-related harm for both internal quality improvement and external reporting. Contemporary hospital systems typically integrate with electronic health records, allowing direct reporting from clinical workflows and supplementation with relevant laboratory and medication data. Some systems incorporate semi-automated detection through trigger tools or rule-based screening to identify potential adverse events for confirmation by clinical reviewers.

Electronic reporting standards enhance interoperability across pharmacovigilance systems by establishing common data elements and transmission formats. The International Conference on Harmonisation E2B standard defines specifications for electronic transmission of individual case safety reports between organizations and regulatory authorities. Implementation of these standards enables more efficient report exchange, reduces duplicate entry requirements, and supports aggregated analysis across multiple data sources while maintaining data privacy requirements.

Literature monitoring constitutes a structured approach to identifying adverse event reports in published medical literature that might not reach spontaneous reporting systems. Pharmaceutical companies and regulatory agencies conduct regular searches of biomedical literature using standardized search strategies designed to identify potential safety signals. Identified publications undergo review to extract reportable information for inclusion in pharmacovigilance databases and analysis. This mechanism proves particularly important for capturing experience in geographic regions with less developed spontaneous reporting infrastructure.

Social media and internet monitoring represent emerging reporting mechanisms leveraging patient discussions in online forums, social networking platforms, and patient communities. Natural language processing and machine learning techniques identify potential adverse effect descriptions in unstructured text, while maintaining appropriate privacy protections. While methodologically challenging due to verification difficulties and selection biases, these approaches potentially capture patient experiences occurring outside formal healthcare encounters and may detect signals earlier than traditional systems, particularly for effects impacting quality of life rather than generating medical interventions.

Vaccine adverse event reporting systems operate as specialized pharmacovigilance mechanisms addressing the unique characteristics of vaccines, including population-wide administration to healthy individuals and complex benefit-risk considerations during public health emergencies. Systems such as the Vaccine Adverse Event Reporting System (VAERS) in the United States employ enhanced surveillance during immunization campaigns and specialized causality assessment systems recognizing the challenges of distinguishing vaccine reactions from coincidental events in mass vaccination programs.

Cross-national reporting networks integrate national pharmacovigilance systems to enhance signal detection capabilities and harmonize safety responses. The World Health Organization's Programme for International Drug Monitoring coordinates the global network of national pharmacovigilance centers, with the Uppsala Monitoring Centre maintaining the VigiBase global database of individual case safety reports. EudraVigilance serves a similar function within the European Union, collecting reports from all member states. These networks enable identification of safety signals too rare to detect within individual countries and support coordinated regulatory responses to emerging safety concerns.

DATA ANALYSIS AND INTERPRETATION

Data analysis and interpretation transform raw pharmacovigilance information into actionable knowledge about medication safety, employing both quantitative and qualitative methodologies to evaluate the strength, consistency, and clinical significance of safety signals. This process navigates numerous methodological challenges including reporting biases, confounding factors, and the inherent limitations of observational data.

Causality assessment systems provide structured approaches to evaluating the likelihood that observed adverse events resulted from medication exposure rather than underlying disease or coincidental occurrence. The World Health Organization-Uppsala Monitoring Centre (WHO-UMC) criteria and the Naranjo algorithm represent widely used systems incorporating factors such as temporal relationship, dechallenge/rechallenge experience, alternative explanations, and known pharmacological properties. More specialized instruments address specific contexts such as vaccine reactions (WHO AEFI causality assessment), hepatotoxicity (RUCAM scale), and cutaneous reactions (ALDEN algorithm). While these systems enhance assessment consistency, they require judicious application with recognition of their limitations in complex clinical scenarios with multiple potential contributing factors.

Quantitative signal detection employs statistical

methodologies to identify disproportionate reporting of specific medication-event combinations. The proportional reporting ratio (PRR) compares the proportion of a specific event among all reports for a medication against the proportion for all other medications. The reporting odds ratio (ROR) uses a case-control conceptualization, comparing the odds of exposure to the medication of interest between cases with and without the specific event. More sophisticated measures such as the information component (IC) and empirical Bayes geometric mean (EBGM) incorporate shrinkage estimation to reduce false signals from small sample sizes. These measures generate signal scores that, when exceeding predefined thresholds, trigger further evaluation.

Table 5.4: Data Analysis Techniques in Pharmacovigilance

Analysis Type	Data Requirements	Limitations	Output Examples
Descriptive Analysis	Aggregate ADR reports Basic demographic data Reporting dates Geographic information Drug exposure data when available	Limited causal inference Subject to reporting biases Data quality dependent May miss important associations Limited by available variables	ADR frequency tables Demographic profiles Time-trend graphs Geographic distribution maps System utilization metrics
Signal Detection and Prioritiz	Large databases of ADR reports Background	False positive signals Masking effects	Signal detection scorecards Prioritized

Analysis Type	Data Requirements	Limitations	Output Examples
ation	frequency data Drug utilization data Historical signal information Structured terminologies	Confounding by indication Variability in clinical coding Resource-intensive validation	signal lists Drug-event combinations Signal threshold reports Comparative signal strength
Case-Level Clinical Assessment	Detailed individual case reports Medical history Concomitant medications Laboratory results Clinical narratives	Subjective assessment Inter-rater variability Missing clinical information Time-consuming process Limited generalizability	Causality assessment scores Case series summaries Expert consensus reports Case narratives Clinical recommendations
Epidemiological Studies	Patient-level clinical data Exposure information Outcome validation Control selection Confounding variable data	Selection bias Information bias Confounding Generalizability concerns Resource requirements	Relative risk estimates Odds ratios Hazard ratios Number needed to harm Population attributable risk
Benefit-Risk	Efficacy data Safety data	Value judgment	Benefit-risk profiles

Analysis Type	Data Requirements	Limitations	Output Examples
Assessment	Indication information Patient preference data Clinical context information	subjectivity Data quality variability Methodological complexity Disease context dependency Stakeholder perspective differences	Decision matrices Visualized benefit-risk balance Stakeholder perspective maps Utility trade-off analyses
Impact Analysis	Longitudinal outcome data Intervention timing information Process metrics Healthcare utilization data Survey or interview data	Causal attribution challenges External factor influence Implementation variability Time lag effects Measurement limitations	Trend impact analyses Process improvement metrics Implementation effectiveness Stakeholder feedback summaries System performance indicators

Signal validation distinguishes genuine safety concerns from statistical artifacts or reporting biases through multifaceted evaluation of detected signals. This process determines signal consistency across subgroups, stability over time, presence of dose-response relationships, biological plausibility based on pharmacological properties, consistency with preclinical data, and potential confounding factors. Triage approaches prioritize signals based on clinical seriousness, signal strength, affected population size, and therapeutic context. Validation outcomes range from signal dismissal as likely artifactual to confirmation requiring risk minimization actions, with intermediate categories prompting continued monitoring or targeted investigation.

Meta-analytic approaches synthesize safety data across multiple studies to enhance statistical power for detecting rare adverse effects. Traditional meta-analysis combines published clinical trial safety data, while individual patient data meta-analysis incorporates raw data from multiple studies to enable more sophisticated modeling and subgroup analysis. Network meta-analysis extends these approaches to situations where direct comparative data are limited, estimating relative safety profiles across multiple treatment options. These methodologies prove particularly valuable for evaluating class effects and comparative safety profiles among therapeutic alternatives.

Observational study designs complement spontaneous reporting analysis by addressing many of its inherent limitations. Cohort studies provide incidence rate estimates and enable direct comparison between exposed and unexposed populations. Case-control designs efficiently evaluate rare outcomes by comparing medication exposure between affected and unaffected individuals. Self-controlled designs use patients as their own controls, comparing event rates during exposed and unexposed periods to control for stable patient characteristics. Each design offers distinct advantages for specific research questions while requiring appropriate methods to address potential bias and confounding.

Risk characterization synthesizes available evidence to describe the nature, frequency, and severity of adverse effects associated with medications. This process defines the affected population through identification of risk factors and vulnerable subgroups, quantifies risk through absolute and relative risk measures with confidence intervals reflecting estimation uncertainty, and contextualizes risk through comparison with therapeutic alternatives and baseline risks in the target population. Effective risk characterization avoids oversimplification while presenting information in formats accessible to various stakeholders, including clinicians, patients, and policymakers.

Benefit-risk assessment integrates safety findings with efficacy data to evaluate the overall value proposition of medications for specific indications and populations. Structured assessment systems such as the Benefit-Risk Action Team (BRAT) framework, the CIRS-BRAT framework, and the FDA's Benefit-Risk Framework incorporate multicriteria decision analysis to systematically compare therapeutic options across multiple domains. Quantitative approaches increasingly complement qualitative judgment, employing quality-adjusted life years (QALYs) or disability-adjusted life years (DALYs) to create common metrics for comparing beneficial and adverse effects. Contemporary approaches emphasize the dynamic nature of benefit-risk balance, recognizing that new safety information or emerging therapeutic alternatives may alter assessments over time.

Real-world evidence integration addresses the frequent divergence between clinical trial safety profiles and post-marketing experience. This approach synthesizes data from diverse sources including electronic health records, claims databases, patient registries, and patient-reported outcomes to develop comprehensive safety profiles reflecting actual usage patterns. Methodological challenges include data quality variation, missing information, selection biases, and confounding by indication. Advanced analytical techniques including propensity score methods, instrumental variable analysis, and high-dimensional propensity score adjustment help address these challenges, though limitations of observational data always require transparent acknowledgment.

Signal communication translates analytical findings into appropriate messages for various stakeholders. Regulatory communications include product labeling changes, safety alerts, and Dear Healthcare Provider letters for urgent concerns. Clinical practice guideline integration ensures safety findings influence treatment recommendations. Patient-directed communications increasingly employ risk visualization techniques, absolute risk presentation, and natural frequency formats rather than relative risks or odds ratios that may distort risk perception. Effective communication strategies consider audience health literacy, risk comprehension capabilities, and information needs while maintaining scientific accuracy and appropriate uncertainty acknowledgment.

Things to Remember

- ☑ Adverse drug reaction monitoring employs multiple methods including spontaneous reporting, active surveillance through established cohorts, and database studies analyzing health records.
- ☑ Signal detection methods use statistical algorithms to identify potential safety concerns through disproportionality analysis, sequence pattern recognition, and multivariate techniques.
- ☑ Reporting mechanisms include national systems (FDA MedWatch, Yellow Card Scheme),

manufacturer requirements, and international networks through WHO's Uppsala Monitoring Centre.

- ☑ Analysis involves causality assessment distinguishing adverse reactions from coincidental events, risk characterization establishing significance, and impact determination driving interventions.
- ☑ Effective pharmacovigilance balances signal detection sensitivity with specificity to prevent both missed safety issues and unnecessary medication abandonment.
- ☑ Communication strategies must ensure appropriate awareness of medication risks while preventing disproportionate concern undermining beneficial therapy.

Multiple Choice Questions

1. Which adverse drug reaction monitoring method involves analyzing large-scale health records for safety signals?
   a) Spontaneous reporting
   b) Active surveillance through established cohorts
   c) Database studies
   d) Case-control studies
2. Signal detection methodologies in pharmacovigilance include:
   a) Exclusively manual review of individual case reports
   b) Statistical algorithms identifying disproportionate reporting patterns
   c) Focus solely on serious adverse events

resulting in hospitalization
d) Analysis limited to medications on market less than one year

3. Which reporting system allows healthcare providers in the United States to submit adverse drug reaction reports?
   a) Yellow Card Scheme
   b) EudraVigilance
   c) FDA MedWatch
   d) Uppsala Monitoring Centre
4. Causality assessment in pharmacovigilance:
   a) Is unnecessary when temporal relationship exists between drug exposure and event
   b) Distinguishes true adverse reactions from coincidental events
   c) Should focus exclusively on previously documented adverse reactions
   d) Is primarily the responsibility of pharmaceutical manufacturers
5. The Uppsala Monitoring Centre:
   a) Regulates medication approval in European countries
   b) Coordinates international adverse reaction data through WHO's global database
   c) Focuses exclusively on adverse reactions in developing countries
   d) Establishes binding regulations for pharmaceutical manufacturers
6. Standardized case definitions in adverse event reporting:
   a) Are primarily used for legal documentation
   b) Limit reporting to previously recognized adverse reactions

c) Enhance data quality by ensuring consistent categorization
d) Are identical across all countries and healthcare settings

7. Effective pharmacovigilance communication strategies must:
   a) Focus exclusively on healthcare providers without patient involvement
   b) Ensure awareness of medication risks while preventing unwarranted abandonment
   c) Emphasize all potential risks equally regardless of frequency or severity
   d) Be limited to package inserts and formal safety communications
8. Which of the following is NOT a typical method of active surveillance in pharmacovigilance?
   a) Pregnancy registries for monitoring medication effects
   b) Cohort studies following specific patient populations
   c) Retrospective chart reviews examining documentation practices
   d) Sentinel site monitoring in selected healthcare facilities
9. Post-marketing surveillance differs from pre-approval clinical trials by:
   a) Having less rigorous methodological requirements
   b) Detecting rare adverse effects through larger patient populations
   c) Focusing exclusively on efficacy rather than

safety

d) Involving only hospitalized patients

10. Benefit-risk evaluation in pharmacovigilance:

a) Should be performed once at medication approval without ongoing reassessment

b) Considers both positive therapeutic effects and potential harms in decision-making

c) Is primarily the responsibility of individual prescribers without systematic approach

d) Should prioritize all potential risks regardless of magnitude or likelihood

Self-Assessment Questions

1. Evaluate the evolution and current state of adverse drug reaction monitoring systems globally, comparing approaches between developed and developing countries.
2. Critically analyze the methodologies used in signal detection for adverse drug reactions, including their statistical foundations and practical applications.
3. Compare and contrast the various reporting mechanisms in pharmacovigilance, evaluating their effectiveness in capturing comprehensive safety data.
4. Discuss the advanced analytical techniques used in pharmacovigilance data interpretation and how they contribute to medication safety decision-making.
5. Evaluate the relationship between pharmacovigilance systems and regulatory actions, using case examples to illustrate the process from signal detection to intervention.
6. Analyze the challenges and opportunities in integrating pharmacovigilance data with electronic health records and other healthcare information systems.
7. Discuss the role of healthcare professionals, patients, and pharmaceutical manufacturers in creating a robust pharmacovigilance ecosystem, with emphasis on their respective responsibilities.
8. Evaluate how risk-benefit assessment is

conducted in pharmacovigilance and its impact on medication availability and usage guidelines.

9. Analyze the application of real-world data and evidence in modern pharmacovigilance systems and their potential to transform safety monitoring.
10. Discuss the ethical considerations in pharmacovigilance, including balancing medical innovation with patient safety, transparency in reporting, and global equity in safety monitoring.

Bibliography

1. World Health Organization. The importance of pharmacovigilance: safety monitoring of medicinal products. Geneva: World Health Organization; 2002.
2. Härmark L, van Grootheest AC. Pharmacovigilance: methods, recent developments and future perspectives. Eur J Clin Pharmacol. 2008;64(8):743-52.
3. Meyboom RH, Egberts AC, Edwards IR, Hekster YA, de Koning FH, Gribnau FW. Principles of signal detection in pharmacovigilance. Drug Saf. 1997;16(6):355-65.
4. Lindquist M. VigiBase, the WHO Global ICSR Database System: basic facts. Drug Inf J. 2008;42(5):409-19.
5. Bate A, Lindquist M, Edwards IR, Olsson S, Orre R, Lansner A, et al. A Bayesian neural network method for adverse drug reaction signal generation. Eur J Clin Pharmacol. 1998;54(4):315-21.
6. Hauben M, Aronson JK. Defining 'signal' and its subtypes in pharmacovigilance based on a systematic review of previous definitions. Drug Saf. 2009;32(2):99-110.
7. Hazell L, Shakir SA. Under-reporting of adverse drug reactions: a systematic review. Drug Saf. 2006;29(5):385-96.
8. Pirmohamed M, James S, Meakin S, Green C, Scott AK, Walley TJ, et al. Adverse drug reactions as cause of admission to hospital: prospective analysis of 18 820 patients. BMJ. 2004;329(7456):15-9.
9. Waller PC, Evans SJ. A model for the future conduct of pharmacovigilance. Pharmacoepidemiol Drug Saf. 2003;12(1):17-29.
10. Almenoff JS, Pattishall EN, Gibbs TG, DuMouchel W, Evans SJ, Yuen N. Novel statistical tools for monitoring the safety of marketed drugs. Clin Pharmacol Ther. 2007;82(2):157-66.

CHAPTER 6

EMBEDDING TECHNOLOGY IN MEDICATION SAFETY

Abstract

Technology integration transforms medication safety through systems addressing human limitations while introducing implementation and workflow considerations requiring careful management. Electronic health records create comprehensive information environments supporting medication decision-making through accurate documentation, integrated historical data, and standardized ordering processes with template-based approaches reducing variation. Clinical decision support systems provide intelligent assistance through interaction checking, dose range verification, laboratory-medication monitoring, and patient-specific risk assessment, requiring careful alert design preventing fatigue while maintaining critical warnings. Automated dispensing systems enhance medication distribution through secure storage, barcode verification during selection, integrated charging capabilities, and controlled access with complete transaction documentation. Barcode medication administration creates point-of-care verification confirming correct medication, patient, dose, route, and timing through systematic scanning processes integrated with documentation systems. Successful implementation requires workflow integration aligning technology with clinical processes, user involvement throughout development, phased introduction with appropriate support, and continuous optimization addressing emerging issues while enhancing safety capabilities.

Keywords: *Clinical decision support, automated dispensing, barcode verification, technology implementation, workflow integration*

Learning Objectives

After completion of the chapter, the learners should be able to:

- Remember the key technological systems used to enhance medication safety.
- Understand how different technologies address specific vulnerabilities in the medication use process.
- Apply principles of effective technology implementation to support medication safety initiatives.
- Analyze the strengths and limitations of various medication safety technologies.
- Evaluate the impact of specific technologies on medication error reduction.
- Create a technology implementation plan addressing workflow integration and user adoption

ELECTRONIC HEALTH RECORDS

Electronic health records (EHRs) have transformed medication management, replacing paper-based processes with integrated digital systems that enhance communication, documentation, and safety monitoring throughout the medication use process. These comprehensive systems serve as the foundational technology infrastructure upon which other medication safety technologies depend, creating interconnected networks of patient information, clinical decisions, and safety checks.

Evolution and Core Functionality

The evolution of EHRs from basic digital documentation to sophisticated clinical information systems reflects the growing recognition of their potential to address medication safety challenges. Early electronic medical records primarily digitized paper charts, offering limited functionality beyond improved legibility and accessibility. Contemporary EHRs integrate medication-specific modules with comprehensive clinical information, creating unified platforms spanning the entire medication use process from prescribing to monitoring.

Core medication management functionality includes computerized provider order entry (CPOE), medication reconciliation tools, allergy documentation, pharmacy verification systems, medication administration records, and documentation of patient response. Integration with laboratory systems enables automated display of relevant physiological parameters alongside medication information, supporting both initial prescribing decisions and ongoing monitoring. Interoperability capabilities facilitate information exchange across care transitions, addressing historical communication gaps that contributed to medication errors during hospital admission, transfer, and discharge.

Safety Benefits and Evidence Base

The safety benefits of EHRs derive from multiple mechanisms, including elimination of transcription processes, improved information access, structured data entry, and automated verification procedures. Research demonstrates substantial reduction in medication errors following well-designed EHR implementation, with particularly strong evidence for error reduction in the prescribing phase. A systematic review of 22 studies found that CPOE implementation was associated with a 48% reduction in medication errors, with greater benefits observed in systems with more sophisticated clinical decision support.

Table 6.1: Electronic Health Record Medication Safety Features and Their Impact

Safety Feature	**Description**	**Unintended Consequences**
Computerized Provider Order Entry (CPOE)	Electronic medication ordering with structured fields, replacing handwritten orders	New error types (e.g., wrong selection) Alert fatigue Copy-paste errors Workarounds Knowledge gaps about system capabilities
Clinical Decision Support (CDS)	Rule-based alerts for drug allergies, interactions, dose checking, and clinical contraindications	Alert fatigue and overrides False positive and false negative alerts Over-reliance on technology Interrupted workflow Potential legal liability concerns
Electronic Medication Administration Record (eMAR)	Electronic documentation of medication administration with workflow support	Device availability issues Delayed documentation Battery/connectivity problems Dual documentation in some settings Time spent on technology vs. patient care
Medication	Electronic tools	Perpetuation of

Safety Feature	Description	Unintended Consequences
Reconciliation Tools	for capturing, comparing, and updating medication lists across transitions	medication errors Incomplete medication histories Fragmented lists across settings Over-reliance on electronic sources Time-consuming processes
Electronic Prescribing/e-Prescribing	Direct electronic transmission of prescriptions to pharmacies	Transmission failures Default selection errors Pharmacy system incompatibilities Patient confusion with multiple systems Automated refill issues
Interoperability and Health Information Exchange	Exchange of medication information across organizations and care settings	Information overload Outdated or incorrect data Incomplete data exchange System downtime impacts Limited standardization across systems

Specific safety advantages include elimination of illegibility issues that historically plagued handwritten orders, incorporation of weight-based dosing calculations that reduce mathematical errors, structured prescription formats that ensure inclusion of essential prescription elements, and improved communication between prescribers, pharmacists, and nurses. EHRs also support population health approaches to medication safety through identification of patients requiring intervention, surveillance for emerging safety issues, and systematic monitoring of high-risk medications across entire patient populations.

Implementation Challenges and Unintended Consequences

Despite their potential benefits, EHR implementation presents significant challenges that must be addressed to realize safety improvements. Financial barriers represent persistent obstacles, particularly for smaller healthcare organizations, despite government incentive programs in many countries. Technical challenges include integration of legacy systems, data migration from paper records, and establishment of interfaces with external systems such as laboratory information systems and pharmacy management software.

Workflow disruption during implementation can temporarily increase error risk, necessitating careful transition planning and adequate support during initial implementation phases. User resistance stemming from increased documentation time, perceived workflow inefficiencies, and technical difficulties requires systematic change management approaches incorporating user engagement in system selection and configuration, comprehensive training programs, and responsive technical support.

Unintended consequences of EHR implementation include new error types specific to electronic environments. Copy-and-paste functionality, while efficient, can perpetuate outdated or incorrect information across multiple documentation instances. Alert fatigue from excessive non-specific warnings leads to routine override behaviors that compromise safety benefits. Screen design limitations may fragment information display, requiring clinicians to navigate multiple screens to assemble a complete clinical picture. System downtime, whether planned or unplanned, creates vulnerability periods requiring robust contingency procedures to maintain medication safety.

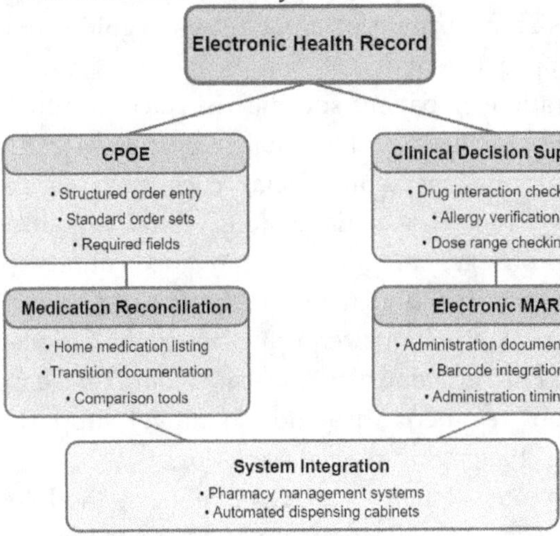

Figure 6.1 Electronic Health Record Safety

Optimization Strategies for Safety Enhancement

Optimization of EHR systems represents an ongoing process of refinement to maximize safety benefits while mitigating unintended consequences. User-centered design principles emphasize alignment with clinical workflows, intuitive interface design, and minimization of unnecessary data entry requirements. Configuration of medication-specific components should prioritize safety over convenience, incorporating appropriate constraints and verification requirements for high-risk medications while streamlining processes for routine orders.

Governance structures for ongoing EHR optimization

should include formal medication safety committees with representation from all disciplines involved in medication use. These committees establish systematic review processes for EHR-related medication safety events, identify improvement opportunities, and evaluate potential configuration changes before implementation. Regular review of override patterns, error reports, and near-miss events provides valuable data to guide targeted system improvements.

Integration of patient-specific risk factors into EHR displays enhances situational awareness during medication management. Visual cues such as color-coding for high-risk patients (e.g., renal impairment, extremes of age, pregnancy) and medications (e.g., anticoagulants, insulin, chemotherapy) create immediate recognition of situations requiring heightened vigilance. Standardized problem lists and care plans for complex medication regimens provide cognitive support for managing challenging clinical scenarios.

Continuous quality improvement methodologies applied to EHR medication modules create systematic approaches to safety enhancement. Regular assessment of medication-related EHR functions using validated tools such as the Leapfrog CPOE Evaluation Tool identifies specific vulnerability areas requiring attention. User feedback mechanisms including structured surveys and direct observation studies provide complementary qualitative information about experienced safety challenges. These continuous improvement processes recognize that EHR safety enhancement represents an evolutionary journey rather than a destination reached at implementation.

CLINICAL DECISION SUPPORT

SYSTEMS

Clinical decision support systems (CDSS) augment human decision-making through automated analysis of patient-specific information and presentation of relevant knowledge at appropriate decision points. These systems range from basic rule-based alerts to sophisticated algorithms employing artificial intelligence, creating layered safety nets throughout the medication use process.

Taxonomy and Core Components

Clinical decision support encompasses diverse interventions classified along several dimensions: timing (preventive vs. reactive), action requirements (informational vs. interruptive), knowledge base (static rules vs. dynamic learning systems), and specificity (general vs. patient-tailored). Core components include a knowledge base containing clinical rules and medication information, an inference engine applying these rules to patient-specific data, input mechanisms gathering relevant clinical information, and output methods communicating recommendations to clinicians.

Basic CDSS functions include drug-drug interaction checking, drug-allergy verification, duplicate therapy detection, dose range verification, and contraindication screening based on documented conditions. More sophisticated systems incorporate pharmacogenomic information, renal dosing adjustments, age-appropriate dosing, pregnancy safety information, and therapeutic drug monitoring guidance. Advanced systems increasingly employ predictive analytics to identify patients at elevated risk for adverse drug events before they occur.

The "five rights" framework for CDSS design emphasizes delivering the right information to the right person in the right format through the right channel at the right time in workflow. This approach recognizes that technical sophistication alone does not ensure safety improvement; rather, effective integration into clinical workflows and decision processes determines practical utility. Systems designed with attention to these principles demonstrate higher acceptance rates and greater safety impact than technically advanced systems that disrupt workflow or present information at inappropriate times.

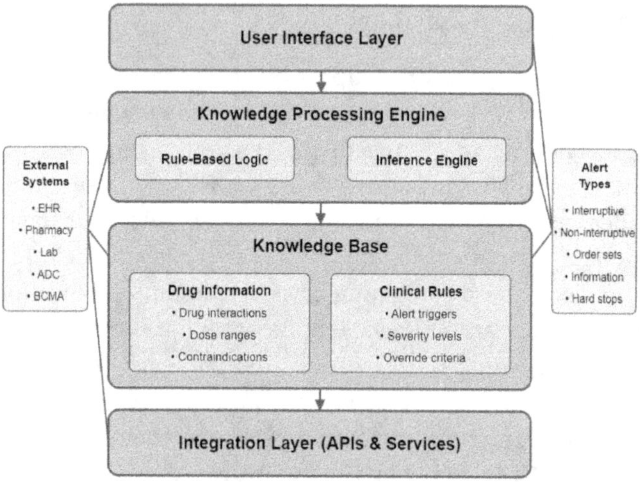

Figure 6.2 Clinical Decision Support System

Evidence Base and Safety Impact

Research demonstrates that well-designed CDSS implementations significantly reduce medication errors and adverse drug events across diverse healthcare settings. A systematic review of 49 randomized controlled trials found that CDSS implementation was associated with a 36-84% reduction in medication errors depending on clinical context and system design. Safety impacts appear strongest for preventable adverse drug events with clear mechanistic pathways, such as renal dosing errors, contraindicated combinations, and therapeutic duplication.

Specific safety domains showing consistent benefits include antibiotic stewardship, anticoagulation management, and geriatric medication safety. In antibiotic management, CDSS tools incorporating local resistance patterns, culture results, and patient-specific factors have demonstrated both safety improvements (reduced adverse drug reactions) and clinical benefits (improved treatment appropriateness). Anticoagulation management systems integrating laboratory monitoring, drug interaction screening, and dose adjustment algorithms show reduced bleeding complications and improved time in therapeutic range. Geriatric-specific systems incorporating screening for potentially inappropriate medications based on Beers criteria or STOPP/START criteria demonstrate reduced adverse drug event rates in elderly populations.

Despite these positive findings, research also indicates substantial variation in effectiveness across implementation contexts. System design characteristics associated with greater impact include provision of actionable recommendations rather than assessment alone, integration into clinical workflow rather than requiring separate access, and automatic provision of decision support rather than requiring user activation. Organizational context factors influencing effectiveness include leadership support, available technical resources, and established quality improvement cultures.

Alert Design and Alert Fatigue Mitigation

Alert design significantly influences CDSS effectiveness, with poorly designed alerts frequently ignored or overridden despite valid safety concerns. Effective alert design incorporates human factors principles including clear, concise language; distinct visual characteristics based on severity; specific actionable recommendations; and provision of sufficient context to enable informed decision-making. Presentation of the specific safety concern, potential consequences, and recommended actions supports appropriate clinical response more effectively than generic warnings.

Table 6.2: Clinical Decision Support Systems for Medication Safety

CDS Type	Primary Functions	Alert Sensitivity/Specificity
Drug Allergy Checking	Screens orders against documented allergies Identifies potential cross-sensitivities Categorizes by severity/reaction type Suggests alternatives	False positives from non-specific reactions Lack of differentiation between intolerance and true allergy Overalerts for class-based cross-reactivity Limited consideration of rechallenge history
Drug-Drug Interaction Checking	Identifies potentially interacting drug pairs Stratifies by severity/evidence Provides mechanism information Suggests	High sensitivity but low specificity Limited context consideration Excessive alerting for common combinations Inadequate timing consideration Limited

CDS Type	Primary Functions	Alert Sensitivity/Specificity
	management strategies	consideration of dose-dependent effects
Dose Range Checking	Validates doses against reference ranges Checks for age/weight-based appropriateness Identifies potential underdosing/overdosing Checks cumulative daily doses	Weight-based calculations require accurate weights Indication-specific dosing challenges Renal/hepatic adjustment complexity Special population reference ranges Limited consideration of combination therapy
Medication-Condition Contraindications	Checks medications against documented conditions Identifies absolute/relative contraindications Provides rationale and alternatives Prioritizes by clinical significance	Dependent on accurate problem list maintenance Limited by non-coded or missing conditions May not consider condition severity/status Overalerts for well-managed conditions Limited consideration of risk-benefit
Medication Monitoring	Prompts for required laboratory	Balance between proactive vs.

CDS Type	Primary Functions	Alert Sensitivity/Specificity
Alerts	monitoring Suggests timing for follow-up tests Identifies missing monitoring parameters Alerts for abnormal results requiring action	reactive alerts Timing precision for monitoring recommendations Consideration of recently ordered tests Limited integration across care transitions Responsibility assignment challenges
Pregnancy/Lactation Alerts	Identifies medications contraindicated in pregnancy/lactation Stratifies risk by trimester/lactation Provides FDA pregnancy category information Suggests safer alternatives	Dependent on documented pregnancy status Limited by pregnancy timing uncertainty Required preemptive documentation Nuanced benefit-risk assessments Limited consideration of disease severity

Alert fatigue—the desensitization to safety warnings due to excessive frequency or perceived irrelevance—represents a significant challenge in CDSS implementation. Studies demonstrate override rates exceeding 90% for certain alert types, undermining the safety value of even well-designed systems. Successful mitigation strategies include tiered alerting based on severity and certainty, contextual filtering using additional clinical parameters, suppression of repeat alerts within appropriate timeframes, and customization based on provider specialty and practice setting.

Evidence-based alert governance establishes systematic processes for alert evaluation and refinement. Effective governance includes regular review of override rates and patterns, assessment of patient outcomes following overrides, solicitation of user feedback regarding alert utility, and structured processes for alert modification based on these data sources. Some organizations implement alert review committees with multidisciplinary representation to evaluate proposed alerts before implementation and periodically review existing alerts for continued relevance and appropriate sensitivity.

Advanced Applications and Emerging Technologies

Advanced CDSS applications extend beyond traditional rule-based alerts to incorporate sophisticated analytics and learning systems. Pharmacogenomic decision support integrates genetic testing results with medication selection and dosing, enabling personalized therapy adjustments based on individual metabolic profiles. These systems demonstrate particular value for medications with narrow therapeutic indices and known genetic influences on metabolism, such as warfarin, clopidogrel, and certain antidepressants.

Predictive analytics employing machine learning algorithms identify subtle patterns in clinical data suggesting elevated risk for adverse drug events before they become clinically apparent. These systems analyze diverse data elements including laboratory trends, vital signs, medication regimens, and comorbidities to generate risk scores that trigger proactive interventions.

Early applications show promise for anticipating adverse events including acute kidney injury, QT interval prolongation, and hypoglycemia, enabling preventive actions before harm occurs.

Natural language processing capabilities extract medication-related information from unstructured clinical notes, identifying potential contraindications, adverse effects, or medication changes not captured in structured data fields. This technology proves particularly valuable for identifying medication changes occurring outside the primary healthcare system or adverse effects mentioned in clinical documentation but not formally coded, enhancing medication reconciliation processes and adverse event detection.

Mobile applications extend decision support beyond traditional clinical environments, providing medication information, interaction checking, and dosing guidance at the point of care regardless of location. These tools prove particularly valuable in settings with limited access to comprehensive electronic health records, such as home care, long-term care facilities, and resource-limited environments. Integration with barcode scanning capabilities enables rapid access to medication information from packaged products, supporting both healthcare professional and patient medication management.

AUTOMATED DISPENSING SYSTEMS

Automated dispensing systems (ADS) represent sophisticated medication management technologies that combine secure storage, inventory control, and dispensing functionality within decentralized locations throughout healthcare facilities. These systems have evolved from basic controlled substance cabinets to comprehensive medication management platforms that interface with electronic health records, barcode verification systems, and clinical documentation tools.

System Types and Core Functionality

Automated dispensing systems encompass several distinct technologies with complementary safety functions. Cabinet-based systems represent the most widespread implementation, featuring electronically controlled compartments containing medications for authorized access at the point of care. These systems typically employ user authentication, automated documentation of medication removal, configurable security features based on medication risk, and interface capabilities with pharmacy information systems and electronic health records.

Carousel technology, typically implemented within central pharmacy operations, provides high-density storage with computerized rotation to present specific medications for retrieval. These systems incorporate barcode verification during stocking and retrieval processes, picking lights to identify specific medication locations, and inventory management software that optimizes storage configuration based on usage patterns. Integration with compounding systems and dispensing robots creates comprehensive pharmacy automation systems spanning medication preparation and distribution functions.

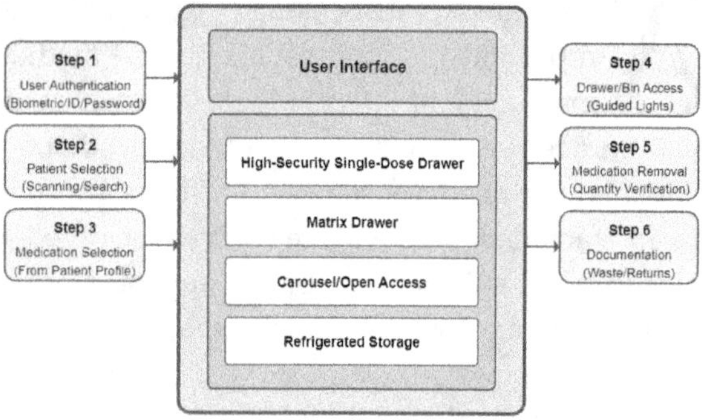

Figure 6.3 Automated Dispensing Cabinet Workflow and Safety

Robotic dispensing systems automate medication picking, packaging, and labeling functions, reducing human manipulation of medications before administration. These systems range from centralized robots handling high-volume medications to sophisticated compounding systems for sterile product preparation. Safety features include barcode verification throughout the preparation process, gravimetric checking of components in compounded products, and automated documentation of preparation parameters for traceability.

Unit-dose packaging systems automate the repackaging of bulk medications into patient-specific doses with appropriate labeling and barcode identification. These systems enhance safety through standardized packaging that reduces manipulation before administration, clear labeling that supports accurate identification, and barcode labeling that enables verification during administration. Integration with dispensing robots and cabinet systems creates closed-loop medication distribution systems with verification at each transfer point.

Table 6.3: Automated Dispensing Systems

Feature	Purpose	Benefits
Profile-Linked Dispensing	Links medication removal to verified pharmacy orders	54-97% reduction in unauthorized medication access Elimination of non-profiled medication use Direct interface with pharmacy verification Reduced verbal order risks
Controlled Substance Management	Secured storage with tracking for controlled drugs	15-59% reduction in controlled substance diversion Complete transaction audit trails Automated inventory reconciliation Waste documentation enforcement Usage pattern analysis
Barcode-Assisted Refill	Verification of medications during cabinet restocking	86-97% reduction in restocking errors Wrong bin placement prevention Expired medication identification Lot/expiration tracking capability Recall management support
Drawer Configuration Options	Various security levels for different medication types	Highest security for high-alert medications High-risk medication segregation Look-alike/sound-alike separation Reduced selection

Feature	Purpose	Benefits
		errors Configurable to risk profile
Integrated Clinical Decision Support	Alerts and warnings during medication removal	5-30% reduction in administration errors High-alert medication warnings Allergy alerts at point of removal Special handling reminders Age/weight-based warnings
Inventory Management	Automated tracking and optimization of medication stock	42-96% reduction in stockouts Expiration date monitoring Par level optimization Usage pattern analysis Recall management
Remote Medication Queuing	Ability to prepare multiple patients' medications remotely	Workflow efficiency improvement Reduced waiting time at cabinet Decreased traffic around ADCs Improved first-dose turnaround Withdrawal organization

Safety Benefits and Evidence Base

Research demonstrates significant safety benefits associated with well-implemented automated dispensing systems across multiple domains. Medication selection errors during dispensing decrease through forced-function design that physically separates look-alike medications and requires barcode verification during restocking processes. Studies demonstrate error reduction rates of 54-97% compared to traditional floor stock systems depending on specific implementation characteristics and baseline error rates.

Controlled substance management represents a particularly important safety domain addressed by automated systems. These technologies create reliable audit trails documenting every transaction, enable automated discrepancy detection through perpetual inventory tracking, implement secure access controls including biometric authentication when appropriate, and generate surveillance reports identifying unusual usage patterns that might suggest diversion. Research demonstrates significant reduction in controlled substance discrepancies following implementation, with associated decreases in diversion opportunities.

Inventory optimization features ensure appropriate medication availability while minimizing expired medication waste and reducing the risk of critical shortages. Automated par level adjustment based on usage patterns, expiration date tracking with removal prompts for soon-to-expire medications, and automated reordering capabilities enhance both operational efficiency and medication safety by ensuring consistent availability of necessary medications. These functions prove particularly valuable during drug shortage situations by enabling optimal allocation of limited supplies.

Emergency medication management benefits from specialized configurations supporting rapid access while maintaining appropriate security and documentation. Emergency override functions allow access to critical medications during emergencies while maintaining complete audit trails. Code cart functionality supports standardized emergency medication organization with automated tracking of expiration dates and usage. Integration with emergency documentation systems creates comprehensive records of medication administration during critical events.

Implementation Considerations and Workflow Integration

Successful implementation of automated dispensing systems requires careful consideration of physical space constraints, workflow patterns, and integration with existing clinical processes. Physical placement should balance accessibility for clinical staff against security considerations and infrastructure requirements. Workspace design around cabinet locations should accommodate medication preparation activities while minimizing congestion and interruptions during critical tasks.

Profiling capabilities that link automated dispensing systems with electronic health records create patient-specific medication profiles that limit access to currently ordered medications. This configuration reduces selection errors by displaying only appropriate medications for each patient and creates an additional verification point against the medication order. Implementation of profiling features requires careful workflow design to address situations requiring urgent medication access before order entry completion.

Override parameters establish balance between accessibility during urgent situations and appropriate verification processes. Properly configured override functions limit unauthorized access while enabling timely care in emergencies through mechanisms including time-limited access to specific medications, mandatory retrospective documentation, automated notifications to pharmacy when overrides occur, and regular review of override patterns to identify improvement opportunities. These parameters require periodic reassessment based on usage patterns and identified safety events.

User interface design significantly influences both efficiency and error potential. Intuitive navigation, clear visual cues for medication location, distinct pathways for routine versus emergency access, and consistent terminology across integrated systems reduce cognitive burden during medication retrieval. Touch screen interfaces with configurable layouts enable optimization based on specific unit needs and user feedback, supporting continuous improvement of human-machine interaction.

Optimization Strategies and Emerging Capabilities

Optimization of automated dispensing systems represents an ongoing process requiring regular assessment and refinement based on usage patterns, error reports, and technological advances. Configuration reviews should determine override frequency by medication and user, discrepancy resolution timeframes, near-miss event patterns, and workflow efficiency metrics. Systematic observation of actual usage patterns often reveals workarounds or efficiency barriers not apparent from system reports alone, informing targeted configuration adjustments.

Advanced inventory management capabilities increasingly incorporate predictive analytics to anticipate medication needs based on patient census, scheduled procedures, seasonal patterns, and historical usage data. These systems optimize par levels dynamically rather than relying on static configurations, reducing both stockouts and excessive inventory. Integration with supply chain management systems creates end-to-end visibility from manufacturer to patient administration, enhancing response capability during shortage situations.

Integration with additional technologies creates synergistic safety benefits beyond those achievable with isolated implementations. Interfacing with smart infusion pumps enables automated documentation of infusion parameters and supports preparation of patient-specific infusions with barcode verification. Connection with medication tracking systems using RFID or other technologies provides real-time location information for high-value or high-risk medications. Integration with temperature monitoring systems ensures proper storage conditions for temperature-sensitive medications.

Remote cabinet monitoring and management capabilities enable centralized oversight of decentralized medication management, creating efficient supervision models that extend pharmacy expertise throughout healthcare facilities. These capabilities prove particularly valuable during night shifts and weekend periods with reduced pharmacy staffing, enabling pharmacist review of medication selection and preparation activities regardless of physical location. Telepresence technologies increasingly support real-time pharmacist consultation during complex medication preparation activities at decentralized locations.

BARCODE MEDICATION ADMINISTRATION

Barcode medication administration (BCMA) systems represent point-of-care verification technology that confirms the "five rights" of medication administration through automated matching of patient, medication, and order information. These systems create the final verification point before medication reaches the patient, addressing administration errors that historically evaded detection by earlier safety systems.

Components and Integration

Comprehensive BCMA implementation requires integration of multiple technological components into a cohesive system supporting the medication administration workflow. Core hardware components include barcode scanners (handheld or hands-free), mobile computers or workstations for accessing electronic records at the bedside, and printers for generating patient identification bands with barcode identifiers. Software components include the medication administration record interface, barcode verification algorithms, documentation tools, and integration engines connecting with pharmacy and electronic health record systems.

Typical workflow begins with scanning the caregiver's identification to establish user authentication and create appropriate documentation trails. The patient's identification band is then scanned to select the correct patient record and medication profile. Individual medication barcodes are scanned before administration, triggering automatic verification against the ordered medications, scheduled administration times, and patient identity. The system provides immediate feedback regarding verification status, prompting the caregiver to proceed with administration or resolve discrepancies before proceeding.

Successful integration requires careful attention to practical workflow considerations including scanner ergonomics, workstation mobility, battery life management, wireless network coverage, and backup procedures for technology failures. Physical design considerations such as placement of medication preparation areas, computer workstation locations, and patient identification band design significantly influence both compliance rates and user satisfaction. Workflow redesign typically accompanies implementation, with elimination of redundant documentation and realignment of medication delivery timing with scanning procedures.

Safety Impact and Evidence Base

Research demonstrates substantial safety benefits associated with well-implemented BCMA systems across diverse healthcare settings. A systematic review of 21 studies found that BCMA implementation was associated with a 50-80% reduction in medication administration errors depending on implementation quality and baseline error rates. The greatest impact appears in prevention of wrong patient, wrong medication, and wrong dose errors, with more modest effects on timing errors and route errors.

Beyond error reduction, BCMA systems create comprehensive documentation of the medication administration process, supporting both quality improvement initiatives and individual case investigations when adverse events occur. Timestamp data enables analysis of medication timing patterns, supporting optimization of medication scheduling and workflow design. Documentation of scan compliance rates and override patterns identifies opportunities for targeted improvement interventions, creating a continuous feedback loop for safety enhancement.

Additional benefits include reduction in missing doses through automated identification of overdue medications, improved charge capture through automated documentation of administered medications, and reduced nursing documentation time when systems are properly configured to minimize redundant entry requirements. Some studies also demonstrate improved communication between nursing and pharmacy departments through more structured notification processes for medication-related issues identified during the administration process.

Table 6.4: Barcode Medication Administration Systems: Implementation and Optimization

System Component	Functions	Challenges
Barcode Infrastructure	Patient wristband barcoding Medication package barcoding Scanner hardware Wireless connectivity Integration with eMAR	Barcode readability issues Wireless dead zones Scanner durability concerns Battery life limitations Integration with existing systems
Workflow Integration	Bedside scanning process Exception handling procedures Documentation workflows Override processes Downtime procedures	Physical space constraints Medication preparation workflows Special medication handling Isolation room procedures Emergency medication processes

System Component	Functions	Challenges
Patient Identification	Wristband scanning Patient verification Alternative ID procedures Multiple ID checks Special population considerations	Difficult-to-band patients Removed/damaged wristbands Unconscious/unidentified patients Multiple wristbands Emergency department challenges
Medication Verification	Medication barcode scanning Product verification Dose verification Special form handling Compounded medication procedures	Nonbarcoded medications Compounded preparations Split/crushed medications Unit-dose packaging issues Partial dose administration
Alert Management	Wrong medication/dose alerts Timing alerts Documentation alerts Override management Alert response	Alert fatigue Alarm soundalike issues Override justification quality Urgent medication delays Multiple alerting systems

System Component	Functions	Challenges
	tracking	
Performance Monitoring	Compliance dashboard Exception reporting Workaround identification Quality improvement process Continuous optimization	Data extraction limitations Performance feedback processes Resource limitations for analysis Identifying root causes Sustained compliance
Training and Support	Initial training programs Ongoing education Super-user development New staff orientation Competency assessment	Staff turnover Training environment limitations Shift coverage for training Complex workflow scenarios Varied technical proficiency

Despite these benefits, research also identifies implementation challenges that can limit effectiveness. Suboptimal implementations characterized by workarounds, inconsistent scanning, and excessive overrides demonstrate substantially reduced safety benefits. Studies of implementation success factors emphasize the importance of workflow optimization, adequate equipment provision, responsive technical support, and clear accountability structures for scanning compliance as critical elements supporting safety improvement.

Challenges and Workaround Prevention

Workarounds—practices that bypass intended safety features of barcode systems—represent a significant threat to BCMA effectiveness. Common workarounds include scanning medication barcodes from lists rather than actual packages, scanning patient identification from room labels rather than wristbands, batch scanning medications before administration to multiple patients, and documenting administration without performing scanning procedures. Research indicates that workarounds occur in response to perceived workflow inefficiencies, technical limitations, and environmental constraints rather than intentional disregard for safety procedures.

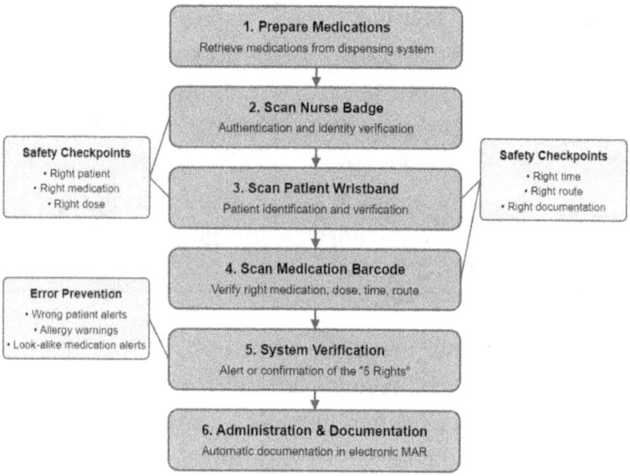

Figure 6.4 Barcode Medication Administration Process

Effective workaround prevention strategies address underlying causes rather than simply enforcing compliance with suboptimal processes. Technical barriers to scanning, such as damaged barcodes, unreadable wristbands, or scanner malfunctions, require systematic remediation through improved printing processes, alternative barcode placement options, and responsive technical support. Environmental factors such as poor wireless network coverage, inadequate workspace for scanning activities, or insufficient battery life for mobile workstations require infrastructure improvements rather than expecting staff adaptation to suboptimal conditions.

Workflow barriers including excessive time requirements, interruption of patient interaction, or requirement for additional steps without perceived value require process redesign with direct involvement of frontline staff. Successful approaches typically involve observation of actual workflow patterns, solicitation of improvement suggestions from users, and iterative refinement of processes to optimize both safety and efficiency. Recognition that safety and efficiency need not conflict, but rather can be complementary when systems are well-designed, guides effective process improvement.

Policy and accountability structures complement technical solutions in preventing workarounds. Clear expectations regarding scanning compliance, regular audit procedures with feedback to individual practitioners, and progressive accountability measures for persistent non-compliance establish normative behavior patterns. Leadership emphasis on the importance of barcode verification, particularly from respected clinical leaders rather than only administrative sources, reinforces cultural expectations for technology utilization as a professional responsibility.

Emerging Capabilities

Technological advances continue to enhance BCMA capabilities beyond basic verification functions. Integration with smart infusion pump systems creates comprehensive verification for intravenous medications, confirming not only the medication identity but also infusion parameters against ordered values. Two-dimensional barcodes enable encoding of additional information including lot numbers, expiration dates, and even preparation instructions, supporting more comprehensive verification and documentation.

Mobile device integration represents an important development enabling more flexible workflows and improved human factors. Smartphone-based scanning applications with secure electronic health record access enable verification procedures without requiring dedicated workstations. Hands-free scanning technologies using wearable devices or fixed scanning infrastructure reduce ergonomic challenges associated with traditional handheld scanners. Voice-confirmation technologies provide audio feedback during scanning processes, enabling clinicians to maintain visual focus on patients and medications rather than computer screens.

Extended verification capabilities beyond the "five rights" incorporate additional safety parameters into the verification process. Systems increasingly verify appropriateness of administration timing in relation to food, other medications, or diagnostic procedures. Laboratory value checking against predefined parameters identifies situations where recent clinical changes might contraindicate scheduled medications. Patient vital sign requirements before specific medication administration create additional safety checks for high-risk medications where physiological parameters significantly affect appropriateness.

Patient engagement features represent an emerging direction in BCMA evolution, with systems increasingly designed to support patient participation in the verification process. Patient-accessible interfaces displaying scheduled and administered medications enable active participation in verification. Automated patient education triggered by scanning events provides contextual information about medication purposes and potential side effects. These features recognize patients as valuable partners in safety verification while supporting informed participation in their own care.

Things to Remember

- ☑ Electronic health records support medication safety through accurate documentation, integrated historical data, and standardized ordering processes with template-based approaches.
- ☑ Clinical decision support systems provide automated safety checks through interaction verification, dose range validation, laboratory-medication monitoring, and patient-specific risk assessment.
- ☑ Alert design must balance comprehensive warnings against alert fatigue through severity stratification, contextual relevance, and appropriate presentation.
- ☑ Automated dispensing systems enhance medication distribution through secure storage, barcode verification, integrated charging capabilities, and controlled access with transaction documentation.
- ☑ Barcode medication administration creates point-of-care verification confirming correct medication, patient, dose, route, and timing through systematic scanning integrated with documentation.
- ☑ Successful implementation requires workflow integration, user involvement, phased introduction with appropriate support, and continuous optimization addressing emerging issues.

Multiple Choice Questions

1. Which component of electronic health records specifically supports medication safety?
   a) Billing documentation
   b) Standardized order sets with embedded safety parameters
   c) Scheduling functionality
   d) Regulatory compliance reporting
2. Clinical decision support systems enhance medication safety through:
   a) Automating all medication decisions without clinician involvement
   b) Providing intelligent assistance including interaction checking and dose verification
   c) Eliminating the need for pharmacist review of medication orders
   d) Restricting prescribing to a limited medication formulary
3. Alert fatigue in clinical decision support systems refers to:
   a) Technical failures causing system crashes
   b) Clinicians becoming desensitized to numerous alerts and potentially ignoring important warnings
   c) Patients receiving too many medication warnings
   d) System slowdowns during periods of high usage
4. Automated dispensing systems enhance medication safety through:
   a) Eliminating the need for pharmacist verification
   b) Secure storage, barcode verification, and

transaction documentation

c) Automatically administering medications to patients

d) Preventing all potential dispensing errors

5. The primary safety benefit of barcode medication administration is:

   a) Reducing medication costs

   b) Eliminating the need for nurse judgment

   c) Point-of-care verification of correct medication, patient, dose, route, and timing

   d) Automated documentation without manual entry

6. Successful technology implementation requires:

   a) Minimal user involvement to ensure efficient deployment

   b) Rapid introduction without pilot testing to ensure quick adoption

   c) Workflow integration aligning technology with clinical processes

   d) Standardized approaches without customization for different clinical areas

7. Which of the following is NOT a typical component of closed-loop medication management systems?

   a) Computerized provider order entry

   b) Pharmacy verification and dispensing

   c) Financial billing processes

   d) Barcode medication administration

8. Human factors engineering in medication safety technology addresses:

   a) Technical infrastructure requirements

   b) Cognitive limitations and workflow

considerations

c) Financial return on investment

d) Regulatory compliance requirements

9. Technology implementation challenges include:

   a) Excessive simplicity of healthcare workflows

   b) Too few available technology options

   c) Workflow disruption and user resistance

   d) Limited potential for medication errors in manual processes

10. After technology implementation, continuous optimization includes:

    a) Eliminating all system customization

    b) Reducing user training requirements

    c) Addressing emerging issues and enhancing capabilities

    d) Freezing system configuration to ensure stability

Self-Assessment Questions

1. Critically evaluate how electronic health records have transformed medication safety practices, analyzing both benefits and unintended consequences.
2. Analyze the design, implementation, and effectiveness of clinical decision support systems in preventing medication errors, including considerations for alert fatigue.
3. Evaluate the impact of automated dispensing systems on medication distribution safety, workflow efficiency, and error prevention.
4. Discuss the implementation challenges and safety outcomes associated with barcode medication administration technology across different healthcare settings.
5. Compare and contrast the effectiveness of various technology solutions across the medication use process, from prescribing to administration and monitoring.
6. Analyze the human factors and ergonomic considerations in designing and implementing medication safety technologies to maximize safety and usability.
7. Evaluate the role of interoperability standards in connecting medication safety technologies and the challenges in achieving seamless integration.
8. Discuss how healthcare organizations should select, implement, and evaluate medication safety technologies to maximize return on

investment and safety improvements.

9. Analyze the evolving role of mobile health technologies, patient portals, and remote monitoring in medication safety beyond traditional healthcare settings.
10. Discuss the ethical and privacy considerations in implementing medication safety technologies, including data security, patient confidentiality, and equitable access.

Bibliography

1. Bates DW, Leape LL, Cullen DJ, Laird N, Petersen LA, Teich JM, et al. Effect of computerized physician order entry and a team intervention on prevention of serious medication errors. JAMA. 1998;280(15):1311-6.
2. Ammenwerth E, Schnell-Inderst P, Machan C, Siebert U. The effect of electronic prescribing on medication errors and adverse drug events: a systematic review. J Am Med Inform Assoc. 2008;15(5):585-600.
3. Kuperman GJ, Bobb A, Payne TH, Avery AJ, Gandhi TK, Burns G, et al. Medication-related clinical decision support in computerized provider order entry systems: a review. J Am Med Inform Assoc. 2007;14(1):29-40.
4. Poon EG, Keohane CA, Yoon CS, Ditmore M, Bane A, Levtzion-Korach O, et al. Effect of bar-code technology on the safety of medication administration. N Engl J Med. 2010;362(18):1698-707.
5. van der Sijs H, Aarts J, Vulto A, Berg M. Overriding of drug safety alerts in computerized physician order entry. J Am Med Inform Assoc. 2006;13(2):138-47.
6. Kaushal R, Shojania KG, Bates DW. Effects of computerized physician order entry and clinical decision support systems on medication safety: a systematic review. Arch Intern Med. 2003;163(12):1409-16.
7. Franklin BD, O'Grady K, Donyai P, Jacklin A, Barber N. The impact of a closed-loop electronic prescribing: a before-and-after study. Qual Saf Health Care. 2007;16(4):279-84.
8. Pedersen CA, Schneider PJ, Scheckelhoff DJ. ASHP national survey of pharmacy practice in hospital settings: Dispensing and administration—2014. Am J Health Syst Pharm. 2015;72(13):1119-37.
9. Chapuis C, Roustit M, Bal G, Schwebel C, Pansu P, David-Tchouda S, et al. Automated drug dispensing system reduces medication errors in an intensive care setting. Crit Care Med. 2010;38(12):2275-81.
10. Ash JS, Sittig DF, Campbell EM, Guappone KP, Dykstra RH. Some unintended consequences of clinical decision support systems. AMIA Annu Symp Proc. 2007:26-30.

CHAPTER 7

SPECIAL POPULATIONS

Abstract

Special populations require tailored medication safety techniques to meet physiological, pharmacokinetic, and practical factors that create distinctive risk profiles. Pediatric medication safety involves weight-based dosing calculations, developmental pharmacology variations, limited therapeutic data, and communication challenges with non-verbal patients, necessitating specialized dosing tools and enhanced verification processes. Geriatric medication safety addresses age-related pharmacokinetic changes, polypharmacy complexities, altered adverse effect profiles, and potential functional limitations affecting medication management, requiring comprehensive regimen reviews and simplified therapeutic approaches. Pregnancy and lactation present unique challenges balancing maternal benefit against fetal or infant risk without robust safety data, requiring careful risk categorization, therapeutic alternatives assessment, and timing optimization throughout reproductive stages. Patients with multiple comorbidities face increased risks from complex regimens, potential drug-disease interactions, competing therapeutic priorities, and involvement of multiple specialists, necessitating coordinated medication management through comprehensive reviews, explicit prioritization, and enhanced monitoring protocols that address the compounded vulnerability created by overlapping conditions and treatments.

Keywords: *Developmental pharmacology, Polypharmacy management, Maternal-fetal risk, Comorbidity interactions, Vulnerable populations*

Learning Objectives

After completion of the chapter, the learners should be able to:

- Remember the distinctive medication safety considerations for pediatric patients, geriatric patients, pregnant/lactating women, and patients with multiple comorbidities.
- Understand how physiological, pharmacokinetic, and practical factors create unique medication risks in special populations.
- Apply appropriate safety strategies addressing specific vulnerabilities in each special population.
- Analyze the complexities of medication management across different vulnerable groups.
- Evaluate the effectiveness of specialized approaches for reducing medication errors in vulnerable populations.
- Create comprehensive safety protocols addressing the unique needs of different special populations.

PEDIATRIC MEDICATION SAFETY

Pediatric patients present unique medication safety challenges requiring specialized knowledge, protocols, and safeguards throughout the medication use process. The physiological, developmental, and communication differences between children and adults create distinct vulnerability patterns necessitating pediatric-specific approaches to medication safety.

Developmental Pharmacology and Dosing Challenges

Developmental pharmacology fundamentally shapes pediatric medication safety, with age-related differences in absorption, distribution, metabolism, and excretion creating dynamic pharmacokinetic profiles that change throughout childhood development. Neonates demonstrate reduced gastric acid secretion affecting absorption of pH-dependent medications, while having higher total body water percentages that alter distribution volumes for water-soluble medications. Immature hepatic enzyme systems, particularly in premature infants, significantly reduce metabolism rates for many medications, creating prolonged half-lives and accumulation risks. Renal tubular function development continues through early childhood, affecting elimination rates for renally cleared medications.

Weight-based dosing represents the standard approach addressing size variation across pediatric populations, but introduces substantial calculation complexity and error potential. Dosing may require multiple mathematical operations involving weight conversion, dose-per-weight calculation, concentration adjustment, and volume determination. Each calculation step introduces error potential, with research demonstrating medication calculation errors in 10-17% of pediatric prescriptions. Electronic health record systems with integrated weight-based dosing calculators significantly reduce mathematical errors but require careful implementation with appropriate range checks and verification processes.

Surface area-based dosing, employed particularly for chemotherapeutic agents and selected other medications, introduces additional complexity requiring both weight and height measurements with application of conversion formulas or nomograms. These calculations prove especially vulnerable to mathematical errors and unit conversion mistakes. Even small calculation errors can result in significant overdoses given the narrow therapeutic indices of many medications dosed by surface area, necessitating multiple independent verification processes before administration.

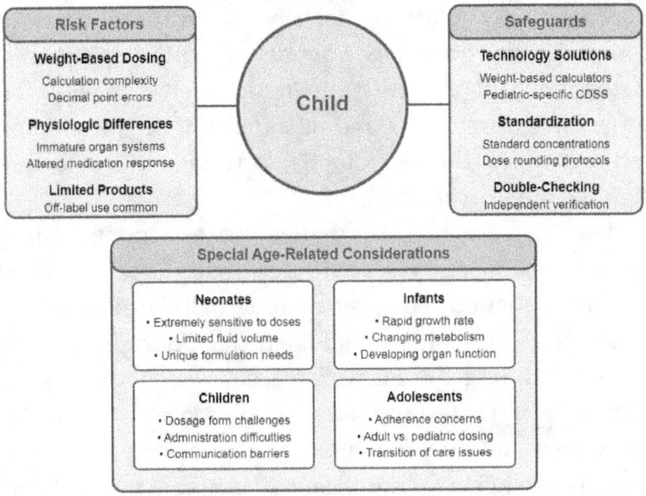

Figure 7.1 Pediatric Medication Safety Risk Factors and Safeguards

Age-appropriate formulation availability significantly influences pediatric medication safety, with many medications lacking commercially available formulations suitable for accurate pediatric dosing. Extemporaneous compounding of liquid formulations from adult dosage forms introduces additional risks including calculation errors, stability uncertainties, bioavailability alterations, and concentration inaccuracies. Standardized compounding protocols, beyond-use dating guidance, and rigorous quality control processes mitigate these risks but require significant pharmacy expertise and resources not universally available across healthcare settings.

Communication and Assessment Challenges

Developmental communication limitations create unique challenges in pediatric medication safety monitoring. Preverbal children cannot directly report adverse effects, making detection dependent on caregiver observation and clinical assessment. Even verbal children may lack vocabulary to describe medication effects or comprehend questions about specific symptoms. Assessment tools must therefore rely heavily on observable parameters and age-appropriate questioning techniques to detect potential adverse effects before significant harm occurs.

Pain assessment exemplifies these communication challenges, with research demonstrating historical undertreatment of pediatric pain partially attributable to assessment difficulties. Validated age-appropriate pain scales including the FLACC (Face, Legs, Activity, Cry, Consolability) scale for preverbal children and faces scales for verbal children enable more consistent assessment, though requiring significant training for reliable application. Inadequate pain assessment can lead to both undertreatment and excessive analgesic administration, each carrying distinct safety risks.

Medication history collection presents particular difficulties with pediatric patients, who frequently receive medications across multiple settings (home, school, childcare, multiple healthcare facilities) with varying caregiver responsibility for administration. Comprehensive history requires gathering information from multiple sources, often with discrepancies requiring reconciliation. Electronic health record systems rarely capture complete cross-setting medication information, necessitating active integration of caregiver-supplied information with documented healthcare prescriptions.

Table 7.1: Pediatric Medication Safety

Risk Factor	Specific Vulnerabilities	Preventive Measures
Weight-Based Dosing	Wide weight variation Rapid growth rates Decimal point sensitivity Multiple concentration options Complex calculations	Standardized weight units (kg only) Independent double-checks Standardized concentrations Dose range checking Calculated doses on orders
Physiological Differences	Immature organ systems Altered absorption/distribution Developing metabolism Reduced drug clearance Variable body composition	Age-specific formularies Specialized pediatric references Enhanced monitoring protocols Excipient screening Age-based medication reviews
Limited Licensed Products	Off-label use common Adult formulation adaptation Limited pediatric data Lack of appropriate concentrations Unsuitable administration forms	Standardized compounding protocols Pediatric-specific formulations Centralized preparation

Risk Factor	Specific Vulnerabilities	Preventive Measures
		Evidence-based off-label guidelines Formulation standardization
Communication Challenges	Multiple caregivers Limited patient self-advocacy Parental anxiety/distress Health literacy variations Language barriers	Standardized communication tools Pictorial medication instructions Caregiver education programs Teach-back methods Child-appropriate education
Administration Challenges	Difficulty swallowing tablets Taste acceptability Need for partial doses Volume limitations Route limitations	Standardized measuring devices Appropriate formulation selection Taste-masking techniques Device dispensing with medication Administration technique education
Developmental Factors	Cognitive developmental stages	Age-appropriate

Risk Factor	Specific Vulnerabilities	Preventive Measures
	Limited understanding of medication Variable cooperation Autonomy development Growth-related dose changes	education Regular weight/growth monitoring Developmental assessment Transitional care planning Adolescent medication education

Developmental understanding of medication purpose and administration instructions varies substantially from infancy through adolescence, requiring age-appropriate education strategies. Adolescents present unique challenges as they develop increasing autonomy in medication management with variable readiness for independent responsibility. Transition planning for adolescents with chronic conditions requires structured assessment of medication management capabilities and gradual responsibility transfer with appropriate supervision, particularly for complex regimens with significant non-adherence consequences.

High-Risk Medications and Error Prevention

High-alert medications in pediatric contexts include many agents not typically categorized as high-alert in adult populations, reflecting children's unique vulnerability patterns. Liquid medications requiring measurement present universal risks, with research demonstrating frequent dosing errors by both healthcare professionals and caregivers. Standard concentration initiatives address this risk by establishing consistent concentrations for commonly used liquid medications throughout healthcare systems, reducing calculation requirements and enabling development of standardized administration tools.

Intravenous fluid therapy carries significant electrolyte and fluid balance risks in pediatric patients due to limited physiological reserves and developing regulatory systems. Standardized maintenance fluid protocols based on weight ranges reduce calculation errors, while integrated electronic documentation tools tracking cumulative fluid volumes and electrolyte administration support appropriate management. Independent double-checks for intravenous fluid orders represent standard practice in many pediatric facilities, reflecting the recognized risk profile.

Opioid safety presents particular challenges in pediatric settings due to respiratory depression risks and weight-based dosing requirements. Standardized pain management protocols with age-appropriate assessment tools, opioid-sparing multimodal approaches, and enhanced monitoring requirements for higher-risk patients (e.g., obstructive sleep apnea, obesity, concurrent central nervous system depressants) create comprehensive safety systems. PCA by proxy—allowing caregivers to activate patient-controlled analgesia devices for children unable to self-administer—requires specific protocols addressing the altered safety profile compared to traditional patient-controlled administration.

Chemotherapeutic agents represent another high-risk category with pediatric-specific considerations beyond those present in adult oncology. Complex roadmap-based protocols with timing-critical sequencing, intrathecal administration risks, and narrow therapeutic windows necessitate specialized verification processes. Many pediatric centers implement comprehensive chemotherapy safety systems including standardized ordering templates, multi-disciplinary verification processes, and enhanced administration protocols with independent verification steps and specialized nursing certification requirements.

System Design and Safety Initiatives

System design for pediatric medication safety requires attention to both technical and human factors dimensions, with recognition that adult-oriented systems rarely adequately address pediatric requirements without significant modification. Electronic health record customization should include pediatric-specific dosing guidance, age-appropriate normal values, weight-based dosing calculators with appropriate range checks, and specialized documentation tools for pediatric assessment parameters. User interface design should clearly differentiate pediatric from adult information to prevent inappropriate application of adult standards to pediatric patients.

Environmental design considerations include storage systems preventing access to high-alert medications without appropriate verification, preparation areas with minimal distractions for pediatric medication measurement, and administration environments supporting caregiver presence and participation during medication administration. Physical separation of neonatal/pediatric medications from adult formulations in similar packaging reduces selection errors, while pediatric-specific administration equipment (oral syringes, calibrated cups, appropriate-sized intravenous catheters) supports accurate delivery.

Specialized pediatric pharmacy services demonstrate significant safety benefits through dedicated expertise in developmental pharmacology, specialized compounding capabilities, and familiarity with age-appropriate formulation selection. These services may include dedicated pediatric pharmacists embedded in patient care areas, centralized pediatric dispensing operations with specialized verification procedures, or hybrid models with distributed expertise throughout medication management systems. Pharmacist participation in pediatric rounds correlates with reduced medication error rates and improved therapy appropriateness, particularly for complex patients.

National and international pediatric safety initiatives have advanced standardization and evidence-based practices across healthcare systems. The Children's Hospitals' Solutions for Patient Safety Network has established collaborative approaches to medication safety improvement through shared protocols, error reporting, and intervention evaluation. The Making Care Safer for Children's Medication (MCS-PEDS) initiative developed standardized concentrations for commonly used medications across pediatric facilities. These collaborative approaches address the historical fragmentation of pediatric medication safety practices while establishing evidence-based standards adaptable across diverse healthcare settings.

GERIATRIC MEDICATION SAFETY

Geriatric patients face distinctive medication safety challenges arising from physiological changes of aging, increased prevalence of multiple chronic conditions, complex medication regimens, and healthcare system fragmentation. These factors collectively contribute to elevated adverse drug event rates requiring specialized approaches throughout the medication use process.

Table 7.2: Geriatric Medication Safety

Risk Domain	Assessment Tools	Evidence-Based Interventions
Polypharmacy	Medication Appropriateness Index ARMOR (Assess, Review, Minimize, Optimize, Reassess) Medication regimen complexity index Number of medications count HIGH-RISK screening tool	Comprehensive medication reviews Deprescribing protocols Medication therapy management Brown bag medication reviews Electronic prescriber coordination
Inappropriate Medication Use	Beers Criteria STOPP/START Criteria Anticholinergic Cognitive Burden Scale Drug Burden Index Medication Appropriateness Index	Computerized decision support Pharmacist-led medication reviews Academic detailing Alternative therapy protocols Geriatric-focused formularies
Altered Pharmacokinetics	Cockcroft-Gault equation MDRD or CKD-EPI formulas Liver function tests Body composition assessment Drug level monitoring	Renal dose adjustment protocols Therapeutic drug monitoring Age-adjusted dosing guidelines Regular renal function monitoring Hepatic function assessment
Altered Pharmacodynami	Orthostatic vital signs Cognitive assessment tools	"Start low, go slow" dosing Lower initial doses

Risk Domain	Assessment Tools	Evidence-Based Interventions
cs	Functional assessments Adverse drug reaction scales QT interval monitoring	Extended titration schedules Enhanced sensitivity monitoring Pharmacodynamic interaction screening
Adherence Challenges	Morisky Medication Adherence Scale Pill counts Medication possession ratio Self-reported adherence Medication Event Monitoring System	Simplified regimens Blister packaging/pill organizers Medication synchronization Electronic reminders Caregiver education and support
Transitions of Care	Care Transitions Measure Post-discharge medication discrepancies Medication reconciliation quality Readmission risk tools Transitional care needs assessment	Pharmacist-led discharge counseling Post-discharge follow-up calls Comprehensive discharge summaries Caregiver education and engagement Medication reconciliation at all transitions

Age-Related Pharmacological Changes

Physiological changes associated with aging significantly alter pharmacokinetic and pharmacodynamic properties of medications, creating safety challenges that extend beyond simple dose adjustments. Absorption changes include reduced gastric acid secretion affecting ionizable drug dissolution, decreased gastrointestinal blood flow potentially reducing absorption rate, and altered gastric emptying time influencing absorption timing. These changes typically produce modest clinical effects compared to more substantial distribution, metabolism, and excretion alterations.

Distribution changes include reduced total body water percentage altering volume of distribution for water-soluble medications, decreased serum albumin affecting highly protein-bound drug availability, and altered body composition with increased adipose tissue proportion affecting lipophilic medication distribution. These changes may significantly alter peak concentrations and elimination half-lives, requiring dosage adjustments to maintain therapeutic effects while avoiding toxicity, particularly for medications with narrow therapeutic indices.

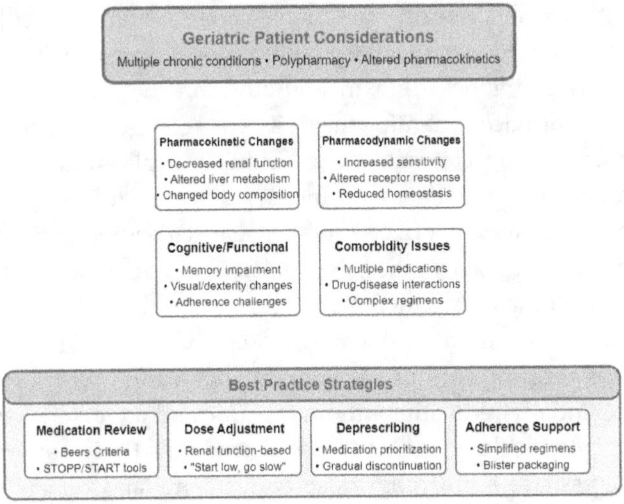

Figure 7.2 Geriatric Medication Safety

Hepatic metabolism changes include reduced liver mass, decreased hepatic blood flow, and diminished activity of certain cytochrome P450 enzymes affecting phase I metabolism. These changes demonstrate substantial inter-individual variability, with some older adults maintaining near-normal hepatic function while others experience significant reduction. Medications undergoing extensive first-pass metabolism show particularly notable age-related pharmacokinetic changes, often requiring dosage adjustment to prevent accumulation toxicity.

Renal excretion represents the most clinically significant age-related pharmacokinetic change, with glomerular filtration rate declining approximately 1% annually after age 40 in many individuals. Serum creatinine measurements often fail to accurately reflect this decline due to concurrent decreased muscle mass, masking significant renal impairment. Medications with primary renal clearance require careful dosage adjustment based on estimated glomerular filtration rate rather than serum creatinine alone, with particular attention to narrow therapeutic index drugs including many antibiotics, digoxin, and lithium.

Pharmacodynamic sensitivity changes independent of altered drug concentrations further complicate geriatric medication management. Increased sensitivity to central nervous system effects appears particularly significant, with benzodiazepines, opioids, and other sedating medications producing exaggerated and prolonged effects even at adjusted doses. Conversely, beta-adrenergic receptor sensitivity decreases with age, potentially reducing both therapeutic and adverse effects of beta-blocking agents. These altered sensitivity patterns necessitate both initial dose adjustments and enhanced monitoring during therapy.

Polypharmacy and Inappropriate Prescribing

Polypharmacy—commonly defined as concurrent use of five or more medications—affects 39-43% of older adults in developed countries, creating substantial medication safety challenges. Multiple medication use intrinsically increases adverse event risk through cumulative side effect burden, complex drug-drug interactions, adherence difficulties, and increased likelihood of prescribing cascades where adverse effects are treated with additional medications rather than recognized as medication consequences.

Potentially inappropriate medication use in older adults has been systematically defined through expert consensus criteria including the Beers Criteria (United States), STOPP/START criteria (Europe), and similar systems in other regions. These criteria identify medications with unfavorable risk-benefit profiles in geriatric populations due to age-related changes in drug effects, high adverse event risks, or availability of safer alternatives. Despite widespread dissemination of these criteria, research indicates that 20-65% of older adults receive at least one potentially inappropriate medication, with higher rates in long-term care settings.

Prescribing cascades represent a particularly insidious form of inappropriate prescribing in which adverse drug effects are misinterpreted as new medical conditions requiring additional medications. Common examples include antihypertensive-induced gout treated with allopurinol, cholinesterase inhibitor-induced urinary incontinence treated with anticholinergics, and NSAID-induced hypertension treated with additional antihypertensives. These cascades increase regimen complexity, cumulative side effect burden, and interaction potential while failing to address the underlying medication issue.

Deprescribing—the systematic process of medication discontinuation when potential harms outweigh benefits—represents a crucial intervention addressing inappropriate prescribing and polypharmacy. Structured deprescribing processes include comprehensive medication review, prioritization of medications for potential discontinuation, gradual dose reduction with monitoring for discontinuation syndromes or disease recurrence, and clear communication with patients regarding rationale and expectations. Evidence-based deprescribing guidelines for specific medication classes including benzodiazepines, proton pump inhibitors, and antipsychotics provide standardized approaches based on systematic reviews of discontinuation outcomes.

Cognitive Impairment and Adherence Challenges

Cognitive impairment significantly complicates medication safety in older adults, affecting both adherence capabilities and adverse effect recognition. Mild cognitive impairment may manifest as difficulty managing complex medication regimens before more generalized functional impairments become apparent. Assessment of medication management capacity represents an important component of functional evaluation in older adults with suspected cognitive changes, providing valuable information for appropriate intervention design.

Adherence support strategies must address the specific cognitive limitations present while maximizing independence when possible. Medication organizers with clear visual cues and compartmentalization reduce working memory demands. Electronic reminder systems provide time-based prompts for administration, though effectiveness depends on consistent response to alerts. Blister packaging with explicit timing indicators supports correct administration sequencing. These interventions should be matched to specific cognitive limitations following formal assessment rather than implemented based on age alone.

More significant cognitive impairment typically requires caregiver involvement in medication management, creating additional safety considerations. Caregiver education regarding proper administration techniques, adverse effect monitoring, and appropriate documentation becomes essential for safety. Structured medication administration records adapted for home use improve communication among multiple caregivers and healthcare providers. Regular caregiver assessment for burden and competence in medication management roles supports early intervention when additional assistance becomes necessary.

Transitions between care settings present particular vulnerability for patients with cognitive impairment, as communication of current medication regimens, recent changes, and special administration requirements may be compromised. Standardized transition documentation including indication for each medication, recent regimen changes, attempted discontinuations with outcomes, and special administration requirements (crushing, timing with meals, etc.) supports safe care transitions. Direct communication between healthcare providers across settings, rather than relying solely on patient or caregiver information transfer, provides additional safety protection for cognitively impaired patients.

Special Considerations and Quality Improvement

End-of-life medication management requires reconsideration of therapeutic goals and risk-benefit profiles as prognosis changes. Medication appropriateness review should consider remaining life expectancy, time to benefit for preventive medications, symptom management priorities, and quality of life impact. Many preventive medications including statins, bisphosphonates, and intensive glycemic control agents offer minimal benefit with continued adverse effect potential in limited life expectancy contexts. Conversely, appropriate symptom management medications should be continued or initiated despite certain risks when they support comfort and quality of life.

Falls risk assessment and mitigation represent crucial components of geriatric medication safety, with numerous medications contributing to fall risk through mechanisms including orthostatic hypotension, sedation, dizziness, vision changes, and altered balance. The Screening Tool of Older Person's Prescriptions in older adults with high fall risk (STOPP-FALL) criteria identify specific medications with elevated fall risk that warrant reconsideration in patients with fall history or high-risk status. Systematic medication review following falls should evaluate potential medication contributions and appropriate adjustments rather than focusing exclusively on environmental factors.

Anticholinergic burden represents a particular concern in geriatric pharmacotherapy due to cumulative effects across multiple medications with varying anticholinergic potency. Adverse effects include cognitive impairment, urinary retention, constipation, dry mouth, blurred vision, and increased fall risk. Validated scales including the Anticholinergic Cognitive Burden Scale and the Anticholinergic Risk Scale quantify cumulative burden across medication regimens, supporting systematic efforts to reduce overall anticholinergic exposure rather than focusing only on obviously anticholinergic agents.

Quality improvement initiatives addressing geriatric medication safety demonstrate greatest impact when combining multiple intervention components in comprehensive programs. Successful models include pharmacist-led medication reviews with structured recommendations, computerized decision support systems incorporating geriatric-specific prescribing guidance, interdisciplinary team approaches to complex medication management, and educational interventions for both healthcare providers and patients/caregivers. Evaluation metrics should include both process measures (reduction in potentially inappropriate medications, appropriate dosage adjustments) and outcome measures (adverse drug event rates, emergency department visits, hospitalizations) to demonstrate comprehensive impact.

PREGNANCY AND LACTATION

Medication use during pregnancy and lactation presents unique safety challenges balancing maternal treatment needs against potential risks to the developing fetus or breastfeeding infant. The ethical complexity, limited research data, and changing physiological context create a particularly challenging domain for evidence-based medication safety practice.

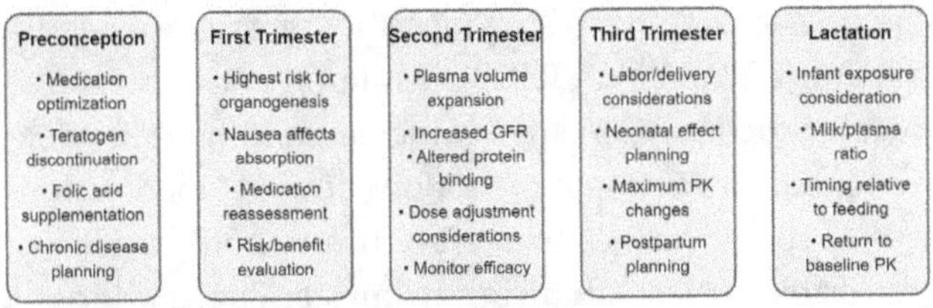

Figure 7.3 Medication Safety Across Pregnancy and Lactation

Physiological Changes and Pharmacokinetic Considerations

Pregnancy induces substantial physiological changes affecting medication pharmacokinetics throughout gestation, with implications for both efficacy and safety. Absorption changes include decreased gastric emptying and intestinal motility potentially delaying absorption, increased gastric pH affecting ionizable drug dissolution, and nausea/vomiting potentially compromising oral medication administration. These changes typically produce modest clinical effects relative to more substantial distribution, metabolism, and excretion alterations.

Distribution changes include increased plasma volume (30-50%) and decreased albumin concentration, significantly affecting highly protein-bound medications through reduced binding and increased free drug concentration. Total body water increases by approximately 8 liters, altering volume of distribution for water-soluble medications. These changes necessitate dosage adjustments for certain therapeutic agents, particularly those with narrow therapeutic indices requiring therapeutic drug monitoring such as anticonvulsants, lithium, and certain antibiotics.

Hepatic metabolism changes with complex and sometimes contradictory effects on medication clearance. Some cytochrome P450 enzymes show increased activity (CYP3A4, CYP2D6, CYP2C9), while others demonstrate reduced function. Concurrent increases in hepatic blood flow enhance clearance of flow-limited medications. These changes vary considerably throughout pregnancy progression, often requiring trimester-specific dosage adjustments to maintain therapeutic effect. Postpartum reversal of these changes necessitates readjustment to pre-pregnancy dosing to avoid toxicity.

Renal function changes include increased glomerular filtration rate (GFR) by approximately 50% beginning in the first trimester, significantly increasing clearance of renally eliminated medications. This enhanced elimination may reduce serum concentrations below therapeutic thresholds for medications including lithium, certain antibiotics, and antiepileptic drugs, potentially compromising treatment efficacy without appropriate dosage adjustment. As with other pregnancy-related changes, postpartum reversal requires careful monitoring and readjustment to avoid toxicity.

Table 7.3: Medication Safety in Pregnancy and Lactation

Pregnancy Stage	Physiological Changes Affecting Medications	Monitoring Recommendations
Preconception	Baseline physiological state Preparation for pregnancy Medication optimization opportunity Chronic condition management Supplementation needs	Chronic disease optimization Medication documentation Genetic screening as indicated Baseline parameters for chronic conditions Preconception counseling documentation
First Trimester	Organogenesis period (highest risk) Nausea and vomiting affecting absorption Minimal changes in drug metabolism	Confirmation of viable pregnancy Detailed medication review Fetal development monitoring Nausea management assessment Chronic disease

Pregnancy Stage	Physiological Changes Affecting Medications	Monitoring Recommendations
	Early plasma volume expansion Altered gastric emptying	monitoring
Second Trimester	Increased plasma volume (30-50%) Increased glomerular filtration rate Enhanced hepatic metabolism Decreased plasma protein concentration Increased cardiac output	Fetal growth monitoring Therapeutic drug monitoring when indicated Blood pressure and glucose monitoring Medication efficacy assessment Adjustment of dose frequency/amount
Third Trimester	Maximal plasma volume expansion Decreased gastric motility Altered drug protein binding Risk of delivery complications Preparation for lactation	Fetal well-being assessment Therapeutic drug levels Delivery planning Potential neonatal monitoring needs Maternal disease stability
Lactation	Drug transfer to	Infant monitoring

Pregnancy Stage	Physiological Changes Affecting Medications	Monitoring Recommendations
	breast milk Infant drug metabolism capacity Maternal metabolism returning to baseline Medication timing optimization Breast milk composition changes	for drug effects Milk supply assessment Maternal disease control Infant growth and development Medication timing relative to feeding
Postpartum (Non-Lactating)	Rapid physiological changes Return to pre-pregnancy metabolism Fluid/electrolyte normalization Hormonal fluctuations Sleep disruption affecting metabolism	Resolution of pregnancy adaptations Chronic disease reassessment Mental health screening Return to pre-pregnancy parameters Adjustment of therapeutic doses

Placental transfer represents the most critical pregnancy-specific pharmacokinetic consideration, determining fetal medication exposure. Factors influencing transfer include molecular weight, protein binding, lipid solubility, ionization state, and placental metabolism capabilities. The placenta expresses numerous transporters including P-glycoprotein that actively exclude certain medications from fetal circulation, providing partial protection. However, most medications cross the placenta to some degree, with lipophilic, non-ionized, and low-molecular-weight compounds generally achieving higher fetal concentrations and potential exposure risk.

Risk Classification and Information Sources

Pregnancy risk classification systems attempt to categorize medications based on available safety information, though all systems have significant limitations reflecting the inherent complexity and limited research base. The former FDA pregnancy category system (A, B, C, D, X) has been replaced with the Pregnancy and Lactation Labeling Rule (PLLR) requiring narrative descriptions of available data rather than simplified categories. This change recognizes that binary "safe/unsafe" categorizations inadequately represent the nuanced risk-benefit considerations necessary for informed decision-making.

Current pregnancy medication information sources include product labeling under PLLR guidelines, pregnancy exposure registries collecting observational data on medication outcomes, specialist-managed teratogen information services providing individualized risk assessments, and databases such as TERIS (Teratogen Information System) and Reprotox synthesizing available literature. These sources collectively support clinical decision-making while acknowledging inevitable limitations including reliance on observational data, potential reporting biases, and inability to control for confounding factors such as underlying maternal conditions.

Risk assessment for specific medications requires consideration of multiple factors beyond simple exposure. Gestational timing significantly influences risk profiles, with organogenesis (weeks 3-8) representing particular vulnerability for structural teratogenesis, while later exposure may affect functional development, growth, or delivery timing. Dose, duration, and concurrent exposures modify risk profiles, as does underlying maternal condition severity which itself may pose risks to fetal development if inadequately treated.

Lactation risk assessment follows similar principles but with distinct physiological considerations. The infant dose received through breast milk depends on medication concentration in maternal plasma, transfer into milk (influenced by molecular weight, protein binding, lipophilicity, and ionization), milk volume consumed, and infant clearance capabilities. The relative infant dose (RID)—the weight-adjusted percentage of maternal dose received by the infant—provides standardized comparison across medications. Medications with RID <10% generally present minimal risk, while those >25% warrant careful consideration of risk-benefit balance.

Clinical Decision-Making and Risk Communication

Therapeutic decision-making during pregnancy requires systematic assessment of treatment options considering maternal benefit, fetal risk, and consequences of untreated maternal conditions. Where feasible, preconception planning allows medication adjustment before pregnancy exposure, substituting medications with established safety profiles for those with unknown or concerning risk profiles. For chronic conditions including epilepsy, depression, and autoimmune disorders, multidisciplinary planning involving relevant specialists optimizes regimens before conception attempts.

When pregnancy occurs without preconception planning or new conditions develop during pregnancy, decision-making follows structured evaluation: Is treatment necessary or can it be safely delayed until after pregnancy? If treatment is necessary, are non-pharmacological options adequate? If medication is required, which option has the most favorable risk-benefit profile based on available evidence? Does the gestational timing influence this decision? This systematic approach ensures appropriate consideration of all relevant factors beyond simplified safety categorizations.

Risk communication with pregnant women requires special attention to both informational and emotional dimensions. Research demonstrates that pregnant women often perceive medication risks as higher than scientific evidence suggests, sometimes leading to non-adherence with needed therapy. Effective communication includes numeric risk presentation with appropriate comparisons to baseline population risks, acknowledgment of evidence limitations, and explicit discussion of risks associated with untreated maternal conditions. Shared decision-making approaches support informed choices aligned with individual values while addressing anxiety through appropriate contextual information.

Psychiatric medication management exemplifies the complexity of pregnancy risk-benefit assessment. Untreated maternal depression and anxiety carry significant risks including poor prenatal care, substance use, preterm birth, low birth weight, and postpartum psychiatric deterioration. Simultaneously, SSRIs and other psychotropic medications have associated risks including potential (though contested) first-trimester cardiac malformation risks, persistent pulmonary hypertension association, and neonatal adaptation syndrome with late-pregnancy exposure. Individualized assessment considering illness severity, prior response to non-pharmacological interventions, and personal risk tolerance guides appropriate management rather than universal recommendations.

Monitoring and Safety Systems

Enhanced monitoring during pregnancy supports early detection of both medication effects and underlying condition changes requiring therapeutic adjustment. Ultrasound surveillance may be indicated for medications with specific structural risk concerns, such as increased nuchal translucency screening with lithium exposure or detailed cardiac evaluation with first-trimester SSRI exposure. Maternal physiological monitoring including renal function assessment, liver function tests, and therapeutic drug level monitoring addresses the changing pharmacokinetic context throughout pregnancy progression.

Documentation systems should clearly identify pregnancy status, gestational age, and planned delivery timing to support appropriate prescribing decisions throughout healthcare systems. Electronic health record modifications including mandatory pregnancy status documentation before teratogenic medication prescribing, specific pregnancy alerts for contraindicated medications, and gestational age-specific dosing guidance for medications requiring pregnancy adjustment enhance systematic safety management beyond individual provider knowledge.

Postpartum monitoring addresses both maternal medication needs and infant effects for breastfeeding mothers. Maternal dosage readjustment may be necessary as pregnancy-induced physiological changes resolve, particularly for medications with substantial clearance changes during pregnancy. For breastfeeding mothers, infant monitoring should address medication-specific concerns; for example, sedation assessment for mothers taking central nervous system agents or thyroid function monitoring for infants whose mothers take antithyroid medications.

Pregnancy exposure registries represent crucial systems for expanding medication safety knowledge through systematic collection of exposure and outcome data. These observational programs enroll pregnant women taking specific medications, following outcomes through delivery and sometimes beyond for long-term developmental assessment. Healthcare providers should routinely inform pregnant patients about relevant registries for their medications, supporting participation to expand the evidence base for future clinical decision-making while respecting individual autonomy regarding participation decisions.

PATIENTS WITH MULTIPLE COMORBIDITIES

Patients with multiple comorbidities present complex medication safety challenges arising from interacting disease processes, complex therapeutic regimens, competing clinical priorities, and care fragmentation across multiple providers. These factors create distinctive vulnerability patterns requiring specialized approaches throughout the medication use process.

Multimorbidity Patterns and Medication Burden

Multimorbidity—the coexistence of multiple chronic conditions within an individual—demonstrates both random and non-random clustering patterns with important implications for medication safety. Concordant conditions sharing pathophysiological pathways frequently co-occur, such as diabetes, hypertension, and coronary artery disease linked through metabolic dysfunction and vascular pathology. Discordant conditions without shared pathophysiology may co-occur randomly or through indirect relationships, creating more complex management challenges due to non-overlapping and potentially conflicting treatment approaches.

Medication regimen complexity grows exponentially rather than linearly with increasing comorbidities, reflecting both multiple medications and complicated administration requirements. The Medication Regimen Complexity Index quantifies this complexity through assessment of dosage forms, frequency schedules, additional administration instructions, and total medication count. High complexity correlates with reduced adherence, increased error potential, and greater healthcare utilization independent of simple medication count, highlighting the importance of complexity reduction as a safety strategy.

Disease-drug interactions represent bidirectional influences between pathophysiological states and medication effects that complicate multimorbidity management. Hepatic or renal dysfunction from one condition alters medication metabolism or elimination for treatments targeting other conditions. Heart failure reduces gastrointestinal perfusion and absorption while increasing sensitivity to fluid retention effects of certain medications. Thyroid dysfunction alters pharmacodynamic responses across multiple medication classes. These interactions often receive less attention than drug-drug interactions despite similar clinical significance, particularly when disease severity fluctuates over time.

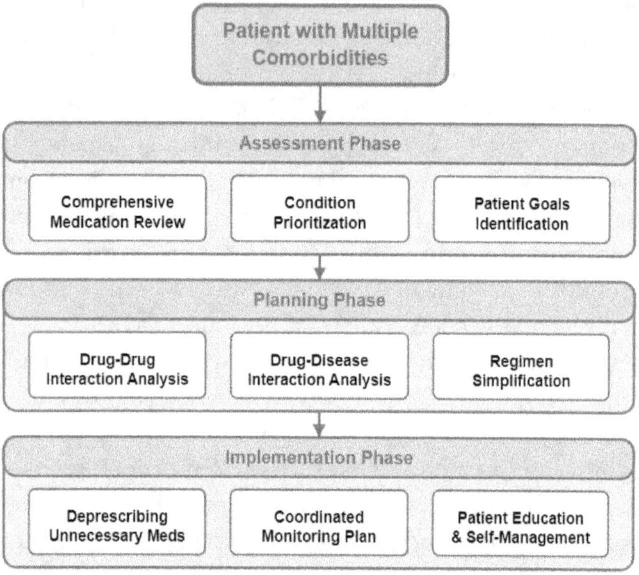

Figure 7.4 Medication Management for Multiple Comorbidities

Treatment burden encompasses the workload demanded of patients in managing their health conditions and the impact on functioning and quality of life. For patients with multiple comorbidities, this burden includes medication management tasks (organizing, remembering, obtaining, paying for, and administering multiple medications), healthcare coordination responsibilities (communicating between specialists, reconciling conflicting advice), self-monitoring requirements (symptoms, vital signs, laboratory values), and lifestyle modifications (often multiple and sometimes conflicting). High treatment burden correlates with reduced adherence, diminished quality of life, and increased healthcare discontinuity when exceeding individual capacity.

Therapeutic Conflicts and Competing Priorities

Guideline conflicts frequently emerge when applying multiple disease-specific guidelines to patients with multimorbidity, creating significant medication safety challenges. These conflicts include direct therapeutic contradictions (e.g., NSAIDs recommended for osteoarthritis but contraindicated in heart failure), conflicting management parameters (e.g., blood pressure targets for diabetes versus chronic kidney disease), cumulative toxicity from recommended combinations (e.g., multiple drugs prolonging QT interval), and practical feasibility limitations when combining multiple guideline-recommended monitoring protocols.

Appropriate guideline application requires recognition that disease-specific guidelines typically derive from studies excluding multimorbid patients, limiting their validity for complex patients. Research demonstrates that strict application of multiple guidelines to patients with common comorbidity patterns frequently results in impractical regimens with high potential for harm through drug interactions and cumulative adverse effect burden. Patient-centered approaches considering condition severity, treatment effectiveness, individual preferences, and life expectancy provide more appropriate guidance than rigid guideline adherence.

Drug-disease interactions create particularly challenging therapeutic conflicts when a medication beneficial for one condition adversely affects another coexisting condition. Common examples include beta-blockers (beneficial for heart failure but potentially worsening asthma or peripheral vascular disease), corticosteroids (effective for inflammatory conditions but exacerbating diabetes and osteoporosis), and anticholinergics (treating overactive bladder but worsening cognitive impairment). These conflicts require explicit trade-off decisions rather than simply avoiding interactions, as some degree of management compromise is often unavoidable.

Prioritization systems support systematic approaches to resolving therapeutic conflicts when perfect adherence to all condition-specific guidelines proves impossible or potentially harmful. Such systems typically consider factors including symptom burden (prioritizing conditions causing greatest current distress), preservation of function (emphasizing treatments supporting independence), condition severity and progression risk, preventable adverse outcomes, and patient-identified priorities. This explicit prioritization supports focused medication regimens addressing highest-value treatments rather than comprehensively treating all conditions regardless of impact.

Table 7.4: Medication Management in Patients with Multiple Comorbidities

Challenge Area	Assessment	Monitoring
Disease-Disease Interactions	Comprehensive condition inventory Condition severity assessment Symptom burden evaluation Disease trajectory mapping Function impact assessment	Disease activity measures Symptom improvement hierarchy Quality of life assessment Functional status trends Patient-reported outcomes
Drug-Disease	Medication impact	Targeted symptom

Challenge Area	Assessment	Monitoring
Interactions	assessment Contraindication screening Risk stratification tools Therapeutic competition analysis Condition-specific considerations	assessment Disease-specific parameters Early warning signs of exacerbation Condition stability indicators Therapeutic response monitoring
Drug-Drug Interactions	Comprehensive interaction screening Drug burden indices Medication timing analysis Side effect inventories Metabolism pathway analysis	Therapeutic drug monitoring Drug effect parameters Adverse effect surveillance Drug levels when indicated Efficacy maintenance assessment
Guideline Conflicts	Guideline applicability assessment Evidence quality evaluation Guideline conflict identification Patient preference incorporation Outcome priority determination	Outcome measures across conditions Guideline adherence balance Priority outcome tracking Unintended consequence monitoring Composite outcome measures
Therapeutic Complexity	Medication regimen complexity index Patient capability assessment	Adherence assessment Medication burden perception Administration

Challenge Area	Assessment	Monitoring
	Support system evaluation Financial impact analysis Administration complexity mapping	error tracking Missed dose patterns Regimen sustainability
Care Coordination	Care coordination assessment Communication network mapping Information transfer evaluation Responsibility assignment clarity Handoff quality assessment	Information consistency Care plan adherence Communication effectiveness Medication discrepancies Provider alignment
Patient-Centered Factors	Treatment burden assessment Goal and preference elicitation Health literacy evaluation Patient activation measure Caregiver assessment	Patient-reported outcomes Goal attainment scaling Quality of life measures Self-efficacy assessment Treatment burden perception

Care Coordination and Medication Reconciliation

Care fragmentation across multiple specialists represents a fundamental challenge for patients with multiple comorbidities, with each provider typically focusing on condition-specific treatments without comprehensive consideration of the complete medication regimen. Research demonstrates that patients seeing four specialists typically receive prescriptions from at least three different prescribers, with limited cross-specialty communication regarding medication changes or observed effects. This fragmentation creates substantial safety risks including therapeutic duplication, unintended drug interactions, and contradictory medication changes.

Medication reconciliation takes on heightened importance in multimorbidity contexts due to frequent care transitions and multiple prescribers. Comprehensive reconciliation requires aggregating information from all treatment sources, resolving discrepancies through direct communication rather than assumption, documenting therapeutic intent for each medication, and capturing recent changes with their rationales. Best practices include designation of a reconciliation responsible provider, structured processes for reconciliation after every care transition, and direct patient involvement to capture self-directed treatments and actual administration patterns that may differ from prescribing records.

Primary care coordination models demonstrate effectiveness in reducing medication-related problems for patients with multiple comorbidities through longitudinal relationship continuity and comprehensive oversight. The Patient-Centered Medical Home model emphasizes care coordination as a core function, with specific medication management responsibilities including maintaining comprehensive medication lists, coordinating consultants' recommendations, performing periodic comprehensive medication reviews, and supporting appropriate deprescribing. These functions reduce duplicate therapy, minimize unintended interactions, and ensure regular reassessment of continuing appropriateness as conditions evolve.

Shared electronic health records with medication

management functionality support coordination across fragmented care systems, though significant limitations remain in current implementations. Beneficial features include flagging potential interactions across prescribers, identifying therapeutic duplications, documenting medication change rationales accessible to all providers, and maintaining problem-medication linkages to clarify therapeutic intent. However, these benefits require consistent use across all care settings, appropriate configuration with clinically meaningful interaction alerts, and integration of non-prescription treatments often omitted from formal records.

Improving Safety for Complex Patients

Comprehensive medication review (CMR) represents a structured approach to evaluating and optimizing medication regimens for patients with multimorbidity. Unlike simple medication reconciliation focusing on verification of current medications, CMR involves systematic assessment of indication appropriateness, effectiveness for intended conditions, safety considering all comorbidities, practical feasibility, and alignment with patient goals. When conducted by clinical pharmacists with physician collaboration, CMR consistently demonstrates reduction in medication-related problems, decreased emergency department visits, and improved therapeutic outcomes for complex patients.

Deprescribing—the systematic process of medication discontinuation when potential harms outweigh benefits—takes on particular importance for patients with multiple comorbidities at risk for polypharmacy-related harm. Structured deprescribing processes include identifying potentially inappropriate medications, assessing actual benefit and harm for individual patients, determining discontinuation priority, implementing gradual dose reduction with monitoring, and documenting outcomes to inform future decisions. For complex patients, deprescribing decisions should consider remaining life expectancy, time to benefit, symptom impact, and overall treatment burden rather than focusing exclusively on condition-specific guidelines.

Patient engagement strategies require adaptation for individuals managing complex regimens with multiple comorbidities. Approaches demonstrating effectiveness include simplified administration systems (blister packs, medication boxes with electronic monitoring), visual medication schedules linking medications to daily routines, explicit indication documentation on medication labels, patient-held medication lists with indication and prescriber information, and technology support including medication reminder applications with education links. These approaches address the cognitive complexity of multimorbidity management while supporting informed participation in treatment decisions.

Quality measurement for medically complex patients increasingly recognizes the limitations of disease-specific quality metrics that may incentivize inappropriate care. Patient-centered quality approaches emphasize outcomes including medication burden reduction, patient-reported functional status, treatment satisfaction, and alignment with individual goals rather than disease-specific surrogate markers. Risk adjustment methodologies accounting for multimorbidity prevent inappropriate comparison between complex and less complex populations, supporting fair evaluation of providers caring for clinically challenging patients. These evolved quality approaches discourage reflexive application of multiple disease guidelines without appropriate individualization, supporting more thoughtful medication management.

Things to Remember

- ☑ Pediatric medication safety requires weight-based dosing tools, age-appropriate formulations, developmental pharmacology considerations, and specialized verification processes for this vulnerable population.
- ☑ Geriatric safety addresses age-related pharmacokinetic changes, polypharmacy issues, altered adverse effect profiles, and functional limitations through regimen reviews and simplified approaches.
- ☑ Pregnancy and lactation necessitate careful risk categorization, therapeutic alternatives assessment, and timing optimization throughout reproductive stages to balance maternal benefit against fetal/infant risk.
- ☑ Patients with multiple comorbidities need coordinated medication management through comprehensive reviews, explicit prioritization, and enhanced monitoring to address complex medication regimens and potential drug-disease interactions.
- ☑ Special populations require tailored approaches recognizing unique physiological, pharmacokinetic, and practical considerations rather than standard medication processes designed for typical adult patients.
- ☑ Context-specific approaches should adapt general safety principles to address the distinctive challenges of each special population.

Multiple Choice Questions

1. Pediatric medication safety challenges include:
   a) Simplified dosing requirements compared to adults
   b) Excessive availability of pediatric-specific formulations
   c) Weight-based dosing calculations increasing error risk
   d) Reduced variation in pharmacokinetics across age groups
2. Age-related pharmacokinetic changes in geriatric patients include:
   a) Increased hepatic metabolism of medications
   b) Enhanced renal clearance of medications
   c) Decreased body fat percentage affecting drug distribution
   d) Reduced gastric acid production potentially affecting drug absorption
3. Which medication safety strategy is particularly important for geriatric patients?
   a) Converting all medications to parenteral forms
   b) Comprehensive regimen reviews addressing polypharmacy
   c) Standardized dosing without individualization
   d) Automated dispensing without pharmacist review
4. Pregnancy risk categories for medications:
   a) Provide absolute certainty about medication safety
   b) Are identical across all regulatory systems

globally
c) Attempt to balance maternal benefit against potential fetal risk
d) Eliminate the need for clinical judgment in prescribing

5. Medication safety for lactating women requires consideration of:
a) Only medication effects on milk production
b) Drug transfer into breast milk and potential infant effects
c) Maternal considerations without regard to infant exposure
d) Only medications specifically approved for breastfeeding women

6. Which of the following represents a particular challenge in managing medications for patients with multiple comorbidities?
a) Simplified medication regimens with few medications
b) Potential drug-disease interactions where treatment for one condition affects another
c) Limited involvement of specialty providers
d) Excessive standardization of treatment approaches

7. Weight-based dosing in pediatric patients:
a) Is unnecessary for most medications
b) Should always use actual body weight regardless of medication
c) Requires appropriate tools and independent verification
d) Is primarily important for oral medications but not intravenous therapy

8. Comprehensive medication reviews for geriatric patients should include assessment of:
   a) Only prescription medications without over-the-counter products
   b) Medications, timing, appropriateness, potential interactions, and adherence barriers
   c) Exclusively medications added within the past month
   d) Only medications treating the primary diagnosis
9. Therapeutic decision-making during pregnancy typically involves:
   a) Avoiding all medications regardless of maternal condition
   b) Using only medications with extensive human pregnancy data
   c) Considering disease risks, medication benefits, alternative treatments, and timing
   d) Relying exclusively on FDA pregnancy categories without clinical judgment
10. Coordinated medication management for patients with multiple comorbidities includes:
    a) Requiring all medications to be prescribed by a single provider
    b) Explicit prioritization of treatment goals across conditions
    c) Treating each condition independently without consideration of interactions
    d) Standardized approaches identical to those used for patients with single conditions

Self-Assessment Questions

1. Analyze the unique challenges in pediatric medication safety, including weight-based dosing, medication formulations, and age-specific risks, providing evidence-based strategies to address these challenges.
2. Evaluate how physiological changes in older adults affect medication safety and discuss comprehensive approaches to reduce adverse drug events in the geriatric population.
3. Critically analyze the ethical and clinical considerations in medication management during pregnancy and lactation, including risk assessment systems and communication strategies.
4. Discuss the challenges of medication safety in patients with multiple comorbidities, including polypharmacy management, drug interactions, and prioritization of therapy.
5. Compare and contrast medication safety considerations across the pediatric age spectrum (neonates, infants, children, adolescents), highlighting unique risks at each stage.
6. Evaluate the role of deprescribing in geriatric medication safety, including assessment tools, implementation strategies, and outcome measures.
7. Analyze the challenges in conducting medication safety research in special populations and strategies to advance

evidence-based practices despite these limitations.

8. Discuss the impact of cognitive impairment on medication adherence and safety, including innovative approaches to support patients and caregivers.
9. Evaluate medication safety considerations in patients with organ dysfunction (renal, hepatic, cardiac) and approaches to dose adjustment and monitoring.
10. Analyze the unique medication safety challenges in patients with communication barriers, including strategies for effective assessment, education, and monitoring.

Bibliography

1. Kaushal R, Bates DW, Landrigan C, McKenna KJ, Clapp MD, Federico F, et al. Medication errors and adverse drug events in pediatric inpatients. JAMA. 2001;285(16):2114-20.
2. Mulherin DW, Zimmerman CR, Chaffee BW. National standards for computerized prescriber order entry and clinical decision support: the case of drug allergies. Am J Health Syst Pharm. 2013;70(7):589-91.
3. Conroy S, Sweis D, Planner C, Yeung V, Collier J, Haines L, et al. Interventions to reduce dosing errors in children: a systematic review of the literature. Drug Saf. 2007;30(12):1111-25.
4. Maher RL, Hanlon J, Hajjar ER. Clinical consequences of polypharmacy in elderly. Expert Opin Drug Saf. 2014;13(1):57-65.
5. Kaufmann CP, Tremp R, Hersberger KE, Lampert ML. Inappropriate prescribing: a systematic overview of published assessment tools. Eur J Clin Pharmacol. 2014;70(1):1-11.
6. American Geriatrics Society 2019 Updated AGS Beers Criteria® for Potentially Inappropriate Medication Use in Older Adults. J Am Geriatr Soc. 2019;67(4):674-94.
7. O'Mahony D, O'Sullivan D, Byrne S, O'Connor MN, Ryan C, Gallagher P. STOPP/START criteria for potentially inappropriate prescribing in older people: version 2. Age Ageing. 2015;44(2):213-8.
8. Tommelein E, Mehuys E, Petrovic M, Somers A, Colin P, Boussery K. Potentially inappropriate prescribing in community-dwelling older people across Europe: a systematic literature review. Eur J Clin Pharmacol. 2015;71(12):1415-27.
9. Schnipper JL, Kirwin JL, Cotugno MC, Wahlstrom SA, Brown BA, Tarvin E, et al. Role of pharmacist counseling in preventing adverse drug events after hospitalization. Arch Intern Med. 2006;166(5):565-71.
10. Lexicomp Inc. Lexi-Drugs: Teratogenicity/Effects in Pregnancy/Breastfeeding [Internet]. Hudson, OH: Wolters Kluwer Clinical Drug Information, Inc.; 2020.

CHAPTER 8

ROLE OF HEALTHCARE PROFESSIONALS

Abstract

Healthcare professionals serve essential medication safety functions through individual competencies and collaborative practice models supporting risk management. Interprofessional collaboration improves safety through team-based approaches leveraging complementary expertise, structured communication methodologies preventing information gaps, collaborative decision-making incorporating diverse perspectives, and shared accountability across traditional boundaries. Effective communication techniques include SBAR framework for structured information transfer, closed-loop verification confirming understanding, standardized terminology preventing ambiguity, and non-punitive questioning encouraging clarification without intimidation. Documentation practices establish information continuity through medication records, standardized formats ensuring consistent capture, appropriate level of detail supporting clinical decisions, and clear intervention documentation preserving rationale beyond immediate care episodes. Professional responsibilities encompass knowledge maintenance through continuous education, competency development matching practice scope, error disclosure supporting transparency and improvement, and advocacy addressing system limitations potentially compromising safety, collectively creating culture where each discipline contributes specialized capabilities while sharing fundamental responsibility for medication safety throughout the healthcare system.

Keywords: *Team-based care, structured communication, interdisciplinary collaboration, professional accountability, safety culture*

Learning Objectives

After completion of the chapter, the learners should be able to:

- Remember the key elements of effective interprofessional collaboration in medication safety.
- Understand how structured communication techniques prevent medication errors across transitions of care.
- Apply appropriate documentation practices to support safe medication management.
- Analyze the professional responsibilities of different healthcare disciplines in medication safety.
- Evaluate the effectiveness of team-based approaches to medication error prevention.
- Create strategies to enhance interprofessional collaboration in medication safety initiatives.

INTERPROFESSIONAL COLLABORATION

Interprofessional collaboration in medication safety transcends traditional role boundaries to create integrated systems where multiple disciplines contribute complementary expertise throughout the medication use process. This collaborative approach recognizes that medication safety challenges exceed the capabilities of any single profession, requiring coordinated efforts across healthcare disciplines with shared accountability for patient outcomes.

Collaborative Practice Models

Team-based care models provide structured systems for interprofessional medication safety collaboration, establishing clear roles while maintaining necessary flexibility for complex clinical scenarios. The interprofessional team typically includes physicians, pharmacists, and nurses as core members, with additional disciplines including physician assistants, nurse practitioners, respiratory therapists, and dietitians participating based on specific patient needs and practice settings. Effective models establish clear domains of responsibility while creating deliberate overlaps that serve as safety redundancies rather than inefficient duplications.

Pharmacist integration within clinical teams represents a particularly significant evolution in medication safety practice. Traditional drug distribution roles have expanded to include clinical services ranging from medication therapy management to collaborative practice agreements with prescribing authority in defined circumstances. Clinical pharmacy specialists with advanced training provide specialized expertise in high-risk areas including anticoagulation management, critical care, oncology, and transplantation, where medication regimen complexity and risk profiles exceed generalist knowledge. Research consistently demonstrates that pharmacist integration reduces medication errors, improves therapy appropriateness, and enhances clinical outcomes across diverse practice settings.

Nurse-led medication safety initiatives leverage nursing's continuous patient presence and administration responsibility to identify safety improvement opportunities and implement practice changes. Medication safety nurse specialists develop expertise in error prevention strategies, system analysis, and improvement methodology while maintaining frontline credibility with nursing colleagues. Unit-based safety champions promote practice consistency and serve as local resources for medication questions. These nursing leadership roles complement formal authority structures with informal influence networks that promote safety culture development at the unit level.

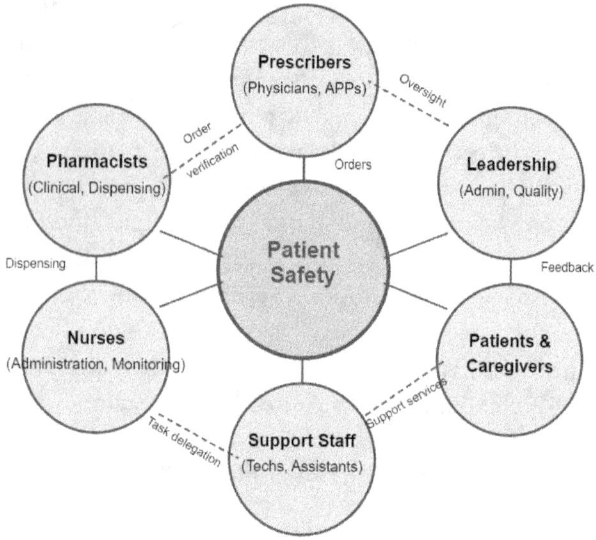

Figure 8.1: Interprofessional Collaboration Model

Interdisciplinary rounding practices provide structured opportunities for prospective medication regimen review and collaborative planning, particularly valuable for complex patients with high-risk medication regimens. Effective models include pharmacist preparation before rounds to identify potential issues, structured medication review during rounds with defined discussion triggers for high-risk situations, and clear documentation of collaborative decisions with assigned accountability for follow-up actions. Research demonstrates that interprofessional rounds reduce preventable adverse drug events by 70-80% when consistently implemented with appropriate team composition and explicit medication safety focus.

Role Delineation and Complementary Expertise

Prescriber responsibilities in collaborative medication safety systems extend beyond accurate order writing to include appropriate patient assessment, clear communication of therapeutic intent, consideration of patient-specific factors affecting medication response, and ongoing evaluation of treatment effectiveness and adverse effects. Prescribers contribute medical diagnosis expertise, integration of treatment approaches across multiple conditions, and ultimate accountability for therapeutic decisions while recognizing the essential contributions of other team members to safe medication use.

Pharmacist contributions include specialized pharmaceutical knowledge regarding medication properties, interactions, and alternatives; system-level medication use oversight; and detailed patient-level medication regimen evaluation. Core safety functions include order verification with appropriate intervention for potential issues, clinical monitoring for adverse effects and therapeutic response, patient education regarding proper medication use, and system-level analysis of medication use patterns to identify improvement opportunities. The pharmacist role increasingly emphasizes proactive involvement in therapeutic decision-making rather than reactive verification of completed orders.

Nursing medication safety responsibilities encompass assessment before administration, accurate medication preparation and administration, monitoring for therapeutic and adverse effects, patient education, and timely communication of medication concerns to other team members. The nursing role provides critical protection at the final stage before medications reach patients, with responsibility for independent verification that the medication remains appropriate given the patient's current condition. Nursing documentation of administration circumstances and subsequent effects creates essential information for ongoing therapy evaluation.

Patient and family participation as active team members represents an evolution in medication safety collaboration, recognizing their unique knowledge of medication experiences, administration challenges, and personal priorities. Patients contribute essential information about actual medication consumption patterns, experienced side effects that may not be apparent during healthcare encounters, and practical barriers to adherence. Collaborative models incorporate structured approaches to eliciting this information through medication reviews, side effect screening tools, and assessment of medication understanding and administration capabilities.

Collaborative Decision-Making Processes

Structured interdisciplinary decision systems support consistent application of collaborative expertise to medication safety challenges. Shared mental models regarding medication safety priorities, common terminology for discussing medication issues, and clear escalation pathways for safety concerns facilitate efficient team functioning without unnecessary conflict. Pre-defined triggers for collaborative consultation recognize situations where multiple perspectives are particularly valuable, including high-alert medication initiation, complex regimen management, significant organ dysfunction affecting medication clearance, and adverse effect evaluation.

Conflict resolution mechanisms address inevitable differences in professional perspective regarding medication decisions. Effective approaches establish communication norms emphasizing patient-centered framing of disagreements, explicit articulation of discipline-specific concerns, focus on information exchange rather than position defense, and clear processes for reaching resolution when consensus proves elusive. These mechanisms recognize that constructive conflict expressing legitimate safety concerns represents a system strength rather than dysfunction, provided appropriate resolution processes exist.

Collaborative technology tools increasingly support asynchronous interprofessional communication when direct interaction proves impractical. Secure messaging integrated with electronic health records enables consultation about medication issues with appropriate clinical context, while shared documentation platforms support coordinated monitoring of high-risk medications. Clinical surveillance systems generate alerts to relevant team members based on predefined triggers such as laboratory abnormalities suggesting adverse drug effects, allowing timely collaborative response across disciplines regardless of physical proximity.

Decision support systems with interprofessional design incorporate multiple disciplinary perspectives rather than reflecting single-profession priorities. Sophisticated systems route different aspects of medication decisions to appropriate team members based on specific expertise—pharmacists for interaction management, nurses for administration timing coordination, prescribers for indication appropriateness. This collaborative technology design recognizes that effective decision support requires both appropriate knowledge content and delivery to the team member best positioned to address specific medication safety issues.

Organizational Support for Collaboration

Formal organizational structures supporting medication safety collaboration include pharmacy and therapeutics committees, medication safety committees, and quality improvement teams with interprofessional membership and explicitly collaborative mandates. These structures establish systematic approaches to formulary management, protocol development, adverse event review, and safety initiative implementation. Effective committees balance necessary profession-specific representation with collective accountability for system improvement, preventing territorial approaches that prioritize professional interests over patient safety.

Educational initiatives supporting collaboration include interprofessional training programs, simulation activities focusing on medication safety scenarios, and shared learning from safety events. Joint education across professions establishes common conceptual systems, develops mutual understanding of complementary roles, and builds collaborative relationships before clinical pressure situations. Team simulation exercises focusing on high-risk medication scenarios develop communication skills and role coordination while identifying system improvement opportunities in a consequence-free environment.

Leadership commitment to collaboration manifests through resource allocation, performance expectations, and reward systems that prioritize team functioning over individual performance. Dedicated time for collaborative activities, physical space supporting team interaction, and information systems enabling shared decision-making demonstrate organizational valuation of interprofessional approaches.

Table 8.1: Interprofessional Roles in Medication Safety

Professional	Core Responsibilities	Development Needs
Physicians/Prescribers	Diagnosis and treatment planning Medication selection and prescribing Risk-benefit assessment Treatment monitoring Patient education	Updated medication safety training Decision support tool utilization Prescribing pattern feedback Error reporting and analysis Interprofessional communication skills
Pharmacists	Medication profile review Clinical verification Medication preparation/dispensing Therapeutic drug monitoring Medication education	Advanced clinical knowledge Technology utilization training Leadership in safety initiatives Research and quality improvement Risk management methods
Nurses	Medication	Specialized

Professional	Core Responsibilities	Development Needs
	administration Patient monitoring Symptom assessment Documentation Patient and family education	medication knowledge Technology competency Patient assessment skills Error prevention strategies Safety culture leadership
Medication Safety Officers/Specialists	Safety program development Safety data analysis Process improvement Education coordination Risk assessment	Advanced safety certification Human factors training Leadership development Project management skills Change management expertise
Information Technology Specialists	Technology implementation System maintenance User support System optimization Integration management	Clinical workflow understanding Human factors principles System safety optimization User

Professional	Core Responsibilities	Development Needs
		experience design Health IT safety certification
Patients and Caregivers	Medication administration at home Symptom monitoring Communication of concerns Adherence management Medication storage	Medication knowledge Self-monitoring skills Communication strategies Problem-solving techniques Health technology literacy
Leadership/Administration	Resource allocation Policy development Accountability systems Strategic planning Regulatory compliance	Safety science knowledge High-reliability principles Financial impact assessment Change leadership Systems thinking

Performance evaluation including collaboration metrics and team-based incentive structures reinforces the essential nature of cross-disciplinary partnerships in medication safety.

Collaborative practice barriers requiring organizational attention include professional licensure limitations, reimbursement structures favoring individual rather than team-based care, hierarchical traditions impeding open communication, and documentation systems designed for single-profession use rather than collaborative work. Progressive organizations address these barriers through advocacy for regulatory changes, innovative payment models, explicit anti-hierarchical communication policies, and health information technology optimized for team-based care. These organizational approaches recognize that interprofessional collaboration requires systematic support rather than merely exhorting professionals to "work together better."

COMMUNICATION TECHNIQUES

Effective communication represents a foundational element of medication safety practice, with communication failures contributing to 50-80% of serious medication errors in analysis of sentinel events. Structured communication techniques create standardized approaches for information transfer across care transitions, professional boundaries, and high-risk situations, reducing reliance on individual communication skills or relationships for safety-critical information exchange.

Standardized Communication

SBAR (Situation-Background-Assessment-Recommendation) methodology provides a structured format for communicating medication concerns across professional boundaries, particularly valuable for hierarchical communications such as nurse-to-physician or resident-to-attending interactions. This framework begins with concise statement of the current situation requiring attention, followed by relevant background information providing context, professional assessment of the medication issue including urgency and safety implications, and specific recommendation for action. SBAR standardization reduces communication variability, ensures inclusion of essential information, and creates explicit opportunity for recommendations from all team members regardless of hierarchical position.

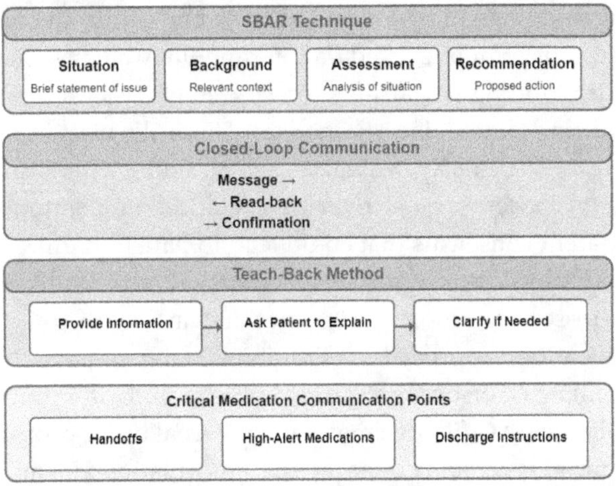

Figure 5.2 Effective Communication Techniques

Closed-loop communication ensures accurate information transfer through a three-step process: sender initiates communication with clear information, receiver acknowledges receipt and repeats key information for verification, and sender confirms accuracy or corrects misunderstandings. This approach prevents assumption of successful communication without verification, particularly valuable during verbal medication orders, critical laboratory value reporting, and high-risk medication adjustment discussions. Research demonstrates that closed-loop implementation reduces medication errors by 42-60% in acute care settings, with particularly strong impact during high-stress situations where communication reliability naturally deteriorates.

Critical language systems establish predefined terminology for safety concerns requiring immediate attention, creating linguistic tools that cut through professional courtesy and hierarchy when serious risks emerge. The "CUS" technique (I'm Concerned, I'm Uncomfortable, This is a Safety issue) provides escalating language signaling increasing urgency while avoiding accusatory framing. "Red flag" terminology creates shared understanding regarding specific high-risk situations requiring immediate response. These linguistic tools prove particularly valuable when subtle medication safety concerns must overcome clinical momentum or apparent consensus that could lead to patient harm.

Medication-specific communication standardization addresses common error mechanisms with tailored prevention approaches. Prohibited abbreviation lists eliminate error-prone expressions such as "U" for units or trailing zeros after decimal points. Verbal order protocols require specific sequences of information including patient identifiers, medication name with spelling clarification for sound-alike drugs, dose with explicit units, and administration route. Telephone order read-back requirements ensure accurate information transfer during indirect communication. These standardized approaches address known communication vulnerability points with consistent preventive strategies.

Table 8.2: Communication Techniques for Medication Safety

Communication Method	Description	Applications
SBAR (Situation-Background-Assessment-Recommendation)	Structured format for communicating critical information in a concise, organized manner	Urgent medication concerns Transfers between units/facilities On-call provider communication Shift-to-shift handoffs Pharmacy-prescriber interactions
Read-Back/Hear-Back	Receiver repeats information to confirm understanding; sender confirms accuracy	Verbal medication orders Critical lab values High-alert medication information Emergency situations Complex instructions
Teach-Back	Asking patients/caregivers to explain in their own words what they need to know or do	Discharge medication instructions New medication education Complex regimen

Communication Method	Description	Applications
		explanations High-risk medication teaching Self-management instructions
Team Huddles	Brief, structured meetings to discuss patient safety concerns and share critical information	Shift transitions High-risk patient reviews Safety alert dissemination Quick problem-solving Real-time coordination
Standardized Handoff Tools	Structured tools (I-PASS, HANDOFF, etc.) for comprehensive information transfer during transitions	Shift changes Unit transfers Service transfers Level-of-care changes Cross-coverage situations
Critical Language/CUS Words	Agreed-upon phrases that signal serious concerns and require immediate attention	Safety concerns Policy violations Escalation situations Wrong-patient/drug situations Time-critical interventions
Closed-Loop Communication	Complete communication cycle ensuring	Critical medication administration

Communication Method	Description	Applications
	message sent, received, understood, and acknowledged	Emergency situations Complex procedures Team-based activities Cross-checking processes
Patient Engagement Techniques	Methods to actively involve patients in safety, including medication lists, questions, and reporting concerns	Medication reconciliation Discharge planning Outpatient management Chronic medication therapy Self-administration programs
Structured Communication Tools	Visual aids, checklists, and standard templates for reliable information transfer	Complex medication instructions Medication reconciliation High-risk processes Multi-step procedures Quality assurance checks

Handoff Communication

Care transitions represent particular vulnerability points for medication safety, with handoff communication quality significantly influencing error risk during these transitions. Structured handoff tools incorporating explicit medication components ensure consistent information transfer regardless of individual communication styles or relationships. The I-PASS handoff bundle (Illness severity, Patient summary, Action list, Situation awareness, Synthesis by receiver) demonstrates 30% reduction in medical errors when consistently implemented, with particular benefit for medication continuity across provider changes.

Medication reconciliation during handoffs requires specific communication elements beyond basic medication lists, including recent changes with rationales, pending monitoring results affecting medication decisions, planned duration for time-limited therapies, previous adverse reactions with specific manifestations, and held medications with resumption criteria. These enriched communication elements provide contextual understanding supporting appropriate continuation of medication plans rather than merely documenting current medication states without underlying therapeutic rationale.

Discharge medication communication presents unique challenges requiring specialized approaches. Effective discharge medication handoffs include clear differentiation between continued, changed, and discontinued medications with explicit rationales; specific monitoring requirements with responsibility assignments; patient education verification regarding critical medications; and follow-up appointment timing linked to medication adjustment needs. Comprehensive discharge communication strategies address both professional-to-professional information transfer and patient/caregiver understanding, recognizing that both elements prove essential for post-discharge medication safety.

Electronic handoff tools increasingly support standardized communication during care transitions while maintaining human interaction for clarification and contextual understanding. Effective tools extract current medication information from electronic health records while providing structured fields for documentation of medication-specific handoff elements, supporting consistency without excessive duplication of existing information. Integration with secure messaging capabilities enables clarification questions after physical handoffs, addressing the inevitable questions arising during subsequent care that might otherwise remain unresolved with safety implications.

Patient Communication Strategies

Medication education for patients requires tailored communication strategies based on health literacy assessment, language proficiency, cultural context, and learning preferences. Teach-back methodology—asking patients to explain medication information in their own words—provides verification of understanding rather than merely documenting information provision. Research demonstrates that teach-back implementation reduces post-discharge adverse drug events by 30-45% while identifying specific misunderstandings requiring clarification before patients assume independent medication management responsibility.

Plain language communication principles address the substantial gap between healthcare professional terminology and patient understanding. These principles include using common words rather than medical terminology, explaining unfamiliar terms when specialized language proves necessary, focusing on action-oriented instructions, and limiting information density to 3-5 key points per communication session. Implementation for medication communication includes developing standardized plain language medication instructions, reviewing existing materials with health literacy experts, and creating simplified counseling approaches for high-risk medications.

Visual communication tools overcome literacy limitations and enhance understanding across language barriers. Pictographic medication schedules displaying administration timing with meal-related visual cues support appropriate administration sequencing. Medication appearance photographs help patients identify specific medications when names prove difficult to remember. Symptom illustration cards assist in adverse effect discussions when vocabulary limitations complicate verbal description. These visual approaches complement verbal and written communication rather than replacing them, recognizing that multimodal communication enhances understanding across diverse patient populations.

Medication risk communication requires special attention to foster informed decision-making without creating unnecessary alarm or non-adherence. Numeric risk presentation using natural frequencies (e.g., "3 in 100 people experience this side effect") rather than percentages or qualitative descriptors improves comprehension. Balanced presentation of both potential benefits and risks supports informed decision-making. Contextual information comparing medication risks to everyday risks or alternative treatment risks provides perspective supporting appropriate risk assessment. These approaches recognize that effective risk communication enables appropriate precaution and monitoring without creating fear-based medication avoidance.

Communication in High-Risk Situations

High-alert medication communication requires enhanced approaches reflecting elevated error consequences with these agents. Specialized protocols for anticoagulants, insulin, opioids, chemotherapy, and other high-alert medications include restricted terminology, mandatory read-back for critical parameters, documentation of dual verification, and explicit communication of monitoring requirements. Independent double-checks for high-alert medications involve structured communication between checking professionals to ensure true independence rather than confirmation bias, with specific role delineation and documentation requirements.

Emergency situation communication presents particular challenges when normal procedures face time pressure. Crisis communication systems establish abbreviated but sufficient medication communication elements for emergent situations, standardized terminology for critical medications, role-defined communication responsibilities, and closed-loop verification for critical information despite time constraints. Simulation training for emergency medication communication develops team capabilities under stress conditions while identifying system improvements that support reliable communication during actual emergencies.

Disclosure communication following medication errors requires thoughtful approaches balancing transparency, appropriate accountability, and sensitivity to both patient and provider emotional responses. Structured disclosure conversations include clear explanation of what happened in understandable language, explicit acknowledgment of resulting harm or potential harm, sincere apology for the error, explanation of corrective actions to prevent recurrence, and appropriate emotional support for both patients and involved healthcare professionals. Training in disclosure communication techniques prepares professionals for these difficult conversations, supporting honest disclosure while minimizing defensive responses that can damage therapeutic relationships and complicate appropriate follow-up care.

Cross-cultural medication communication addresses the influence of cultural perspectives on medication understanding, acceptance, and use. Culturally responsive approaches include ascertaining cultural beliefs regarding specific medication classes, identifying traditional treatments that might interact with prescribed medications, recognizing cultural factors affecting adherence, and adapting education approaches to cultural communication norms. Professional interpreter utilization for limited English proficiency patients, rather than reliance on family members or bilingual staff without interpreter training, ensures accurate medication information transfer while respecting confidentiality and technical complexity.

DOCUMENTATION

Documentation practices significantly influence medication safety through their impact on information transfer, decision support, and accountability throughout the medication use process. Comprehensive, accurate, and accessible documentation creates an essential foundation for safe medication management while supporting both individual patient care and system-level quality improvement.

Documentation Standards and Requirements

Legal and regulatory documentation requirements

establish minimum standards for medication-related documentation across healthcare settings. These requirements address essential elements including patient identification, medication details (name, dose, route, frequency), ordering provider information, administration timing, and clinician accountability through appropriate authentication. Regulatory systems including Conditions of Participation for Medicare/Medicaid, accreditation standards from organizations such as The Joint Commission, and state practice acts for individual professions create overlapping requirements necessitating comprehensive documentation practices.

Table 8.3: Documentation Requirements for Medication Safety Across the Medication Use Process

Process Stage	Essential Documentation Elements	Documentation Systems
Prescribing	Patient identifiers Allergies and adverse reactions Complete medication information (name, dose, route, frequency, duration) Indication for use Special instructions Weight/BSA for dose calculation Prescriber identification	Electronic prescribing systems Computerized provider order entry Electronic health records Standardized order sets Paper order forms (limited settings)
Medication Reconciliation	Complete pre-admission medication list Sources of medication information Continued, discontinued, and changed medications Rationale for changes	Dedicated reconciliation forms Electronic reconciliation tools Admission/discharge documentation

	Patient/caregiver involvement Reconciliation completion verification Responsible provider identification	Transfer documentation Medication histories Patient provided medication lists
Dispensing and Preparation	Verification of order appropriateness Pharmacist clinical checks Preparation details Compounding records Beyond-use dating Verification processes Final product inspection Special storage requirements	Pharmacy information systems Verification documentation Compounding worksheets Preparation logs Quality assurance documentation Electronic workflow systems Automated dispensing records
Administration	Pre-administration verification (right patient, medication, dose, route, time) Time of administration Administration site/route Patient response Patient education Reason for any deviations Administrator identification Independent verification for high-alert medications	Electronic medication administration record (eMAR) Barcode medication administration systems Paper medication administration records Specialty documentation (e.g., chemotherapy) Smart pump documentation Controlled substance records

Monitoring	Assessment of therapeutic response Adverse effect monitoring Laboratory test results Vital sign monitoring Patient-reported outcomes Follow-up plans Medication changes based on monitoring Monitoring frequency documentation	Progress notes Flow sheets Specialty monitoring forms Patient diaries/logs Telehealth monitoring records Remote monitoring systems Home health documentation
Adverse Events and Near Misses	Event description Medications involved Contributing factors Patient impact Immediate actions taken Notification documentation Follow-up plan Reporting compliance	Incident reporting systems Safety learning systems Risk management documentation Patient safety organization reports Root cause analysis documentation Regulatory reporting forms Disclosure documentation

Electronic documentation standardization initiatives address historical inconsistencies that complicated information retrieval and exchange. The Consolidated Clinical Document Architecture (C-CDA) establishes standard formats for medication-related documentation exchange between electronic systems, including structured medication lists with essential elements in standardized terminology. RxNorm provides standardized nomenclature for medication documentation, reducing confusion from varied naming conventions. Implementation of these standards supports both internal consistency within healthcare organizations and external information exchange across care settings.

Specific high-risk scenarios require enhanced documentation beyond standard practice. Controlled substance documentation includes perpetual inventory tracking, witnessed waste verification, chain of custody documentation for transfers, and reconciliation documentation at defined intervals. Chemotherapy documentation incorporates body surface area calculations, cumulative dose tracking, special handling verification, and verification signatures at multiple preparation steps. Investigational medication documentation adds protocol adherence verification, informed consent confirmation, and research-specific monitoring parameters beyond standard clinical documentation.

Documentation timing requirements address the patient safety implications of delayed or retrospective documentation. Contemporary standards emphasize contemporaneous documentation whenever possible, particularly for medication administration, vital patient assessment parameters, and critical decision points. When contemporaneous documentation proves impossible due to emergent patient care requirements, clear institutional policies should establish maximum acceptable time intervals between clinical activities and documentation, with requirements for explicit identification of delayed entries to maintain documentation integrity.

Electronic Health Record Documentation

Electronic health record (EHR) medication documentation offers significant safety advantages through structured data capture, automated cross-checking, integrated decision support, and enhanced information accessibility. Structured medication order entry eliminates illegibility issues, enables automated screening against allergies and interactions, and ensures inclusion of required elements through forced-function design. Administration documentation with barcode verification creates transaction records confirming the "five rights" at the point of care. Laboratory integration enables automated presentation of relevant physiological parameters alongside medication information, supporting both initial prescribing decisions and ongoing monitoring.

Template design significantly influences documentation quality and safety impact. Well-designed templates guide clinicians through appropriate assessment parameters for specific medications, incorporate relevant monitoring guidelines, and include decision support triggers for potential safety issues. Conversely, poorly designed templates can introduce new risks through excessive auto-population creating inaccurate documentation, clipboard functionality perpetuating outdated information, or excessive structured fields creating documentation burden that reduces attention to patient care. User-centered design principles with clinician involvement in template development optimize the balance between standardization benefits and documentation burden.

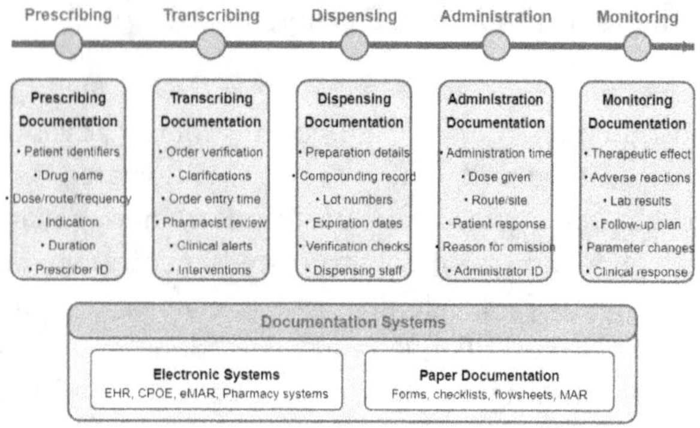

Figure 8.3 Documentation Requirements Across Medication Use

Alert documentation presents particular challenges in electronic systems, balancing the need for verification that safety information was considered against creating excessive documentation requirements that contribute to alert fatigue. Progressive approaches include tiered documentation requirements based on alert severity, structured response options capturing clinical rationale for alert overrides, and streamlined documentation workflows minimizing additional steps for appropriate responses to alerts. Review of override documentation patterns provides valuable information for alert optimization, identifying alerts requiring refinement based on override frequency and documented rationales.

Metadata capture represents an important but often overlooked documentation aspect in electronic systems, automatically recording contextual information including documentation timing, author, modifications, information sources, and system status. This metadata creates an auditable documentation trail supporting both individual case review and system-level pattern analysis. From a safety perspective, metadata enables identification of documentation patterns associated with increased error risk, such as retrospective documentation clusters suggesting memory-based rather than contemporaneous recording, or frequent record access without modification suggesting information retrieval challenges.

Documentation Across Care Transitions

Medication reconciliation documentation requires specific elements beyond simply recording current medications, creating a comprehensive foundation for safe continuation or appropriate modification of therapy during care transitions. Essential documentation components include verification sources for each medication, resolution documentation for identified discrepancies, explicit decisions regarding continuation or modification of previous regimens with clinical rationales, and accountability assignment through reconciliation authentication. Structured reconciliation documentation tools supporting these elements demonstrate 35-50% reduction in transition-related medication errors compared to unstructured approaches.

Discharge medication documentation addresses the particularly vulnerable transition from healthcare facility to home or post-acute care settings. Comprehensive discharge documentation includes clear differentiation between new, continued, and discontinued medications; specific administration instructions including timing, food considerations, and administration techniques; duration expectations for time-limited therapies; monitoring requirements with responsibility assignments; and follow-up plans for dose adjustments or efficacy evaluation. Integration of this documentation with patient-directed materials in appropriate literacy levels and languages supports safe medication management after discharge.

Referral documentation between providers requires specific medication-related elements to support care coordination and prevent fragmentation-related safety issues. Effective referral documentation includes current medication lists with initiation dates, recent medication changes with rationales, previous medication trials with reasons for discontinuation, monitoring results guiding current therapy, identified adverse effects with specific manifestations, and pending medication decisions requiring specialist input. This comprehensive medication context supports appropriate specialist recommendations considering the full medication experience rather than isolated current regimen information.

Transfer documentation between healthcare facilities presents unique requirements related to continuity of complex medication regimens. Beyond basic medication lists, essential transfer documentation includes next dose timing to prevent missed or duplicated doses during transition, administration details for complex medications (e.g., infusion rates, titration parameters), recent dose adjustments with clinical rationales, held medications with resumption criteria, and patient-specific response patterns to as-needed medications. Standardized transfer documentation tools incorporating these elements demonstrate significant reduction in transition-related medication errors, particularly for complex regimens requiring precise timing or specialized administration.

Documentation for Quality Improvement

Medication error documentation systems support both individual incident response and aggregate analysis for system improvement. Effective documentation includes objective event description without assignment of blame, patient impact assessment using standardized harm scales, contributing factor identification across system components, immediate actions taken to protect the patient, and planned improvement actions addressing identified system vulnerabilities. Standardized taxonomies such as the NCC MERP medication error classification system and the Institute for Safe Medication Practices (ISMP) error reporting categories enable consistent categorization supporting meaningful aggregate analysis.

Near-miss documentation captures valuable safety information from errors detected before reaching patients, providing opportunities for system improvement without patient harm. Effective near-miss documentation systems emphasize the positive nature of interception rather than negative focus on potential errors, employ streamlined documentation processes minimizing burden for reporting, and provide systematic feedback regarding resulting improvements to reinforce reporting value. Organizations with robust near-miss documentation typically identify 10-15 system vulnerabilities for each harm event, enabling proactive improvement rather than reactive response to actual patient harm.

Performance measurement documentation supports systematic assessment of medication safety across various dimensions. Structure measures document safety system components such as technology implementation, staffing patterns, and policy development. Process measures capture compliance with evidence-based safety practices such as independent double-checks, barcode scanning rates, and appropriate monitoring completion. Outcome measures document actual medication safety performance through metrics such as adverse drug event rates, harm per 1000 doses, and intercepted error rates. Comprehensive measurement documentation enables longitudinal tracking, comparative assessment, and focused improvement initiatives addressing identified opportunities.

Root cause analysis documentation provides structured assessment of serious medication events to identify fundamental system vulnerabilities rather than superficial causes. Effective documentation includes detailed event chronology without interpretation, multidisciplinary team composition and process, thorough investigation of contributing factors across system components, clear distinction between proximate and root causes, specific improvement recommendations with responsibility assignments and timelines, and follow-up assessment of implementation effectiveness. This structured documentation transforms individual error events into organizational learning opportunities with system-wide safety implications beyond the specific case

PROFESSIONAL RESPONSIBILITIES

Professional responsibilities in medication safety extend beyond technical competence to encompass ethical obligations, leadership functions, continuous development, and system improvement contributions. These responsibilities derive from professional codes of ethics, regulatory requirements, organizational expectations, and societal trust in healthcare professions as guardians of patient wellbeing.

Ethical and Legal Obligations

Duty of care establishes fundamental professional responsibility for medication safety regardless of specific role within the medication use process. This duty includes maintaining appropriate competence for assigned responsibilities, practicing within scope limitations, seeking assistance when encountering unfamiliar situations, and prioritizing patient safety above competing concerns including productivity pressures, interpersonal relationships, and personal convenience. Courts have consistently upheld that all healthcare professionals involved in medication management share non-delegable responsibility for basic safety verification, regardless of hierarchical position or primary role assignment.

Error disclosure responsibilities reflect both ethical obligations and evolving legal standards requiring transparency with patients following medication errors. Professional responsibilities include prompt notification of patients about clinically significant errors, honest explanation of occurrences without deflection or minimization, sincere apology for mistakes, and clear communication about corrective actions both for the individual patient and system improvement. These responsibilities apply regardless of personal discomfort, liability concerns, or potential reputational impact, reflecting the profession's fundamental commitment to patient autonomy and truth-telling.

Privacy and confidentiality obligations apply to medication safety activities including error reporting, root cause analysis, and quality improvement initiatives. These obligations include maintaining patient confidentiality in safety discussions while ensuring appropriate information sharing for clinical care, limiting access to error investigation information to individuals with legitimate need for improvement purposes, and protecting the privacy of involved professionals during safety investigations to encourage reporting while maintaining accountability. Balancing these privacy concerns with transparency needs requires thoughtful approaches recognizing both values rather than prioritizing either exclusively.

Documentation integrity represents both legal

requirement and ethical obligation, with particular importance in medication contexts where documentation serves as critical communication vehicle across providers and care transitions. Professional responsibilities include contemporaneous recording whenever possible, accurate representation of clinical events without embellishment or omission, appropriate correction of errors through organizationally defined procedures rather than alteration, and authentication limited to personally verified information. These practices maintain documentation as reliable foundation for clinical decision-making rather than retrospective justification or defensive construction.

Professional Development and Competency

Core competency maintenance requires ongoing education and assessment regarding evolving medication safety standards, emerging safety technologies, and updated medication information relevant to practice area. Professional responsibilities include regular self-assessment of knowledge gaps, proactive pursuit of educational opportunities addressing identified needs, and willing participation in organizational competency verification processes. These activities should extend beyond minimum continuing education requirements to encompass specific high-risk medications, new safety systems, and emerging best practices relevant to individual practice responsibilities.

Specialty certifications increasingly recognize medication safety expertise as distinct professional competency beyond general practice qualifications. Certifications including Certified Professional in Patient Safety (CPPS), Certified Specialist in Poison Information (CSPI), and medication safety certifications within pharmacy and nursing specialties establish recognized credentials for advanced safety expertise. Pursuit of these certifications demonstrates professional commitment to safety specialization while creating recognized qualification standards for leadership positions with substantial medication safety responsibilities.

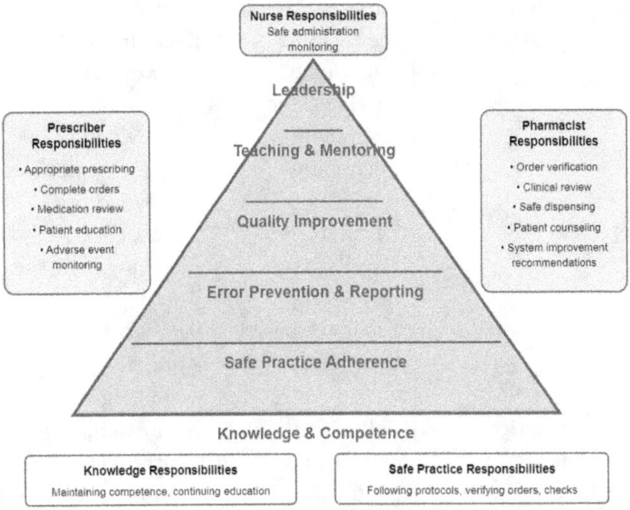

Figure 8.4: Healthcare Professional Responsibilities in Medication Safety

Simulation participation provides experiential learning opportunities for high-risk medication scenarios without patient risk, supporting competency development through deliberate practice. Professional responsibilities include active engagement in simulation exercises despite potential performance anxiety, honest reflection on identified improvement opportunities, and application of simulation learning to actual practice situations. Organizations increasingly incorporate medication safety simulation into both initial competency verification and ongoing assessment, recognizing the value of performance demonstration beyond knowledge testing alone.

Table 8.4: Professional Responsibilities in Medication Safety

Professional Responsibility	Components	Individual Accountability
Continuous Professional Development	Maintaining current medication knowledge Safety science competency Technology proficiency Regulatory requirement awareness Evidence-based practice updates	Meeting certification requirements Addressing personal knowledge gaps Applying new knowledge to practice Seeking feedback on performance Reflecting on practice challenges
Safe Practice Standards Adherence	Following established protocols Adhering to best practices Maintaining competencies Completing required documentation Following safety checks	Knowledge of current standards Refusing to bypass safety systems Seeking help when uncertain Maintaining focus during tasks Self-checking practices
Error and Near-Miss Reporting	Recognizing reportable events Completing accurate reports Participating in analysis Supporting improvement	Overcoming reporting barriers Providing thorough information Focusing on system improvement

Professional Responsibility	Components	Individual Accountability
	Maintaining transparency	Supporting peers after events Maintaining confidentiality
Interprofessional Collaboration	Respectful team communication Role clarity and respect Shared decision-making Cross-disciplinary learning Collaborative problem-solving	Active listening Speaking up with concerns Respecting others' expertise Sharing critical information Supporting team members
Patient Engagement and Education	Medication education provision Shared decision-making Patient preference incorporation Family/caregiver education Self-management support	Assessing patient understanding Adapting to literacy/language needs Documenting education provided Involving caregivers appropriately Respecting patient autonomy
Quality Improvement Participation	Data collection and analysis Improvement initiative involvement Testing and implementing changes Measuring	Identifying improvement opportunities Suggesting process changes Participating in improvement teams Adopting new

Professional Responsibility	Components	Individual Accountability
	outcomes Sharing learnings	practices Evaluating change effectiveness
Leadership and Mentorship	Setting safety expectations Modeling safe behaviors Providing feedback and coaching Supporting new staff Advocating for safety resources	Modeling safety practices Providing constructive feedback Supporting struggling colleagues Speaking up about safety concerns Advocating for system improvement
Ethical Practice	Disclosure of errors Maintaining confidentiality Addressing impaired colleagues Managing conflicts of interest Allocating resources ethically	Ethical decision-making Courage to address issues Accountability for actions Transparency in practice Patient advocacy

Peer review participation constitutes an essential professional responsibility for maintaining collective medication safety standards. Effective peer review requires willingness to both provide constructive feedback to colleagues and receive evaluation of personal practice without defensiveness. Professional responsibilities include objective assessment based on established standards rather than personal preference, specific recommendations for improvement rather than general criticism, and appropriate escalation of significant safety concerns while maintaining collegial relationships. These activities maintain professional self-regulation as alternative to external control while supporting continuous practice improvement.

Leadership and Advocacy

Safety culture leadership represents a professional responsibility extending beyond formal authority positions to encompass informal influence opportunities available to all healthcare professionals. This leadership includes consistently modeling safety-focused behaviors such as using available safety systems, speaking up about concerns, acknowledging personal mistakes, and prioritizing thoroughness over efficiency when safety requires. It further encompasses active reinforcement of colleagues' safety behaviors through recognition and appreciation, creating social norms supporting safe practices rather than workarounds or shortcuts despite production pressures.

Policy and procedure development participation ensures that medication safety guidelines reflect practical clinical realities while maintaining necessary safety standards. Professional responsibilities include volunteering for safety committee service when opportunities arise, providing constructive feedback during policy development and review processes, identifying potential unintended consequences of proposed procedures before implementation, and supporting evidence-based standardization even when requiring personal practice changes. This participation bridges the frequent gap between administrative policy perspective and frontline implementation challenges.

Patient advocacy regarding medication safety requires willingness to navigate potentially difficult conversations with both colleagues and patients. Professional responsibilities include appropriate escalation of safety concerns when initial communication proves insufficient, persistence in addressing identified risks despite resistance, providing patients with necessary information to participate in safety verification, and supporting patients expressing medication concerns rather than dismissing them as non-adherence. This advocacy recognizes that safety vulnerabilities often become apparent at the point of care, requiring immediate professional response rather than deferral to formal safety systems.

System improvement advocacy extends professional responsibility beyond individual practice to address organizational and policy factors affecting medication safety. This advocacy includes identifying system-level improvement opportunities from frontline experience, participating in formal improvement initiatives despite competing time demands, sharing safety insights across departmental and organizational boundaries, and engaging with professional organizations addressing medication safety at policy level. These activities recognize that sustainable safety improvement requires system-level change beyond individual vigilance, with professionals bearing responsibility for translating practice observations into improvement momentum.

Interdisciplinary Role Respect and Collaboration

Scope of practice understanding across professions supports appropriate collaboration while respecting disciplinary expertise boundaries. Professional responsibilities include recognizing both capabilities and limitations of each involved discipline, appropriate consultation when encountering issues beyond personal expertise, and receptivity to input from other professionals regardless of hierarchical position. This understanding allows efficient deployment of specialized expertise while maintaining appropriate accountability within collaborative systems, avoiding both territorialism that rejects valuable input and inappropriate deference that fails to exercise professional responsibility.

Psychological safety promotion enables essential communication across professional boundaries despite hierarchical traditions or interpersonal dynamics. Professional responsibilities include receptivity to questions or concerns regardless of source, non-punitive response to information sharing even when revealing potential errors, explicit invitation of input from all team members, and appropriate acknowledgment of valuable contributions regardless of professional background. These behaviors create environments where medication safety concerns receive attention based on clinical significance rather than originator status.

Conflict resolution skills enable productive management of inevitable professional disagreements regarding medication decisions without compromising safety or professional relationships. Professional responsibilities include focusing discussions on patient-centered outcomes rather than professional prerogatives, separating medication issues from interpersonal conflicts, employing appropriate escalation pathways when consensus proves elusive, and maintaining respectful dialogue regardless of outcome. These skills prevent medication disagreements from creating ongoing interprofessional tension that might inhibit future safety communication.

Interprofessional education participation supports development of collaborative capabilities while enhancing understanding of complementary professional contributions to medication safety. Professional responsibilities include active engagement in educational activities involving multiple professions, willingness to learn about other disciplines' perspectives and priorities, and openness to examining traditional practices that may impede optimal collaboration. These educational experiences establish foundations for effective teamwork in actual practice settings while developing mutual respect for distinct professional contributions to comprehensive medication safety systems.

Things to Remember

- ☑ Interprofessional collaboration enhances safety through team-based approaches leveraging complementary expertise, structured communication, and shared accountability transcending traditional boundaries.
- ☑ Effective communication techniques include SBAR framework for information transfer, closed-loop verification confirming understanding, standardized terminology preventing ambiguity, and non-punitive questioning.
- ☑ Documentation practices establish information continuity through comprehensive medication records, standardized formats, appropriate detail, and clear intervention documentation preserving rationale.
- ☑ Professional responsibilities include knowledge maintenance through continuous education, competency development, error disclosure supporting transparency, and advocacy addressing

system limitations.

- ☑ Each discipline contributes specialized capabilities while sharing fundamental responsibility for medication safety throughout the healthcare system.
- ☑ Successful collaboration requires mutual respect for different professional perspectives, clear role definition, and established communication pathways

Multiple Choice Questions

1. Which communication technique structures information transfer using situation, background, assessment, and recommendation components?
   a) Closed-loop verification
   b) SBAR framework
   c) Readback protocol
   d) Standardized handoff
2. Interprofessional collaboration enhances medication safety through:
   a) Eliminating the need for individual accountability
   b) Restricting information sharing to within specific disciplines
   c) Leveraging complementary expertise from different professions
   d) Centralizing all medication decisions with a single provider
3. Closed-loop communication in medication safety:
   a) Restricts information to a limited group of providers

b) Confirms that critical information has been received and understood

c) Eliminates the need for documentation

d) Focuses exclusively on electronic rather than verbal communication

4. Which of the following is NOT an essential component of effective medication documentation?

   a) Standardized formats ensuring consistent information capture

   b) Comprehensive medication histories including over-the-counter products

   c) Narrative explanations rather than structured data fields

   d) Clear intervention documentation preserving clinical rationale

5. Professional responsibilities in medication safety include:

   a) Restricting error disclosure to avoid confusing patients

   b) Maintaining knowledge through continuous education

   c) Delegating safety concerns to designated specialists

   d) Focusing exclusively on individual practice without system advocacy

6. Non-punitive questioning in healthcare communication:

   a) Avoids challenging potential errors in any circumstance

   b) Encourages clarification without intimidation

   c) Is only appropriate between professionals of

the same discipline
d) Eliminates accountability for serious mistakes

7. Team-based approaches to medication safety:
   a) Are most effective when responsibilities are ambiguous
   b) Require standardized roles without flexibility for adaptation
   c) Create shared accountability transcending traditional boundaries
   d) Work best when communication follows strict hierarchical patterns
8. Which of the following most accurately describes the concept of safety culture as it relates to healthcare professionals?
   a) A culture where errors are never tolerated regardless of circumstances
   b) An environment where professionals share values supporting open communication and continuous improvement
   c) A system where safety responsibilities are assigned exclusively to designated specialists
   d) A framework where regulatory compliance is the primary focus of all activities
9. Error disclosure responsibilities of healthcare professionals include:
   a) Limiting information to prevent patient concerns
   b) Communicating openly about errors while maintaining appropriate professionalism
   c) Delegating all disclosure to risk management departments

d) Discussing errors only when patients specifically inquire

10. Effective medication safety advocacy by healthcare professionals:

    a) Should focus exclusively on individual practice improvement

    b) Is best conducted through anonymous reporting only

    c) Addresses system limitations potentially compromising safety

    d) Should avoid challenging established practices regardless of safety concerns

Self-Assessment Questions

1. Analyze the evolving roles and responsibilities of different healthcare professionals in ensuring medication safety, highlighting both unique and shared accountabilities.
2. Evaluate models of interprofessional collaboration that optimize medication safety, including team structures, workflow integration, and outcome measures.
3. Critically analyze evidence-based communication techniques that improve medication safety across care transitions and between healthcare team members.
4. Discuss the documentation requirements across the medication use process and how they contribute to safety, continuity of care, and regulatory compliance.
5. Analyze the professional, ethical, and legal responsibilities of healthcare providers related to medication safety, including disclosure of errors and participation in improvement efforts.
6. Evaluate strategies for building effective interprofessional medication safety teams, including training approaches, role clarity, and leadership development.
7. Discuss how scope of practice variations across healthcare professions impact medication safety practices and collaborative care models.
8. Analyze the role of simulation and team-based training in developing effective

communication and collaboration skills for medication safety.

9. Evaluate the impact of workload, staffing, and workplace environment on healthcare professionals' ability to maintain medication safety practices.
10. Discuss the role of healthcare professionals as advocates for system-level medication safety improvements and policy changes.

Bibliography

1. Kohn LT, Corrigan JM, Donaldson MS, editors. To Err Is Human: Building a Safer Health System. Washington, DC: National Academies Press; 2000.
2. Manias E, Kinney S, Cranswick N, Williams A. Medication errors in hospitalised children. J Paediatr Child Health. 2014;50(1):71-7.
3. Lingard L, Espin S, Whyte S, Regehr G, Baker GR, Reznick R, et al. Communication failures in the operating room: an observational classification of recurrent types and effects. Qual Saf Health Care. 2004;13(5):330-4.
4. Leonard M, Graham S, Bonacum D. The human factor: the critical importance of effective teamwork and communication in providing safe care. Qual Saf Health Care. 2004;13 Suppl 1:i85-90.
5. Haig KM, Sutton S, Whittington J. SBAR: a shared mental model for improving communication between clinicians. Jt Comm J Qual Patient Saf. 2006;32(3):167-75.
6. Manojlovich M, DeCicco B. Healthy work environments, nurse-physician communication, and patients' outcomes. Am J Crit Care. 2007;16(6):536-43.
7. Resar RK, Rozich JD, Classen D. Methodology and rationale for the measurement of harm with trigger tools. Qual Saf Health Care. 2003;12 Suppl 2:ii39-45.
8. Gandhi TK, Sittig DF, Franklin M, Sussman AJ, Fairchild DG, Bates DW. Communication breakdown in the outpatient referral process. J Gen Intern Med. 2000;15(9):626-31.
9. Leape LL, Cullen DJ, Clapp MD, Burdick E, Demonaco HJ, Erickson JI, et al. Pharmacist participation on physician rounds and adverse drug events in the intensive care unit. JAMA. 1999;282(3):267-70.
10. Kaboli PJ, Hoth AB, McClimon BJ, Schnipper JL. Clinical pharmacists and inpatient medical care: a systematic review. Arch Intern Med. 2006;166(9):955-64.

CHAPTER 9

QUALITY MANAGEMENT SYSTEMS

Abstract

Quality management systems establish integrated approaches to medication safety through structured systems supporting consistent excellence rather than isolated improvement initiatives. Quality assurance programs implement proactive standards compliance through policy development, routine assessment against established criteria, variance management addressing identified gaps, and documentation systems maintaining performance evidence. Performance improvement methodologies employ systematic approaches including PDSA cycles testing interventions before full implementation, Lean processes eliminating unnecessary complexity, Six Sigma reducing variation through statistical analysis, and change management addressing human factors affecting adoption. Audit procedures provide objective evaluation through systematic sampling of medication processes, structured assessment using standardized tools, comparative analysis against internal and external benchmarks, and formal reporting creating accountability for identified issues. Continuous monitoring establishes ongoing awareness through automated data collection from electronic systems, real-time dashboard display highlighting critical metrics, trend analysis detecting emerging patterns, and threshold-based alerting identifying significant deviations requiring intervention.

Keywords: *Integrated quality systems, Performance improvement, Standards compliance, Continuous monitoring, Systematic auditing*

Learning Objectives

After completion of the chapter, the learners should be able to:

- Remember the core components of quality assurance programs in medication safety.
- Understand how different performance improvement methodologies support medication safety enhancement.
- Apply appropriate audit procedures to evaluate medication safety processes.
- Analyze continuous monitoring data to identify medication safety improvement opportunities.
- Evaluate the effectiveness of quality management approaches in various healthcare contexts.
- Create an integrated quality framework addressing both compliance verification and continuous advancement.

QUALITY ASSURANCE PROGRAMS

Quality assurance programs provide systematic approaches to ensuring medication safety through standardized processes, preventive measures, and ongoing verification activities. These programs establish organizational infrastructure supporting consistent application of safety principles throughout medication management systems.

Program Structure and Governance

Formal quality assurance structures create

organizational systems supporting systematic medication safety oversight. Effective structures typically include a medication safety committee with multidisciplinary representation, direct reporting relationships to organizational leadership, defined authority for safety intervention, and clear delineation of roles and responsibilities across departments. Governance documents including committee charters, reporting structures, and authority statements establish legitimacy and accountability for medication safety oversight while preventing fragmentation of responsibility across multiple organizational entities.

Leadership engagement represents an essential component of effective medication safety programs, with senior leader involvement extending beyond nominal support to active participation in safety governance. This engagement includes regular review of medication safety metrics in leadership meetings, executive participation in serious event analyses, resource allocation decisions supporting safety initiatives, and visible prioritization of safety over competing organizational priorities when necessary. Organizations demonstrating exemplary medication safety performance typically feature governance models where senior leadership maintains direct connection with medication safety activities rather than complete delegation to quality departments.

Policy systems establish clear expectations, standardized processes, and accountability mechanisms supporting medication safety throughout organizational operations. Comprehensive policy structures address high-risk processes (e.g., high-alert medications, chemotherapy, anticoagulation), vulnerable populations (e.g., pediatrics, geriatrics, obstetrics), and system components (e.g., storage, preparation, dispensing, administration). Effective policies balance sufficient specificity to ensure standardization of critical safety elements with appropriate flexibility for clinical judgment in patient-specific situations. Regular policy review cycles ensure continued relevance as practices, technologies, and evidence evolve.

Table 9.1: Components of Medication Safety Quality Assurance Programs

Component	Purpose	Elements
Structure Assessment	Evaluate resources, systems, and infrastructure	Staffing levels Policies/procedures Technology Physical environment
Process Evaluation	Assess medication-use workflow adherence	Workflow compliance Protocol adherence Documentation Safety checks
Outcome Measurement	Determine medication safety results	Adverse drug events Medication errors Near-miss events Patient harm
Risk Assessment	Identify potential failure points	Proactive analysis Safety prioritization Vulnerability assessment

Quality assurance plans establish systematic approaches to safety verification through defined monitoring activities, assessment methodologies, and response mechanisms for identified issues. Comprehensive plans include proactive process assessments before safety events occur, reactive investigation procedures for adverse events, targeted monitoring of high-risk areas, and systematic surveillance of key safety indicators. These plans explicitly connect monitoring findings with improvement mechanisms, creating closed-loop systems where quality assurance activities directly inform quality improvement rather than existing as separate organizational functions.

Risk Assessment and Prevention

Failure mode and effects analysis (FMEA) provides structured methodology for proactive identification and mitigation of potential failure points before actual safety events occur. Applied to medication processes, FMEA involves multidisciplinary teams systematically analyzing each process step to identify potential failure modes, their potential effects, probability of occurrence, likelihood of detection, and severity of consequences if undetected. These assessments generate risk priority numbers guiding resource allocation for preventive interventions. Proactive application to high-risk processes before implementation, such as new technology introduction or novel therapy protocols, demonstrates particular preventive value compared to reactive application after problems emerge.

Safety design reviews establish formal evaluation processes for new medications, technologies, or procedures before implementation, ensuring proactive safety consideration rather than reactive mitigation of problems after introduction. Structured review methodology typically includes standardized assessment criteria, multidisciplinary evaluation teams, documentation of identified risks with mitigation strategies, and formal approval processes incorporating safety evaluation results. Organizations with mature quality assurance programs require safety design review completion before implementation approval for any significant medication system change, recognizing that prevention through design proves more effective than post-implementation correction.

Standardization initiatives reduce unnecessary variation in medication processes, eliminating error opportunities created by process inconsistency while creating predictable work environments supporting reliable performance. High-impact standardization targets include medication concentrations (particularly for high-alert medications), dosing protocols for weight-based medications, administration timing systems, and infusion practices. Effective standardization balances safety benefits of consistency against necessary clinical flexibility, standardizing aspects with clear safety implications while preserving appropriate variation for patient-specific clinical judgment.

High-reliability principles adapted from industries with exemplary safety records despite high-risk operations (aviation, nuclear power) provide systems for medication safety program development beyond traditional healthcare approaches. These principles include preoccupation with failure (actively seeking weak signals suggesting potential problems), reluctance to simplify interpretations (maintaining awareness of system complexity), sensitivity to operations (attention to frontline realities rather than work-as-imagined), commitment to resilience (developing capacity to detect and recover from inevitable problems), and deference to expertise (valuing knowledge over hierarchy in safety decisions). Implementation transforms traditional quality assurance from compliance orientation to dynamic safety management addressing evolving risks.

Verification and Assessment Mechanisms

Independent verification protocols establish systematic double-checking processes for high-risk medications and vulnerable points in medication processes, creating redundant safety layers without excessive resource utilization. Effective protocols clearly define verification elements requiring confirmation, specify appropriate independence between initial preparation and verification steps, establish documentation requirements capturing both verification completion and discrepancy resolution, and identify specific high-risk situations requiring additional verification beyond standard processes. Research indicates that verification effectiveness depends on true independence between performance and checking rather than superficial verification that may perpetuate initial errors.

Self-assessment programs enable organizations to systematically evaluate medication safety systems against established best practice standards, identifying improvement opportunities without external inspection requirements. Tools such as the Institute for Safe Medication Practices (ISMP) Medication Safety Self Assessment and the Agency for Healthcare Research and Quality (AHRQ) Patient Safety Culture Survey provide structured methodologies for comprehensive internal review. Effective implementation includes multidisciplinary teams conducting honest assessment without defensive justification of current practices, gap analysis comparing current performance against optimal standards, prioritization of identified opportunities based on risk assessment, and development of specific action plans addressing high-priority gaps.

External quality certification provides independent validation of medication safety program effectiveness through evaluation against established standards by qualified external reviewers. Programs including The Joint Commission Medication Management Certification,

URAC Specialty Pharmacy Accreditation, and Foundation for the Accreditation of Cellular Therapy (FACT) certification for organizations handling cellular therapies establish minimum safety standards while recognizing exemplary performance through commendation or center of excellence designation. While requiring significant preparation resources, external certification creates accountability pressure supporting comprehensive program implementation while providing external validation useful for stakeholder confidence in safety systems.

Technology verification systems provide automated surveillance of medication processes, creating continuous monitoring capabilities beyond human observation limitations. Bar code verification systems confirm medication selection accuracy during preparation and administration. Automated dispensing cabinet reports identify discrepancies requiring investigation. Smart infusion pump databases capture programming errors intercepted by safety limits. Electronic health record reports identify orders bypassing clinical decision support or overriding critical alerts. These technological verification systems complement human checking processes with particular value for high-volume processes where human verification of every instance proves impractical.

Documentation and Reporting Systems

Adverse event reporting systems establish formal mechanisms for capturing information about medication-related harm, creating essential data sources for both individual event response and aggregate pattern analysis. Comprehensive systems include voluntary reporting pathways for near-miss events and minor harm, mandatory reporting requirements for serious events, anonymous reporting options for safety concerns that might not otherwise be reported, and specific classification taxonomies supporting meaningful aggregation and analysis. Effective systems emphasize learning purpose rather than punitive orientation, demonstrate responsive investigation of reported concerns, and provide feedback to reporters about resulting improvements to reinforce reporting value.

Standardized documentation systems create consistent information capture supporting both individual patient safety and system-level quality assurance. Medication administration records with standardized formats ensure complete documentation of essential elements including administration timing, dose verification, patient response, and reasons for any omissions. Electronic health record templates for medication reconciliation capture information sources, discrepancy resolution, and verification completion rather than merely listing current medications. Infusion therapy documentation includes preparation verification, administration parameters, site assessment, and patient response monitoring. This standardized documentation supports both clinical care and quality review processes.

Medication use evaluation (MUE) programs systematically assess medication use patterns against established standards, identifying both appropriate practice patterns and deviation requiring intervention. Traditional drug use evaluation focused primarily on cost and utilization patterns has evolved to comprehensive medication use evaluation addressing appropriateness, safety, effectiveness, and efficiency. Sophisticated programs employ both retrospective review of completed therapy and concurrent review during active treatment, enabling real-time intervention for identified issues rather than solely retrospective learning. Integration with electronic health records increasingly supports automated data collection for high-volume medications while preserving focused manual review for complex or high-risk therapies.

Safety alert management systems provide structured oversight of clinical decision support warnings, addressing the critical balance between sufficient alerting for genuine safety issues and excessive alerting leading to override fatigue and ignored warnings. Effective management includes alert inventory maintenance documenting all active alerts with their triggering criteria and expected responses, regular review of override patterns identifying alerts with low specificity or poor clinical value, systematic processes for alert modification based on performance data, and governance structures ensuring appropriate clinical input before alert implementation or modification. These systems recognize that unmanaged alerting often defeats safety purposes through excessive overrides of even important warnings.

PERFORMANCE IMPROVEMENT

Performance improvement methodologies transform quality assurance findings into actionable changes that enhance medication safety outcomes. These approaches establish systematic processes for identifying improvement opportunities, designing effective interventions, implementing sustainable changes, and evaluating impact on patient safety and clinical outcomes.

Improvement Systems and Methodologies

The Model for Improvement provides a fundamental framework combining three essential questions (What are we trying to accomplish? How will we know that a change is an improvement? What changes can we make that will result in improvement?) with Plan-Do-Study-Act (PDSA) cycles for testing and implementing changes. Applied to medication safety, this approach establishes clear safety targets, defines specific measurement strategies confirming improvement rather than simply change, identifies potential interventions based on causal understanding, and tests changes in progressive cycles before broader implementation. The structured yet flexible nature of this framework allows application across diverse medication safety challenges from simple process refinements to complex system redesigns.

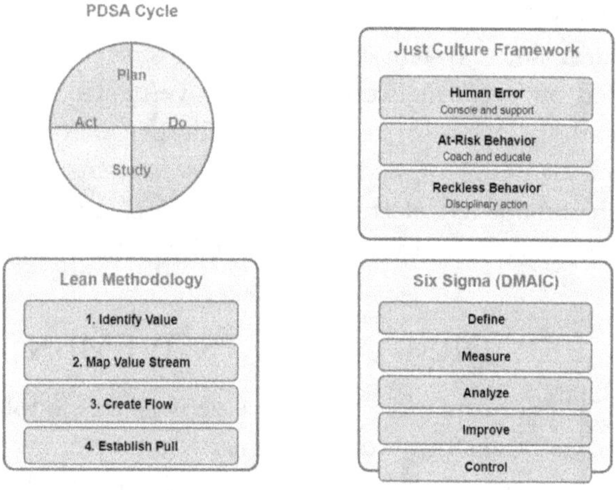

Figure 9.1: Performance Improvement Methods for Medication Safety

Lean methodology focuses on eliminating waste and improving flow within medication processes, addressing safety implications of unnecessary complexity, redundancy, and workflow interruptions. Applied to medication management, Lean approaches identify value-added steps from the patient perspective, map current processes to distinguish value from waste, establish continuous workflow with minimal handoffs and interruptions, create standardized work for consistent performance, and develop visual management systems supporting adherence to designed processes. Safety benefits include reduced error opportunities from process simplification, decreased cognitive burden allowing greater attention to critical safety tasks, and enhanced detection of abnormal conditions through standard work expectations.

Six Sigma methodology employs statistical analysis to reduce variation in critical processes, addressing the safety implications of inconsistent performance in medication management. The DMAIC framework (Define, Measure, Analyze, Improve, Control) provides structured approach to improvement through precise problem definition, collection of baseline performance data, analysis identifying root causes of variation, implementation of targeted interventions addressing identified causes, and establishment of control mechanisms maintaining improvements. Applied to medication safety, Six Sigma proves particularly valuable for high-volume, standardized processes where reduction in performance variation directly enhances safety outcomes. factors engineering applies scientific knowledge about human capabilities and limitations to medication system design, addressing the reality that human performance varies under different conditions and system designs significantly influence error likelihood. This approach helps understand interactions between people, technologies, procedures, and environments to identify design elements contributing to error potential. Medication safety applications include workstation design reducing interruptions during critical tasks, user interface improvements for technologies like computerized provider order entry and automated dispensing cabinets, procedure redesign aligning with natural cognitive workflows, and environmental modifications supporting safety-critical activities such as dedicated medication preparation areas with appropriate lighting and minimal distraction.

Improvement Selection and Prioritization

Data-driven prioritization establishes objective selection processes for improvement initiatives, focusing limited organizational resources on opportunities with greatest safety impact. Effective approaches combine quantitative data including event frequency, harm severity, and detection probability with qualitative information such as near-miss patterns, staff safety concerns, and external safety alerts. Formal prioritization matrices incorporating these multiple dimensions support transparent decision-making while balancing reactive response to identified problems with proactive addressing of potential risks before harm occurs. This structured prioritization prevents scattered improvement efforts addressing high-visibility but lower-impact issues at the expense of less apparent but more consequential safety risks.

Return on investment analysis applied to medication safety initiatives supports appropriate resource allocation by quantifying both implementation costs and expected benefits in comparable terms. Comprehensive analysis includes direct implementation costs (technology, staffing, training), indirect costs (workflow disruption, productivity impact), tangible benefits (reduced adverse events, shortened lengths of stay, decreased liability costs), and intangible benefits (enhanced reputation, improved staff satisfaction, reduced psychological impact of harmful errors). While acknowledging the ethical imperative of safety improvement regardless of financial return, this analysis supports strategic allocation of limited resources among competing safety priorities while building business cases for necessary investments.

Table 9.2: Performance Improvement Models for Medication Safety

Model	Concept	Strengths
Plan-Do-Study-Act (PDSA)	Iterative testing of changes on small scale	Simple structure Rapid cycles Data-driven
Lean	Eliminate waste and maximize value	Workflow focus Staff engagement Visual management
Six Sigma	Reduce variation and defects	Statistical rigor Root cause focus Structured approach
Just Culture	Balance accountability and system improvement	Reduces blame Encourages reporting Consistent response

External standard alignment ensures that improvement initiatives address recognized safety priorities beyond internal organizational perspectives. Sources including National Patient Safety Goals, professional society guidelines, regulatory requirements, and published safety alerts from organizations such as the Institute for Safe Medication Practices provide external validation of improvement priorities. Systematic processes for reviewing these external sources, comparing against current organizational performance, and incorporating applicable recommendations into improvement planning ensure comprehensive safety approaches rather than solely internal focus that might miss emerging safety concerns recognized in broader healthcare contexts.

Stakeholder engagement in prioritization enhances both selection quality and implementation success through incorporation of diverse perspectives on improvement needs and feasibility. Effective engagement includes frontline staff input regarding practical improvement opportunities observed during daily work, patient and family perspectives on experienced safety concerns, and leadership viewpoints on strategic alignment and resource implications. Structured engagement mechanisms such as safety committees with broad representation, regular frontline safety rounds, patient safety advisory councils, and systematic review of safety suggestions create continuous input channels beyond formal improvement planning cycles.

Implementation Strategies

Implementation science systems recognize that improvement effectiveness depends on both intervention design and implementation approach, addressing the frequent gap between evidence-based safety practices and actual clinical implementation. The Consolidated Framework for Implementation Research (CFIR) determines intervention characteristics, implementation context (inner and outer setting), individual characteristics, and process elements affecting implementation success. Applied to medication safety improvements, these systems guide strategy selection addressing specific implementation barriers rather than assuming that well-designed interventions automatically achieve successful adoption in complex healthcare environments.

Multi-faceted intervention design addresses the reality that significant safety improvements typically require changes across multiple system components rather than single-element interventions. Comprehensive approaches combine technological elements (e.g., computerized order entry, barcode verification), procedural components (e.g., standardized processes, verification requirements), educational interventions (e.g., training, simulation exercises), and cultural elements (e.g., leadership engagement, psychological safety). Research demonstrates that such multi-component interventions typically achieve greater and more sustainable improvements than single-element approaches, reflecting the complex, sociotechnical nature of medication safety challenges.

Pilot implementation with iterative refinement enables controlled testing and improvement of interventions before organization-wide deployment, reducing risks associated with large-scale changes while enhancing design quality through practical experience. Effective pilot implementations include careful site selection representing diverse practice environments, explicit evaluation criteria established before implementation, structured feedback mechanisms capturing both quantitative metrics and qualitative experience, and systematic refinement processes addressing identified limitations before broader deployment. This approach recognizes that even carefully designed interventions typically require adaptation based on implementation experience, particularly for complex interventions affecting multiple workflow components.

Sustainability planning addresses the frequent challenge of improvement degradation over time, establishing mechanisms for maintaining gains beyond initial implementation period. Essential elements include transition from special project status to standard operations, integration of new processes into routine performance expectations and evaluation systems, ongoing monitoring systems detecting performance drift, refresher training maintaining competency as staff changes occur, and designated accountability for sustained performance. Organizations with mature improvement programs incorporate sustainability planning from project initiation rather than addressing sustainability as afterthought following initial implementation, recognizing that design choices significantly influence long-term sustainability potential.

Evaluation and Spread

Comprehensive evaluation designs provide objective assessment of improvement effectiveness, supporting both intervention refinement and decisions regarding potential spread to additional settings. Robust evaluation includes baseline measurement establishing pre-intervention performance, process measures confirming implementation as designed, outcome measures assessing actual safety impact, balancing measures identifying potential unintended consequences, and sustainability measures tracking performance maintenance over time. Beyond simple pre-post comparison, sophisticated evaluation employs time-series analysis distinguishing actual improvement from random variation, statistical process control methodology identifying significant performance changes, and when feasible, controlled comparison with non-intervention areas to account for external factors affecting outcomes.

Return on investment evaluation provides post-implementation assessment of actual financial and operational impacts compared to projected benefits, supporting both accountability for resource utilization and planning for future initiatives. Effective approaches compare actual implementation costs against projections, quantify realized safety benefits through metrics such as adverse event reduction or decreased monitoring requirements, and calculate actual return timeframes compared to projections. Beyond financial analysis, comprehensive evaluation includes operational impacts such as workflow efficiency changes, staff satisfaction effects, and patient experience implications, recognizing that medication safety improvements frequently generate benefits beyond direct adverse event reduction.

Systematic spread methodologies support effective dissemination of successful interventions beyond initial implementation sites, addressing the frequent challenge of localized improvements that fail to achieve organization-wide impact. The Institute for Healthcare Improvement's Framework for Spread identifies key elements including leadership commitment to spread goals, identification of target populations and sites, development of initial spread strategy, measurement and feedback systems supporting spread, and knowledge management systems sharing implementation experience. Applied to medication safety improvements, effective spread requires both technical content transfer (intervention design details) and implementation knowledge transfer (experience regarding implementation challenges and solutions), recognizing that contextual adaptation rather than rigid replication typically proves necessary for successful spread.

Knowledge dissemination beyond organizational boundaries represents professional responsibility for sharing successful medication safety improvements with broader healthcare community. Dissemination mechanisms include publication in peer-reviewed journals, presentation at professional conferences, participation in collaborative improvement networks, and submission to patient safety organizations supporting information sharing across institutions. Effective dissemination includes transparent reporting of both successes and challenges, detailed methodology supporting replication, and contextual factors influencing outcomes rather than simply reporting positive results. This knowledge sharing accelerates safety improvement across healthcare systems while reducing duplication of effort in developing similar interventions across multiple organizations.

AUDIT PROCEDURES

Audit procedures provide systematic assessment of medication practices against established standards, identifying compliance gaps, potential safety vulnerabilities, and improvement opportunities through structured evaluation methodologies. These processes create essential feedback mechanisms verifying that safety systems function as designed while detecting emerging issues before patient harm occurs.

Audit Program Design

Comprehensive audit programs establish systematic oversight across the entire medication use process rather than focusing on isolated components, recognizing the interconnected nature of medication safety systems. Well-designed programs include coverage of prescribing appropriateness, order verification processes, preparation accuracy, administration procedures, monitoring practices, and documentation completeness. Audit scope typically employs risk-based approaches concentrating resources on high-alert medications, vulnerable populations, and complex processes with elevated error potential. This approach balances resource limitations against the need for system-wide safety assurance.

Table 9.3: Medication Safety Audit Types and Methodology

Audit Type	Methods	Frequency
Medication Process Audit	Direct observation Documentation review Workflow analysis	Monthly or quarterly
High-Alert Medication Audit	Tracer methodology Documentation review Storage inspection	Monthly
Regulatory Compliance Audit	Policy review Documentation audit Environment inspection	Annually or biannually
Event Response Audit	Chart review Interview Root cause analysis	After significant events

Sampling methodology significantly influences audit validity and resource efficiency, requiring careful design based on specific audit objectives and medication process characteristics. Random sampling provides representative assessment of overall system performance while targeted sampling focuses on known high-risk areas or suspected problem points. Sample size determination balances statistical validity against resource constraints, with approaches ranging from continuous monitoring of highest-risk processes to periodic sampling of lower-risk activities. Stratified sampling ensures appropriate representation of different patient populations, medication classes, or care settings within heterogeneous organizations, preventing misleading conclusions from unrepresentative samples.

Audit tools development establishes standardized evaluation instruments supporting consistent assessment across different auditors, time periods, and organization locations. Effective tools clearly define audit parameters with objective criteria distinguishing compliant from non-compliant performance, include data collection mechanisms capturing both quantitative metrics and qualitative observations, and incorporate severity classification for identified issues supporting appropriate prioritization. Tool development should include validation processes ensuring inter-rater reliability, content validity covering critical safety elements, and usability testing confirming practical field application. Regular tool refinement based on implementation experience and evolving safety standards maintains relevance while ensuring detection of emerging safety concerns.

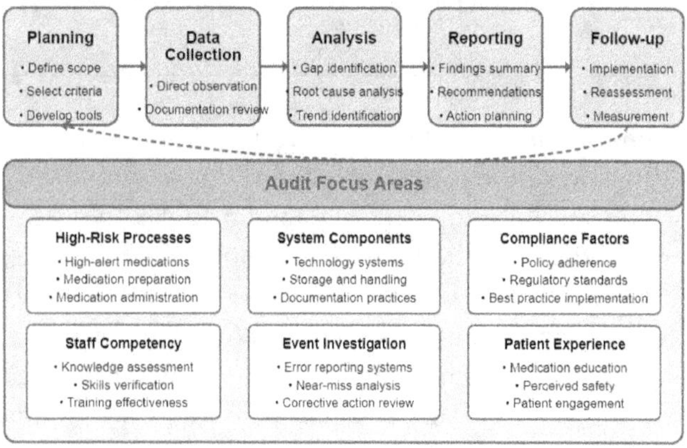

Figure 9.2 Medication Safety Audit Process

Auditor training and qualification establish consistent interpretation and application of audit standards, addressing the significant influence of auditor knowledge and perspective on findings validity. Comprehensive training includes both technical content regarding medication safety standards and methodological training in objective assessment, evidence collection, and finding classification. Qualification processes typically include supervised practice audits, inter-rater reliability assessment comparing findings against experienced auditors, and continuing education requirements maintaining knowledge currency as practices evolve. Organizations with mature audit programs typically establish formal auditor certification processes ensuring qualified personnel for this safety-critical function.

Audit Types and Methodologies

Process audits estimate adherence to established procedures throughout the medication use system, verifying that safety practices occur consistently as designed. These audits typically employ direct observation methodologies capturing actual practice patterns rather than relying solely on documentation review that may not reflect actual performance. Focus areas include compliance with independent double-check procedures for high-alert medications, adherence to sterile compounding standards, proper execution of medication reconciliation processes, and consistent performance of barcode verification procedures. Process audits prove particularly valuable for detecting drift from established procedures before resulting in actual safety events, enabling proactive intervention rather than reactive response to adverse outcomes.

Documentation audits assess completeness, accuracy, and timeliness of medication-related documentation, addressing both legal requirements and communication quality supporting safe care transitions. These reviews typically determines medication orders for required elements (dose, route, frequency, duration), administration records for administration time documentation and appropriate response monitoring, medication reconciliation forms for verification completion and discrepancy resolution, and controlled substance records for inventory accuracy and chain of custody documentation. Beyond simple presence or absence of required elements, sophisticated documentation audits assess quality dimensions including clarity, internal consistency, and alignment with observed practice patterns.

Outcome audits determine actual medication safety performance through retrospective review of adverse events, near-misses, and clinical outcomes associated with medication therapy. These reviews employ methodologies including chart audit using trigger tool approaches to identify possible adverse drug events, structured analysis of reported medication incidents, and focused review of high-risk scenarios such as naloxone administration potentially indicating opioid adverse events. Outcome audits provide ultimate validation of safety system effectiveness beyond process compliance, identifying situations where processes function as designed yet safety events still occur due to unrecognized vulnerabilities or interaction effects across system components.

Technology utilization audits assess appropriate use of medication safety technologies, addressing the frequent gap between technology availability and effective utilization supporting safety improvement. Focus areas include computerized provider order entry utilization rates and override patterns, clinical decision support alert response appropriateness, barcode medication administration scanning compliance, automated dispensing cabinet override frequency and documentation, and smart infusion pump drug library utilization with override analysis. These audits recognize that technology safety benefits depend on proper utilization rather than mere presence, identifying both individual practice variations requiring correction and system design issues contributing to workarounds or inconsistent use.

Conducting Effective Audits

Transparent communication regarding audit purpose and methodology establishes appropriate expectations while promoting acceptance of findings as improvement opportunities rather than punitive evaluation. Effective communication includes advance notice of audit timing and focus areas when appropriate, clear explanation of evaluation standards and methodology, explicit statement of improvement-oriented purpose, and appropriate confidentiality protection for involved individuals. This transparency differentiates safety-focused audits from punitive investigations, supporting honest process examination rather than defensive showcase performances during announced audit periods that may not reflect typical practice patterns.

Just culture principles applied to audit processes support identification of system vulnerabilities without inappropriate individual blame, creating psychological safety essential for honest practice evaluation. These principles distinguish human error requiring support and system redesign from at-risk behavior requiring coaching and risk awareness development, and from reckless behavior requiring appropriate accountability measures. Application to audit processes includes focusing findings on system improvement opportunities rather than individual identification, appropriate confidentiality for findings discussions, and proportional response to identified issues based on behavior category rather than outcome severity alone. This balanced approach supports thorough examination of actual practices rather than idealized versions that conceal potential safety vulnerabilities.

Real-time feedback during audit processes provides immediate learning opportunities while demonstrating improvement focus rather than simply documenting deficiencies for later reports. Immediate feedback proves particularly valuable for process issues presenting actual patient safety risk requiring prompt intervention, educational opportunities where correct practice can be immediately reinforced, and positive practices deserving recognition and spread to other areas. This real-time communication complements rather than replaces formal reporting, adding immediate safety intervention and learning value beyond documentation of findings.

Interdisciplinary perspectives incorporated throughout audit processes enhance both finding validity and improvement potential through diverse professional viewpoints on medication safety requirements. Effective approaches include multidisciplinary audit teams combining pharmacy, nursing, physician, and quality perspectives; review of draft findings by representatives from involved disciplines before finalization; and collaborative development of improvement recommendations drawing on varied professional expertise regarding feasible solutions. This interdisciplinary approach recognizes that medication safety spans professional boundaries, with comprehensive assessment requiring multiple viewpoints rather than single-profession perspective that may miss important safety elements outside discipline-specific focus.

Audit Findings Management

Systematic categorization of audit findings supports appropriate prioritization and response based on safety implications rather than treating all identified issues with equal urgency. Effective categorization systems typically include critical findings requiring immediate intervention to prevent imminent patient harm, major findings indicating significant system vulnerabilities with serious potential consequences, minor findings representing improvement opportunities without immediate safety threat, and positive findings identifying exemplary practices deserving recognition and potential spread. This structured classification supports resource allocation proportional to safety impact while ensuring appropriate attention to highest-risk issues.

Corrective action planning transforms audit findings from identified problems to implemented solutions through structured improvement processes. Comprehensive planning includes root cause analysis identifying fundamental contributing factors rather than superficial issues, corrective action development addressing identified causes rather than symptoms, responsibility assignment with clear accountability for implementation, realistic timeframes balancing urgency against implementation complexity, and verification mechanisms confirming effective implementation. Organizations with mature quality systems typically establish standardized corrective action planning templates ensuring consistent response quality while maintaining documentation trails supporting regulatory compliance.

Trending and aggregate analysis extract broader improvement opportunities from individual audit findings by identifying patterns across multiple audits, locations, or time periods. Sophisticated analysis show the common factors in recurrent findings, correlation between audit results and actual safety events, performance differences across organizational units suggesting local practice variations, and longitudinal trends indicating improving or deteriorating performance over time. This aggregate perspective identifies system-level improvement opportunities that might remain obscured when viewing individual findings in isolation, supporting strategic improvement initiatives addressing fundamental system characteristics rather than isolated process corrections.

Closing the loop through verification of corrective action effectiveness represents an essential audit program component frequently overlooked in less mature quality systems. Effective verification includes follow-up audits specifically examining previously identified issues, review of performance data indicating actual practice change rather than simply confirmed policy updates, and when appropriate, direct observation verifying sustained implementation in actual practice environments. This verification transforming the traditional linear audit process into a continuous improvement cycle ensuring that identified issues receive effective resolution rather than merely documented response without practical implementation or sustained change.

CONTINUOUS MONITORING

Continuous monitoring systems provide ongoing surveillance of medication safety performance, enabling real-time detection of emerging issues, prompt intervention before harm occurs, and longitudinal tracking of safety trends. These systems complement periodic audit processes with persistent vigilance, creating comprehensive safety oversight spanning both proactive surveillance and responsive intervention.

Monitoring Program Development

Metric selection establishes the foundation for effective monitoring by identifying key indicators providing meaningful insight into medication safety performance. Comprehensive selection includes structure measures assessing safety system components (e.g., technology implementation percentages, staffing ratios), process measures capturing compliance with safety practices (e.g., barcode scanning rates, independent verification completion), outcome measures documenting actual safety events (e.g., adverse drug events, severity-categorized medication errors), and balancing measures detecting unintended consequences (e.g., turnaround time impacts, staff satisfaction effects). Selection should emphasize high-sensitivity metrics capable of detecting safety changes before serious events occur, supporting proactive intervention rather than reactive response to harm.

Data collection infrastructure development establishes reliable information pipelines supporting consistent monitoring without excessive manual effort that proves unsustainable over time. Effective infrastructure includes automated extraction from electronic systems where feasible (e.g., barcode scanning compliance from medication administration records, override rates from automated dispensing cabinets), standardized manual collection processes where automation proves impractical, validation procedures ensuring data accuracy before analysis, and appropriate security protections for sensitive safety information.

Table 9.4: Continuous Monitoring for Medication Safety

Metric Category	Example Metrics	Data Sources
Safety Events	Medication errors per 1,000 doses Harm events by category Near-miss reporting rate	Incident reports, chart review, trigger tools
Process Compliance	Barcode scanning compliance Double-check documentation Medication reconciliation completion	Electronic systems, chart audits, observations
Patient Outcomes	ADEs per 100 admissions Medication-related readmissions Antidote use rates	Chart review, administrative data, pharmacy data
Culture Assessment	Safety culture survey scores Reporting rates by unit Safety suggestion implementation	Surveys, reporting systems, improvement tracking

Organizations with mature monitoring programs typically implement medication safety dashboards integrating multiple data sources into unified displays supporting both executive overview and detailed analysis capabilities.

Statistical methodology selection ensures appropriate interpretation of monitoring data, differentiating genuine safety signals from random variation that might prompt unnecessary intervention or mask important trends. Basic approaches including run charts and statistical process control charts establish visualization methods distinguishing special cause variation requiring investigation from common cause variation representing expected system performance fluctuation. More sophisticated methodology including risk-adjusted analysis accounts for patient population differences affecting expected event rates, time-series analysis detects subtle trends over extended periods, and multivariate techniques identify complex relationships between system factors and safety outcomes. These analytical approaches prevent both overreaction to normal variation and underresponse to genuine safety signals requiring intervention.

Alert threshold establishment creates trigger mechanisms converting continuous monitoring into actionable information through predefined intervention points. Effective threshold development balances sensitivity (detecting genuine safety issues) against specificity (avoiding false alarms), typically through multi-level alert structures including watch-level thresholds indicating potential emerging issues warranting increased attention, warning-level thresholds triggering initial investigation activities, and critical-level thresholds requiring immediate intervention to prevent harm. Threshold determination methods range from statistical approaches based on historical performance variation to consensus-based clinical judgment regarding acceptable performance levels, with sophisticated systems often combining both approaches.

Technology-Enabled Monitoring

Computerized surveillance systems employ rule-based algorithms to continuously scan clinical data for patterns suggesting potential medication safety issues, creating automated detection capabilities extending human monitoring capacity. These systems analyze multiple data elements including laboratory values, medication orders, vital signs, and antidote administration to identify situations requiring investigation. Common surveillance targets include warfarin patients with supratherapeutic INR values, patients receiving nephrotoxic medications with rising creatinine levels, QTc interval prolongation in patients receiving multiple QT-prolonging medications, and naloxone administration potentially indicating opioid overdose. Advanced systems incorporate machine learning algorithms identifying subtle patterns human observers might miss, creating increasingly sensitive detection capabilities as systems analyze larger datasets.

Smart infusion pump analytics leverage data generated during medication administration to identify both individual safety events and system improvement opportunities. Basic analytics include frequency of soft limit overrides by medication and care unit, hard limit override attempt patterns potentially indicating dosing confusion or knowledge gaps, and programming error correction rates demonstrating pump safety feature effectiveness. Advanced analytics estimates relationships between override patterns and specific patient populations, temporal patterns suggesting workflow or shift-related factors, and correlation between pump alerts and subsequent adverse events. These analyses support both immediate intervention for critical safety issues and system-level improvement addressing underlying causes of detected patterns.

Electronic health record safety reports provide standardized monitoring of medication-related electronic system functions, addressing the safety implications of system design, configuration, and usage patterns. Focus areas include alert override frequencies by alert type and provider, order set utilization patterns, medication reconciliation completion rates and discrepancy resolution documentation, and medication-related order entry errors corrected during the ordering process. Sophisticated monitoring includes periodic structured review of patient charts specifically examining electronic health record safety issues such as wrong patient selection, incorrect medication selection from similar options, and copy-forward errors perpetuating outdated information. These monitoring activities recognize electronic systems as both safety solution and potential risk source requiring specific oversight.

Automated dispensing cabinet reports provide continuous monitoring of medication storage and retrieval activities, supporting both diversion surveillance and general medication safety oversight. Standard reports include discrepancy tracking identifying mismatches between recorded and actual medication counts, override utilization patterns highlighting medications frequently removed without pharmacist review, expired medication tracking preventing administration of outdated products, and restocking accuracy verification ensuring correct medication loading. Advanced monitoring employs user-specific utilization pattern analysis identifying unusual transaction patterns potentially indicating diversion activity. Integration with electronic health record data enables verification that removed medications correspond to actual ordered therapy, creating closed-loop monitoring capabilities spanning prescribing through administration.

Human Surveillance Systems

Safety rounds conducted by leadership, quality personnel, and subject matter experts provide direct observational monitoring of medication practices in actual clinical environments, detecting issues electronic monitoring might miss while demonstrating organizational commitment to safety oversight. Effective rounds employ structured observation tools focusing attention on high-risk processes, create non-threatening environments encouraging honest discussion of safety concerns, include direct interaction with frontline staff regarding experienced safety challenges, and establish clear follow-up mechanisms ensuring identified issues receive appropriate response. Advanced approaches include targeted rounds addressing specific high-risk medications or processes, simulation scenarios during rounds testing response to safety challenges, and involvement of patients and families providing unique perspective on experienced medication practices.

Real-time safety coaches provide human monitoring and immediate intervention addressing medication practices before errors occur, functioning as safety resources rather than punitive oversight. These roles typically combine medication expertise with exceptional interpersonal skills, enabling supportive coaching rather than critical evaluation. Activities include providing immediate feedback on observed practice variations, offering assistance during complex medication situations, serving as readily available resource for medication questions, and identifying system issues contributing to observed workarounds. Organizations implementing safety coach programs typically report both immediate error prevention through direct intervention and lasting practice improvement through educational influence, creating sustainable safety culture enhancement beyond transient surveillance benefit.

Patient and family reporting systems engage care recipients as active safety monitors with unique perspective on medication administration, experienced effects, and potential errors. Structured approaches include bedside reporting mechanisms allowing immediate concerns expression, post-discharge safety surveys capturing safety issues becoming apparent after hospitalization, specific medication side effect screening during follow-up contacts, and dedicated communication channels for medication concerns requiring investigation. Advanced programs provide specific education regarding appropriate safety vigilance without creating excessive anxiety, guidance on constructive concern expression, and explicit encouragement viewing safety partnership as valuable contribution rather than challenging healthcare providers. These patient-centered monitoring approaches detect issues traditional surveillance might miss while empowering patients as active participants in their medication safety.

Staff reporting systems establish structured mechanisms for frontline personnel to identify safety concerns observed during routine work, creating distributed surveillance networks extending formal monitoring programs. Beyond traditional incident reporting systems capturing actual errors and adverse events, comprehensive approaches include near-miss reporting capturing potential errors intercepted before reaching patients, safety suggestion systems for identified improvement opportunities, and anonymous reporting channels for concerns staff might hesitate to express through official pathways. Successful systems demonstrate non-punitive response to reported concerns, provide feedback to reporters about resulting actions, and celebrate positive identification enabling prevention rather than merely documenting errors after occurrence. This frontline engagement creates monitoring capability extending far beyond dedicated quality personnel resources.

Response Systems and Performance Feedback

Escalation protocols establish standardized response pathways converting monitoring findings into appropriate action based on safety urgency and organizational responsibility. Comprehensive protocols define criteria for various response levels, specify required notifications for different finding categories, establish expected response timeframes proportional to safety risk, and clearly delineate authority for intervention decisions. Organizations with mature response systems typically implement tiered approaches including unit-level response for routine findings, medication safety specialist involvement for more significant issues, and executive engagement for critical safety concerns potentially requiring major system changes or resource allocation. These structured pathways prevent both delayed response to serious safety signals and excessive escalation overwhelming leadership with routine matters appropriately handled at operational levels.

Performance feedback systems close communication loops by providing monitoring results to relevant stakeholders throughout the organization, creating awareness supporting both accountability and improvement. Effective feedback includes executive-level safety dashboards providing organizational perspective supporting strategic decisions, department-level reports enabling operational management oversight and resource allocation, unit-level displays supporting local improvement initiatives, and individual-level feedback supporting professional development and practice improvement. Feedback design should consider audience information needs, appropriate comparison benchmarks providing context, and presentation formats maximizing comprehension while minimizing misinterpretation risk. Regular feedback cadences establish expected review cycles ensuring monitoring information receives appropriate attention rather than collection without utilization.

Continuous learning systems transform monitoring findings from retrospective performance documentation to forward-looking improvement drivers through structured analysis and knowledge dissemination. Beyond basic trending identifying performance changes, sophisticated learning approaches include correlation analysis examining relationships between safety outcomes and potential contributing factors, comparative assessment identifying practice differences between high and low-performing units, and root cause analysis of significant events providing deeper understanding of system vulnerabilities. Knowledge dissemination mechanisms include safety alerts for urgent findings requiring immediate awareness, regular safety newsletters sharing trends and improvement opportunities, focused education addressing identified knowledge gaps, and modification of training programs based on recurring issues identified through monitoring.

Integration with improvement methodologies creates closed-loop systems connecting monitoring findings directly to systematic enhancement of medication safety processes. Effective integration includes regular review of monitoring data by improvement teams identifying intervention opportunities, prioritization mechanisms selecting highest-impact issues for improvement focus, structured improvement projects addressing identified vulnerabilities, and follow-up monitoring verifying sustained performance improvement after intervention. Organizations with mature quality systems typically establish formal connections between monitoring and improvement functions through shared committee structures, integrated data systems, and coordinated planning processes ensuring aligned effort rather than parallel activities with limited connection. This integration transforms monitoring from passive observation to active catalyst for continuous medication safety enhancement.

Things to Remember

- ☑ Quality assurance programs implement proactive standards compliance through policy development, routine assessment, variance management, and documentation systems maintaining performance evidence.
- ☑ Performance improvement methodologies include PDSA cycles testing interventions, Lean processes eliminating unnecessary complexity, Six Sigma reducing variation, and change management addressing human factors.
- ☑ Audit procedures provide objective evaluation through systematic process sampling, structured assessment, comparative analysis against benchmarks, and formal reporting creating accountability.
- ☑ Continuous monitoring utilizes automated data collection, real-time dashboard display, trend

analysis detecting patterns, and threshold-based alerting identifying significant deviations requiring intervention.

- ☑ Effective quality systems balance reactive response to identified issues with proactive improvement addressing potential vulnerabilities before events occur.
- ☑ Integration between quality initiatives prevents fragmented approaches addressing similar issues through different methodologies or organizational structures

Multiple Choice Questions

1. Quality assurance programs implement proactive standards compliance through:
   a) Retrospective review of adverse events only
   b) Policy development, routine assessment, and variance management
   c) Focus exclusively on regulatory requirements without clinical considerations
   d) Individual provider monitoring without system evaluation
2. Which performance improvement methodology employs rapid cycle testing of interventions before full implementation?
   a) Six Sigma
   b) Lean processes
   c) Plan-Do-Study-Act (PDSA) cycles
   d) Root cause analysis
3. Audit procedures provide objective evaluation through:
   a) Annual regulatory inspections only
   b) Self-reporting by department managers

c) Systematic sampling and structured assessment using standardized tools
d) Focus exclusively on documentation practices

4. Continuous monitoring in medication safety includes:
   a) Manual data collection on selected high-risk medications only
   b) Annual comprehensive reviews of all processes
   c) Automated data collection with dashboard display and trend analysis
   d) Focus exclusively on adverse events without process metrics
5. Which of the following is NOT typically a component of performance improvement using Lean methodology?
   a) Identifying and eliminating non-value-adding steps
   b) Focusing on process flow and efficiency
   c) Requiring complex statistical analysis for all improvements
   d) Reducing unnecessary complexity in workflows
6. Threshold-based alerting in continuous monitoring:
   a) Replaces the need for human review of quality data
   b) Identifies significant deviations requiring intervention
   c) Should be applied equally to all metrics regardless of clinical significance

d) Functions best with frequently changing threshold values

7. Balanced quality metrics in medication safety should include:

   a) Focus primarily on outcome measures with limited process assessment

   b) Emphasis on regulatory compliance with minimal clinical measures

   c) Equal consideration of outcome, process, and structural measures

   d) Priority on financial measures above clinical indicators

8. The relationship between quality assurance and performance improvement is best described as:

   a) Completely separate functions requiring different organizational structures

   b) Sequential activities with quality assurance always preceding improvement

   c) Complementary approaches with quality assurance ensuring standard compliance while performance improvement drives advancement

   d) Identical processes with different terminology

9. Change management in quality improvement addresses:

   a) Exclusively technological aspects of implementation

   b) Human factors affecting adoption of new processes

   c) Only formal leadership approval processes

d) Documentation requirements for regulatory compliance

10. Comparative analysis against benchmarks in audit procedures:

    a) Is only valuable when comparing similar departments within one organization

    b) Should focus exclusively on national averages without consideration of facility context

    c) Provides context for performance evaluation and goal-setting

    d) Is primarily useful for marketing purposes rather than improvement

Self-Assessment Questions

1. Analyze the key components of comprehensive medication safety quality assurance programs and how they integrate with broader healthcare quality systems.
2. Evaluate different performance improvement methodologies (e.g., PDSA, Lean, Six Sigma) and their application to medication safety improvement initiatives.
3. Critically analyze the design, implementation, and effectiveness of medication safety audit procedures, including selection of indicators and interpretation of findings.
4. Discuss the role of continuous monitoring systems in medication safety, including real-time surveillance, trigger tools, and automated detection systems.
5. Evaluate how quality management principles can be applied to create a culture of continuous improvement in medication safety.
6. Analyze the relationship between quality management systems for medication safety and regulatory compliance requirements, discussing strategies to align these priorities.
7. Discuss the governance structures necessary to support effective medication safety quality management systems, including committee functions and leadership roles.
8. Evaluate how medication safety data should be collected, analyzed, and presented to drive improvement at different organizational levels.

9. Analyze how quality management approaches to medication safety differ across healthcare settings (hospitals, ambulatory care, long-term care) and strategies for each context.
10. Discuss the economic considerations in implementing and maintaining robust quality management systems for medication safety, including return on investment and resource allocation.

Bibliography

1. Deming WE. Out of the Crisis. Cambridge, MA: MIT Press; 2000.
2. Juran JM, Godfrey AB. Juran's Quality Handbook. 5th ed. New York: McGraw-Hill; 1999.
3. Berwick DM. Continuous improvement as an ideal in health care. N Engl J Med. 1989;320(1):53-6.
4. Batalden PB, Davidoff F. What is "quality improvement" and how can it transform healthcare? Qual Saf Health Care. 2007;16(1):2-3.
5. Institute of Medicine. Crossing the Quality Chasm: A New Health System for the 21st Century. Washington, DC: National Academies Press; 2001.
6. Langley GJ, Moen RD, Nolan KM, Nolan TW, Norman CL, Provost LP. The Improvement Guide: A Practical Approach to Enhancing Organizational Performance. 2nd ed. San Francisco: Jossey-Bass; 2009.
7. Taylor MJ, McNicholas C, Nicolay C, Darzi A, Bell D, Reed JE. Systematic review of the application of the plan-do-study-act method to improve quality in healthcare. BMJ Qual Saf. 2014;23(4):290-8.
8. Pronovost PJ, Berenholtz SM, Goeschel CA, Needham DM, Sexton JB, Thompson DA, et al. Creating high reliability in health care organizations. Health Serv Res. 2006;41(4 Pt 2):1599-617.
9. Dixon-Woods M, McNicol S, Martin G. Ten challenges in improving quality in healthcare: lessons from the Health Foundation's programme evaluations and relevant literature. BMJ Qual Saf. 2012;21(10):876-84.
10. Berwick DM, Nolan TW, Whittington J. The triple aim: care, health, and cost. Health Aff (Millwood). 2008;27(3):759-69.

CHAPTER 10

MEDICATION RECONCILIATION

Abstract

Medication reconciliation establishes information accuracy throughout care transitions through systematic comparison between information sources, verification of discovered discrepancies, and documentation ensuring appropriate continuity. Admission reconciliation creates accurate foundation for inpatient therapy through various information collection from multiple sources, systematic verification against objective records, specialized approaches for vulnerable populations, and clear documentation connecting home medications to admission orders. Transfer reconciliation addresses internal transition vulnerabilities through active medication profile review during unit or service changes, order set transitions preventing unintended duplications, structured handoff communication beyond written orders, and technology support enabling information synchronization between care areas. Discharge reconciliation provides critical verification before transitioning to self-management through pre-discharge medication review, explicit documentation comparing pre-admission and discharge regimens, integrated prescription generation preventing transcription errors, and effective patient education ensuring understanding beyond simple information provision. Best practices include dedicated personnel resources, interdisciplinary accountability systems, standardized documentation formats supporting consistent information capture, risk stratification directing enhanced efforts toward highest-risk situations, and technology integration embedding reconciliation.

Keywords: *Care transitions, Information accuracy, Discrepancy resolution, Discharge planning, Medication continuity*

Learning Objectives

After completion of the chapter, the learners should be able to:

- Remember the key components of effective medication reconciliation at different transition points.
- Understand how reconciliation processes prevent medication errors during care transitions.
- Apply appropriate reconciliation techniques for admission, transfer, and discharge situations.
- Analyze the challenges in obtaining accurate medication information across different care settings.
- Evaluate the effectiveness of various reconciliation strategies in preventing transition-related errors.
- Create a comprehensive reconciliation program incorporating best practices for different care transitions.

ADMISSION RECONCILIATION

Medication reconciliation at admission establishes an accurate foundation for inpatient medication management, addressing the substantial safety risks associated with incomplete or inaccurate medication information during care transitions. This critical process bridges the information gap between pre-admission medication regimens and inpatient therapy decisions, preventing unintended discontinuations, duplications, and dosing errors that could compromise patient safety.

Information Collection Strategies

Comprehensive information sources form the foundation of effective admission reconciliation, with reliance on single sources frequently resulting in significant omissions. Patient interviews remain essential despite technological advances, providing information about actual consumption patterns that may differ from prescribed regimens, self-administered medications not captured in prescription records, and recently discontinued therapies still influencing physiological status. Structured interview techniques employing open-ended questions, specific prompts for commonly omitted medications (e.g., over-the-counter products, inhalers, injectable medications), and focused queries about recent changes enhance information quality beyond basic medication lists.

Caregiver interviews provide essential supplementary information when patients have cognitive limitations, complex regimens, or medication management assistance at home. Effective approaches identify the specific caregiver most knowledgeable about medication management, distinguish between multiple caregivers' responsibilities if applicable, and gather specific information about administration patterns and observed effects rather than merely duplicating patient-provided lists. These interviews reveal practical details about medication administration timing, adherence challenges, and symptom patterns that patients themselves may not fully articulate, particularly for individuals with memory impairments or limited health literacy.

Community pharmacy records offer valuable verification sources, particularly for prescription medications filled consistently at the same pharmacy. Most valuable when obtained directly from pharmacy systems rather than patient-provided medication lists, these records provide accurate medication names, prescribed doses, dispensing dates, and refill patterns offering insight into potential adherence issues. The increasing prevalence of pharmacy benefit managers consolidating prescription records across multiple pharmacies enhances this information source, though significant limitations remain regarding over-the-counter medications, prescriptions filled outside insurance networks, and actual consumption patterns versus dispensed supplies.

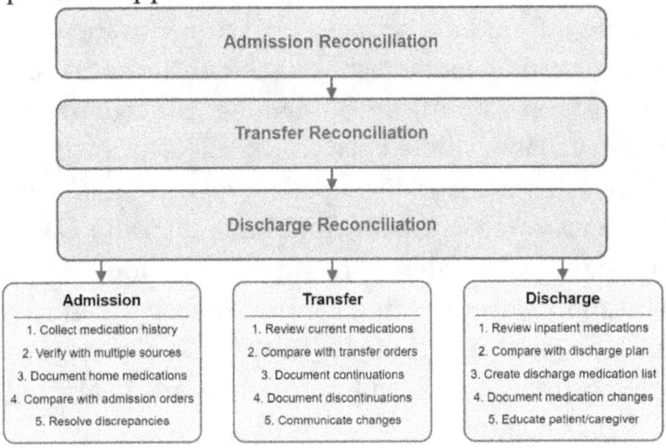

Figure 10.1 Medication Reconciliation Process

Electronic health record reconciliation tools increasingly facilitate information aggregation from multiple sources, including organizational prescription records, previous hospitalization medication lists, and in some cases, health information exchange data incorporating records from other healthcare organizations. Advanced systems employ medication fill data from insurance claims, outpatient visit documentation, and medication administration records from previous hospitalizations to construct comprehensive medication history profiles. While offering significant efficiency improvements over manual information gathering, these systems require careful supplementation through direct patient assessment to capture medications not documented in accessible electronic records.

Verification and Resolution Processes

Verification against multiple sources establishes confidence in medication list accuracy before making inpatient therapy decisions. Progressive verification levels include confirmation of medication presence across multiple information sources, dosage verification across sources, brand/generic reconciliation ensuring consistent identification regardless of naming conventions, and when available, adherence verification through refill pattern assessment or direct patient report. Organizations with mature reconciliation programs typically establish minimum verification requirements for different medication categories, with more extensive verification for high-risk medications such as anticoagulants, immunosuppressants, and anticonvulsants compared to lower-risk therapies.

Discrepancy resolution processes systematically address inevitable differences between information sources, preventing perpetuation of inaccurate information into inpatient medication orders. Effective resolution begins with explicit documentation of identified discrepancies rather than undocumented selection between conflicting sources, proceeds through structured investigation determining the most reliable information for each specific medication, and concludes with clear documentation of resolution decisions with supporting rationale. Common discrepancies requiring resolution include dosage differences between patient report and prescription records, timing variations between prescribed and actual administration schedules, and presence of medications in one information source but not others.

Specialized population approaches address unique reconciliation challenges presented by specific patient groups. Pediatric reconciliation requires particular attention to weight-based dosing information, liquid medication concentrations, and administration techniques used at home. Geriatric reconciliation often involves multiple prescribers, extensive over-the-counter supplement use, and medication management systems requiring documentation to maintain continuity. Transplant recipient reconciliation demands precise immunosuppressant regimen verification including exact timing, brand specifications, and recent monitoring results. These specialized approaches recognize that standard reconciliation processes may require significant modification to address population-specific complexities.

Home medication retrieval programs enhance reconciliation accuracy by examining actual medication containers rather than relying on recall or secondary documentation. These programs employ various mechanisms including encouraging patients or families to bring medications from home, offering medication bag programs at pre-admission testing, and in some cases, conducting home visits for highest-risk patients to directly observe medication supplies and administration systems. Beyond simple verification of medication names and doses, physical medication review enables identification of multiple containers of the same medication suggesting duplicate therapy, expired medications potentially causing therapeutic failure, and administration devices requiring specific technique instruction during hospitalization.

Documentation and Communication

Standardized documentation formats establish consistent information capture supporting both individual patient care and system-level reconciliation quality assessment. Essential documentation elements include medication name using both brand and generic designations when applicable, complete dosage information including strength and quantity, route of administration with specific device information when relevant, administration frequency including specific timing patterns, last dose timing establishing continuity for scheduled medications, and therapy duration for limited-term treatments. Advanced documentation incorporates additional elements including indication linking medications to specific conditions, prescriber information identifying responsible providers for follow-up questions, pharmacy information for verification purposes, and patient-reported adherence patterns.

Linkage between home medications and admission orders creates explicit documentation of reconciliation decisions rather than simply capturing historical information without clear connection to current therapy. This linkage establishes clear disposition for each pre-admission medication with standard categories including continued with same regimen, continued with modified regimen (with specific change documentation), temporarily held (with resumption criteria), or discontinued (with discontinuation rationale). Complete linkage ensures that each pre-admission medication receives explicit consideration rather than unintentional omission through oversight, creating both patient safety protection and clear communication to all providers regarding therapeutic intent.

Interaction with admission medication orders establishes reconciliation as integral to the ordering process rather than parallel documentation without direct clinical impact. Effective integration includes reconciliation completion before non-urgent medication ordering, automated presentation of home medication information during order entry, capability to convert home medications directly to inpatient orders with appropriate modifications for institutional formulary and protocols, and clinical decision support comparing ordered medications against reconciled home medications to identify potential unintended discrepancies. This integration transforms reconciliation from documentation exercise to clinical decision support tool directly influencing prescribing decisions.

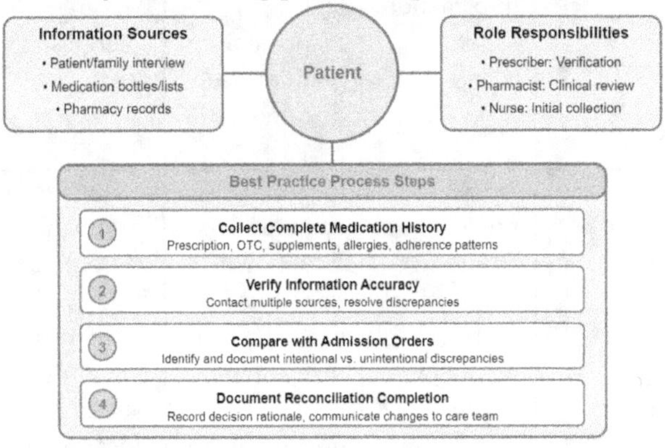

Figure 10.2 Admission Reconcillation

Communication to the care team extends reconciliation value beyond documentation to active clinical information sharing influencing ongoing care decisions. Effective communication includes making reconciled medication information prominently available in electronic health records, explicitly identifying unresolved discrepancies requiring further investigation,

Table 10.1: Elements of Admission Medication Reconciliation

Element	Description	Best Practices	Common Pitfalls
Information Sources	Data used to create medication history	Minimum of 2-3 sources Patient/family interview Outpatient pharmacy records	Relying on single source Missing OTC medications Outdated information
Medication History Collection	Process of gathering complete medication information	Structured interview approach Dedicated staff responsibility Standardized documentation	Rushed collection Incomplete questioning Missing allergies
Comparison with New Orders	Aligning pre-admission medications with inpatient orders	Side-by-side comparison Intentional decisions for each medication Clear documentation of changes	Assuming automatic discontinuation Incomplete comparison Missing dose/route changes
Discrepancy Resolution	Process for addressing unintentional differences	Defined resolution process Clear responsibility assignment Prescriber communication protocol	Delayed resolution Unclear responsibility Undocumented resolutions

highlighting recent medication changes preceding admission that might influence clinical presentation, and communicating specific verification limitations when incomplete information necessitates ongoing medication history refinement during hospitalization.

Organizations with mature reconciliation programs typically include structured communication about reconciliation findings during handoff procedures, ensuring that key medication information influences clinical assessment beyond simple documentation completion.

10.1.4 Timing and Accountability

Timing requirements establish expectations for reconciliation completion, balancing the urgency of medication information needs against practical constraints during the admission process. Most organizations establish tiered timing expectations with shortened timeframes for high-risk situations, matching clinical urgency with reconciliation priority. Common approaches include requiring immediate reconciliation for critically ill patients or those receiving high-alert medications, establishing short timeframes (typically 4-8 hours) for general admission reconciliation, and allowing extended timeframes only for specific situations such as overnight admissions with stable patients not receiving time-critical medications. These timing standards recognize that delayed reconciliation creates vulnerability periods where clinical decisions proceed without complete medication information.

Responsibility assignment establishes clear accountability for reconciliation completion while recognizing the multidisciplinary nature of comprehensive medication history development. Organizations employ various assignment models including physician responsibility with pharmacy verification, pharmacy responsibility with physician review, or shared responsibility with specific elements assigned to different disciplines based on expertise. Regardless of specific model, effective approaches include explicit responsibility designation rather than assumed accountability, clear delineation between information collection and clinical decision responsibilities, and appropriate authentication requirements documenting each involved provider's specific contribution to the reconciliation process.

Compliance monitoring creates accountability mechanisms ensuring reconciliation completion according to organizational standards rather than variable attention based on individual provider patterns or workload pressures. Monitoring typically includes reconciliation completion rates by time interval, quality assessment through sample review of completed reconciliations, discrepancy identification rates suggesting thoroughness of information gathering, and appropriate authentication verification ensuring accountability documentation. Advanced monitoring estimates correlation between reconciliation quality and medication safety outcomes including unintended discrepancies and potential adverse events, providing direct evidence of reconciliation impact rather than simple process measurement.

Escalation protocols establish standardized response pathways when reconciliation cannot be completed within required timeframes due to information limitations, patient condition constraints, or resource availability. Effective protocols include interim reconciliation expectations documenting available information while acknowledging limitations, required notifications to responsible providers and pharmacy personnel when complete reconciliation proves impossible, specific documentation requirements regarding reconciliation status and remaining information needs, and handoff procedures ensuring ongoing reconciliation responsibility across shift changes or service transfers. These protocols prevent situations where reconciliation simply remains incomplete without appropriate awareness and response.

TRANSFER RECONCILIATION

Transfer reconciliation addresses the substantial medication safety risks occurring during internal transitions between care settings, service teams, or levels of care within healthcare facilities. These internal handoffs involve significant information transfer challenges, provider knowledge discontinuities, and technological interface issues that collectively create vulnerability for medication errors without appropriate reconciliation processes.

Transfer Types and Specific Challenges

Critical care transitions between intensive care and general care units present distinct reconciliation challenges related to therapy intensity changes, monitoring capability differences, and specialization transitions. Medications requiring reconciliation attention during these transitions include vasoactive agents requiring tapering rather than abrupt discontinuation, continuous infusions needing conversion to intermittent administration, temporary therapies appropriate only during critical illness, and medications held during hemodynamic instability requiring reassessment for resumption. Effective reconciliation addresses both therapy continuation decisions and administration method transitions, ensuring appropriate adaptation to the receiving unit's capabilities while maintaining therapeutic intent.

Table 10.2: Transfer Reconciliation Considerations by Care Setting

Transfer Type	Critical Considerations	Safety Techniques
Unit-to-Unit	Continuation of specialized therapies Monitoring requirement transfer IV to oral conversions	Structured handoff tools Pharmacist review Standardized transfer orders
ICU to Floor	Medication dose adjustments Monitoring frequency changes Discontinued critical care meds	ICU step-down protocols Medication therapy review Monitoring parameter transfer
Perioperative	Resumption of home medications Anticoagulation management Pain management transition	Perioperative medication protocols Standardized order sets Documented resumption plan
Facility Transfer	Formulary differences Coverage/payment changes Medication availability	Advance communication Formulary reconciliation Complete transfer documentation

Perioperative transitions encompass multiple transfer points surrounding surgical intervention, each presenting unique reconciliation requirements. Pre-operative reconciliation focuses on identifying medications requiring continuation through surgery (e.g., antiseizure medications, cardiac therapies), medications needing temporary discontinuation with specific timing (e.g., anticoagulants, certain antihypertensives), and chronic medications requiring postoperative resumption planning. Intraoperative to post-anesthesia care reconciliation addresses anesthetic agents with lingering effects, intraoperative medication responses influencing recovery monitoring, and analgesic transitions between surgical and recovery phases. Post-anesthesia to inpatient reconciliation manages pain control regimen transfers, prophylactic therapy initiation, and resumption timing for temporarily discontinued chronic medications.

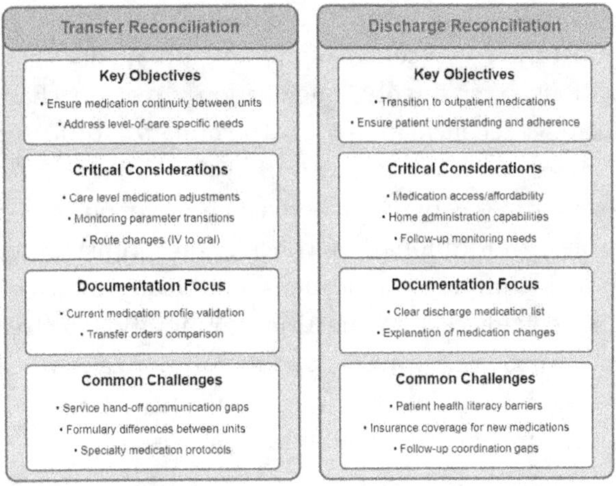

Figure 10.3 Comparison between Transfer and Discharge Reconcilation

Service transfers between clinical specialties or provider teams within the same physical location create reconciliation challenges related to different treatment perspectives, documentation system variations, and communication discontinuities. Key reconciliation elements during these transitions include clearly documenting therapeutic intent for medications initiated during previous service management, establishing explicit continuing or tapering plans for temporary therapies, resolving multiple consultant recommendations that may create unintended interactions, and ensuring appropriate handoff of monitoring responsibilities for medications requiring specialized follow-up. Effective reconciliation prevents both unintended therapy discontinuation due to unfamiliarity with rationale and inappropriate continuation of therapies intended for short-term use.

Level of care transitions including movement between observation status and inpatient admission or transitions to rehabilitation units involve both clinical and administrative reconciliation requirements. These transitions often involve medication coverage changes requiring reconciliation of formulary differences, adjustment to new administration scheduling systems, and sometimes conversion between intravenous and oral therapies. Additional reconciliation considerations include identifying medications potentially affected by payment status changes, ensuring continuity of restricted medications requiring special authorization, and addressing home medications that may have different handling under changed admission status.

Reconciliation Processes and Accountability

Active medication profile review forms the foundation of transfer reconciliation, involving systematic assessment of all current medications rather than simply continuing existing orders without evaluation. This review includes verification of continued indication for each medication, assessment of effectiveness based on available monitoring parameters, evaluation of potential adverse effects requiring regimen modification, and consideration of potential interactions with planned new therapies in the receiving unit. Beyond technical order verification, comprehensive review incorporates clinical judgment regarding therapeutic appropriateness in the new care context, ensuring that medication regimens adapt appropriately to changing clinical circumstances rather than continuing by default.

Order set transitions require particular reconciliation attention when transfers involve movement between standardized order groupings with potential duplicate therapy or contraindicated combinations. Effective reconciliation includes systematic comparison between previous and new order sets identifying therapeutic overlaps in different medication combinations, automatic discontinuation of previous orders when new order sets are activated rather than layering new orders over existing therapy, and clinical decision support alerting to potential unintended discrepancies between previous and new medication regimens. These safeguards prevent compound prescribing errors where individually appropriate order sets create unsafe combinations when applied sequentially without comprehensive reconciliation.

Handoff communication protocols establish standardized medication information transfer during transitions, ensuring that critical therapy details extend beyond written orders to include contextual understanding essential for appropriate continuation. Structured handoff tools typically include sections for high-risk medications requiring special attention, recent medication changes that might influence current clinical status, pending monitoring results that might necessitate dosage adjustments, medications being actively titrated with specific targets, and scheduled regimen modifications planned for upcoming days. This verbal information transfer complements electronic order review with situational details and therapeutic reasoning that might not be fully captured in documentation systems.

Responsibility transfer documentation establishes clear accountability transition for medication management during handoffs, preventing situations where responsibility becomes ambiguous during transition periods. Effective documentation includes explicit acceptance of medication management responsibility by receiving providers, specific notation of medications requiring immediate attention versus stable therapies, documentation of information received regarding medication-related monitoring responsibilities, and contact information for previous providers should questions arise regarding therapy rationale. This formal responsibility acceptance transforms medication lists from passive information transfer to active care transition with clear accountability throughout the transfer process.

Technology Support and Integration

Electronic health record continuity across care transitions provides technical infrastructure supporting medication information transfer, though requiring specific design features addressing unique transfer reconciliation needs. Essential capabilities include visibility of complete medication history regardless of originating care area, clear differentiation between active and discontinued medications during transition periods, ability to maintain original ordering information with prescriber identification while transferring management responsibility, and status tracking showing verification completion by receiving providers. Advanced systems provide specialized transfer reconciliation interfaces explicitly comparing current medication profiles with receiving area standard practices, identifying potential discrepancies requiring clinical review before transfer completion.

Status synchronization between sending and receiving units addresses the common reconciliation vulnerability of temporary dual responsibility during transitions. Effective synchronization includes real-time visibility of medication administration in the sending unit while transfer orders are being prepared, automated timing adjustments for scheduled medications to prevent unintended duplications or extended intervals during physical transfer, clear electronic designation of medication administration responsibility at each transition point, and automated checks for administration gaps or overlaps during transition periods. This synchronization prevents the common reconciliation error of duplicated or missed doses during physical transfer when administrative responsibility precedes or lags behind actual patient movement.

Medication administration record transfer establishes appropriate documentation continuity while maintaining clear differentiation between activities in different care areas. Effective transfer includes automated creation of administration records matching new scheduling patterns in the receiving unit, clear visual differentiation between previous and current administration records to prevent confusion, appropriate carrying forward of relevant administration history such as pain medication response patterns or titration history, and automated closing of previous administration records to prevent documentation in obsolete records. These capabilities support both historical information continuity and appropriate documentation separation, preventing the medication safety risks associated with fragmented or duplicative administration records.

Decision support during transfers provides automated

verification enhancing manual reconciliation processes, particularly valuable during complex transitions or high-workload periods with elevated error risk. Useful support functions include automatic identification of restricted medications requiring special authorization in the receiving unit, alerts for medications requiring adjustment based on level of care changes (e.g., intensive care to general care), suggestions for intravenous to oral conversion when appropriate for the transition, and verification of therapeutic duplication when multiple order sets are applied during transitions. These support functions serve as safety nets supplementing clinical judgment rather than replacing professional review, providing systematic verification that becomes particularly valuable during complex transitions involving multiple medication changes.

Special Transfer Considerations

Timing-critical medications require specific reconciliation attention during transfers to prevent dangerous administration interruptions or unintended discontinuation. Medications needing specialized transfer planning include anticoagulants with specific dosing intervals, immunosuppressants with narrow therapeutic windows, anti-seizure medications with serum level dependencies, and cardiovascular medications where rebound effects from missed doses could cause significant deterioration. Effective reconciliation includes explicit identification of timing-critical medications requiring administration during transition periods, specific transfer orders addressing administration responsibility during physical movement, and verification of first administration timing in the receiving unit to prevent unintended extended intervals.

Continuous infusion management presents particular

challenges during transfers, requiring explicit reconciliation of infusion rates, concentration standardization differences between units, pump programming responsibilities, and monitoring parameter transitions. Comprehensive reconciliation includes documented handoff of critical infusion parameters including current rate, recent adjustments, titration protocols in effect, and monitoring triggers for rate changes. Physical transfer of infusions requires explicit verification of pump settings against transfer orders, concentration verification when moving between units with different standard dilutions, and clear documentation of infusion continuity or intentional modifications during transition. These specialized procedures address the high-risk nature of continuous medication therapy where administration errors during transitions can have rapid and significant consequences.

Implanted or patient-controlled devices require specific reconciliation attention during transitions, addressing both device management responsibility and integration with new care environments. Device types requiring specialized reconciliation include patient-controlled analgesia pumps, insulin pumps, implanted medication delivery systems, and transdermal delivery systems with specific monitoring requirements. Effective reconciliation includes documented transfer of device management protocols, explicit responsibility assignment for device monitoring and adjustment, verification of appropriate device function after physical transfer, and integration with new care area medication administration systems to prevent duplicate therapy when transitioning between device and conventional administration.

Pain management transitions represent a particularly challenging reconciliation domain, requiring careful attention to maintaining analgesia while adapting to different unit capabilities and monitoring intensities. Effective reconciliation includes documented transfer of recent pain scores and response patterns, conversion guidance between different analgesic modalities when level of care changes necessitate delivery method changes, specific rescue dose availability planning during transitions, and clear communication of patient-specific response information beyond standardized protocols. Organizations with mature reconciliation programs typically implement specialized pain management transfer protocols recognizing both the clinical importance of analgesia continuity and the significant safety risks associated with opioid management transitions.

DISCHARGE RECONCILIATION

Discharge reconciliation represents the critical final medication safety verification before patients transition from structured healthcare environments to self-management or care settings with significantly reduced professional oversight. This process addresses the substantial risks associated with medication regimen changes during hospitalization, coordination between multiple prescribers, and communication across care boundaries to establish safe therapy continuation after discharge.

10.3.1 Discharge Medication Planning

Proactive discharge medication planning begins well before actual discharge, establishing medication regimens appropriate for post-discharge environments rather than making hurried adjustments during the discharge process. Effective planning includes early identification of medications requiring special discharge arrangement such as prior authorization, specialty pharmacy dispensing, or patient assistance programs; transition from intravenous to oral therapy when clinically appropriate to establish regimen stability before discharge; and progressive patient education throughout hospitalization rather than concentrated at discharge. Organizations with mature reconciliation programs typically initiate discharge medication planning at admission for scheduled admissions and at stabilization for emergency admissions, recognizing that successful post-discharge therapy requires anticipatory planning rather than reactive arrangements.

Regimen simplification represents an important discharge planning component, addressing the reality that complex regimens developed during hospitalization with professional administration often prove difficult for patients to manage independently after discharge. Simplification strategies include consolidating multiple daily doses into once-daily alternatives when therapeutically equivalent, eliminating unnecessary medications added during hospitalization without clear ongoing indication, standardizing administration times to establish consistent daily patterns supporting adherence, and when possible, selecting combination products reducing total pill burden. This simplification recognizes that the most therapeutically sophisticated regimen provides limited benefit if patients cannot realistically maintain adherence in home environments.

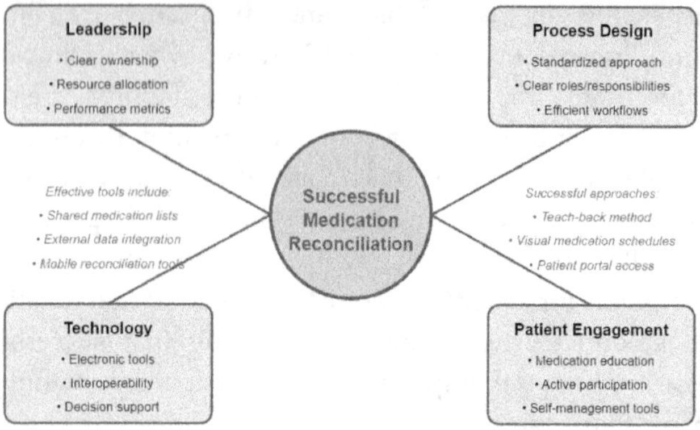

Figure 10.4 Best Practices for Medication Reconciliation

Post-discharge environment assessment establishes medication management capabilities in the planned care setting, ensuring that discharge regimens remain feasible after hospitalization. Assessment elements include physical ability to manage medication administration (e.g., opening containers, splitting tablets, operating delivery devices), cognitive capacity for appropriate self-administration decision-making, availability of necessary caregiver support for patients with functional limitations, access to required monitoring services for medications requiring ongoing parameter assessment, and financial resources for medication acquisition. This realistic assessment prevents discharge with medication regimens that cannot be practically continued, requiring either regimen modification or additional support arrangement before discharge rather than therapy failure after transition.

Continuity planning for restricted medications addresses the common discharge challenge of medications readily available in hospital but restricted in outpatient settings due to cost, distribution limitations, or authorization requirements. Effective planning includes identifying insurance coverage limitations necessitating alternative agent selection, arranging prior authorization initiation before discharge for restricted medications, establishing transitional supply provisions bridging between discharge and outpatient prescription availability, and when necessary, identifying patient assistance programs or alternative resources for uncovered essential medications.

Table 10.3: Discharge Reconciliation Components and Strategies

Component	Purpose	Implementation
Discharge Medication List	Provide complete list of medications to continue	EMR-generated lists Clear format with purpose Medication calendar format
Medication Changes	Clearly communicate medication changes	Highlighting new/stopped medications Documented reasons for changes Before/after comparison
Patient Education	Ensure patient understanding and ability to self-manage	Teach-back method Focused education on high-risk medications Caregiver inclusion
Follow-up Planning	Establish ongoing medication management	Follow-up appointment timing Monitoring requirements Pharmacy communication

This proactive approach prevents therapy interruptions commonly occurring when discharge prescriptions require authorization processes or prove prohibitively expensive in outpatient settings.

Reconciliation Process and Documentation

Comprehensive medication review before prescription generation establishes the foundation for accurate discharge reconciliation, ensuring that all medication decisions receive explicit consideration rather than automated continuation of admission or hospital regimens. This review systematically addresses four medication categories: pre-admission medications requiring decisions regarding resumption, continuation, or discontinuation; new medications started during hospitalization requiring determination of continued necessity; hospital-specific medications requiring conversion to outpatient equivalents; and additional medications needed based on newly diagnosed conditions or treatment plan changes. This structured approach prevents both unintended omissions of necessary therapy and inappropriate continuation of medications intended only for inpatient management.

Reconciliation documentation establishes clear comparison between pre-admission, inpatient, and discharge medication regimens with explicit rationale for all modifications. Essential documentation includes final disposition of each pre-admission medication (resumed, modified, or discontinued with specific rationale), status of each hospital-initiated medication (continued, converted to outpatient equivalent, or discontinued with rationale), and complete details for all discharge medications including dose, route, frequency, duration, and purpose. This comprehensive documentation creates both clear guidance for patients and accountability trail demonstrating intentional consideration of all medication changes rather than accidental omissions or duplications.

Prescription generation integrates reconciliation decisions into actual discharge orders, preventing discrepancies between reconciliation documentation and prescriptions actually provided to patients. Effective processes include systematic verification that each medication identified for continuation appears on discharge prescriptions with correct details, appropriate prescription format selection based on medication type and patient circumstances (e.g., electronic, printed, or direct pharmacy communication), and practical considerations including prescription quantity sufficient to reach follow-up appointments. Organizations with advanced reconciliation systems typically implement technical connections between reconciliation documentation and prescription generation, allowing direct conversion of reconciliation decisions into prescription format to eliminate transcription errors.

Communication to outpatient providers establishes information continuity essential for safe ongoing medication management after direct hospital oversight ends. Comprehensive communication includes complete discharge medication lists with clear differentiation between continued, modified, and new medications; explicit rationale for medication changes occurring during hospitalization; relevant monitoring results influencing medication selection or dosing; specific follow-up recommendations for dose adjustments or medication changes requiring post-discharge evaluation; and when applicable, limited-duration intent for medications not intended for indefinite continuation. This detailed communication transforms simple medication lists into clinically valuable information supporting appropriate continuing care decisions beyond discharge.

Patient Education and Engagement

Teach-back methodology represents best practice for discharge medication education, providing verification of actual understanding rather than simply documenting information provision. This approach involves providing clear medication information in appropriate language and literacy level, asking patients to explain key information in their own words, identifying and addressing gaps in understanding through targeted re-education, and repeating the process until satisfactory comprehension is demonstrated. Research indicates that teach-back implementation reduces post-discharge medication errors by 30-45% compared to conventional education, with particular benefit for complex regimens and high-risk medications requiring specific administration techniques or monitoring.

Written materials supporting verbal education provide ongoing reference after discharge when patients can no longer access direct healthcare professional guidance for medication questions. Effective materials include complete medication lists in patient-friendly format with clear administration instructions, visual differentiation between newly prescribed and continuing medications, specific information about medication purposes connecting therapy to health conditions, explicit duration information for time-limited treatments, and plain-language side effect information with appropriate response guidance. Materials should address health literacy considerations including appropriate reading level (typically 5th-6th grade), adequate font size, use of visual cues supporting text information, and when necessary, non-English language versions matching patient preferences.

Specific high-risk medication education addresses the elevated safety concerns associated with certain medication classes commonly involved in post-discharge adverse events. Medications typically requiring enhanced education include anticoagulants (with specific bleeding risk information and monitoring requirements), insulin and oral diabetes medications (with hypoglycemia recognition and management guidance), opioid analgesics (with safety precautions and appropriate tapering expectations), heart failure medications (with weight monitoring instructions and diuretic adjustment guidance when applicable), and antibiotics (with completion importance and specific timing requirements). This targeted education prioritizes safety-critical information about highest-risk medications when limited education time precludes comprehensive discussion of all therapies.

Post-discharge support arrangements establish continuing medication management assistance beyond hospitalization, particularly valuable for patients with complex regimens, cognitive limitations, or limited home support systems. Support mechanisms include scheduled follow-up telephone contact reviewing medication understanding and adherence, home care services with medication management components, referral to community pharmacy medication therapy management programs, specialized transition clinics with medication review focus, and when available, telehealth monitoring for highest-risk patients or medications. These arrangements recognize that discharge education alone may prove insufficient for complex medication management, with continuing support often necessary for successful therapy continuation.

Coordination and Follow-up

Prescription fulfillment coordination addresses the critical gap between discharge prescription provision and actual medication availability, a transition point where therapy discontinuity frequently occurs. Effective approaches include direct transmission of prescriptions to patient-identified pharmacies before physical discharge, medication bedside delivery programs bringing prescribed medications to patients before leaving the hospital, follow-up verification of prescription filling for highest-risk medications or vulnerable patients, and transitional supply provision bridging between discharge and community pharmacy acquisition. These coordination efforts prevent the common scenario of patients leaving hospitals with prescriptions but without actual medications, creating dangerous therapy gaps particularly problematic for condition-stabilizing medications.

Follow-up appointment coordination integrates medication management into post-discharge care planning, ensuring appropriate clinical oversight during therapy transition periods. Comprehensive coordination includes scheduling follow-up appointments with appropriate timing based on medication risk profiles, explicit communication of medication review expectations to follow-up providers, specific laboratory testing arrangements for medications requiring monitoring, and when possible, medication-related visit preparation helping patients articulate therapy questions or concerns during limited appointment times. Organizations with sophisticated discharge programs increasingly implement specialized post-discharge medication review appointments specifically focused on therapy adjustment and adherence support during the vulnerable transition period.

Readmission prevention through medication management recognizes that medication-related problems contribute to 10-28% of hospital readmissions, representing a significant opportunity for both quality improvement and cost reduction. Effective prevention strategies include identifying high-risk patients for enhanced medication transition interventions, implementing "meds to beds" programs ensuring actual medication possession before discharge, conducting post-discharge telephone follow-up specifically addressing medication understanding and adherence, and establishing urgent medication problem response systems providing assistance without requiring emergency department utilization. These approaches recognize appropriate medication management as fundamental readmission prevention rather than simply focus on disease management alone.

Post-discharge monitoring programs provide structured surveillance during the high-risk period following hospitalization, enabling early detection and intervention for medication-related problems before serious complications develop. Monitoring may include remote tracking of physiologic parameters affected by medication therapy (e.g., blood pressure, weight, glucose levels), structured assessment of medication adherence through telephone contact or electronic monitoring devices, patient-reported symptom tracking identifying potential adverse effects requiring intervention, and when available, serum level monitoring for narrow therapeutic index medications. These monitoring approaches create safety nets during transition periods between the highly supervised hospital environment and routine outpatient care, addressing the elevated risk immediately following discharge before stable outpatient management is established

BEST PRACTICES

Best practices in medication reconciliation reflect evidence-based approaches and operational experiences that consistently demonstrate superior outcomes across diverse healthcare settings. These practices establish benchmarks for reconciliation program development while providing practical implementation guidance addressing common challenges throughout the medication reconciliation process.

Organizational Infrastructure

Dedicated reconciliation personnel represent a fundamental best practice addressing the reality that reconciliation responsibilities added to existing workflow without dedicated resources frequently receive inadequate attention during high-workload periods. Personnel models demonstrating effectiveness include pharmacy technicians specially trained in medication history collection, nurses with dedicated reconciliation time separate from direct patient care responsibilities, and clinical pharmacists with specific reconciliation focus complementing broader clinical pharmacy services. Research indicates that dedicated personnel models achieve 70-85% reduction in unintended medication discrepancies compared to shared-responsibility models without dedicated resources, with favorable return on investment through prevented adverse events and reduced rework requirements.

Interdisciplinary accountability systems establish appropriate responsibility distribution while preventing reconciliation gaps from unclear ownership. Effective systems explicitly define discipline-specific responsibilities matching professional expertise (e.g., pharmacy personnel for medication history collection, physicians for clinical decision-making regarding therapy continuation), establish clear handoff procedures between disciplines for different reconciliation stages, implement shared documentation systems making reconciliation status visible to all team members, and create escalation pathways for unresolved discrepancies requiring additional expertise. These systems recognize that effective reconciliation requires multiple professional perspectives while preventing diffusion of responsibility that allows reconciliation completion to become secondary to competing priorities.

Educational programs develop and maintain the specialized knowledge required for effective reconciliation beyond basic professional education. Comprehensive programs include initial competency development through structured training in interviewing techniques, common medication class familiarity, administration formulation identification, and documentation systems; ongoing education addressing frequently encountered reconciliation challenges; competency verification through direct observation rather than solely knowledge assessment; and specialized training for high-risk scenarios including multiple pharmacy utilization, complex medication regimens, and limited patient communication capabilities. Organizations with mature reconciliation programs typically implement tiered competency models with progressive expertise development moving from basic reconciliation to complex case management.

Information technology integration establishes reconciliation as fundamental medication management component rather than parallel documentation process, creating workflow efficiency while enhancing clinical impact. Optimal integration includes embedding reconciliation tools within electronic health record medication management modules rather than separate systems, implementing single sign-on access preventing authentication barriers to reconciliation information, establishing bidirectional information flow between reconciliation documentation and ordering systems, and incorporating reconciliation status into clinical dashboards creating visibility equal to other essential clinical activities. This integration transforms reconciliation from documentation burden to clinical decision support tool, enhancing both completion rates and quality through workflow incorporation.

Table 10.4: Medication Reconciliation Best Practices by Role

Role	Responsibilities	Tools and Resources
Physicians	Prescribing decisions Intent documentation Clinical assessment	Standardized order sets Clinical decision support Prescribing protocols
Pharmacists	Medication history verification Clinical review Discrepancy resolution	Structured interview tools External medication history sources Pharmacy dispensing records
Nurses	Initial medication history Patient education Medication administration continuity	Bedside reconciliation tools Education materials Administration scheduling tools
Patients/Care givers	Accurate information provision Medication list maintenance Understanding changes	Personal medication lists Medication apps Education materials

Risk Stratification and Prioritization

Medication risk stratification directs enhanced reconciliation resources toward situations presenting greatest safety vulnerability, enabling appropriate resource allocation when comprehensive high-intensity reconciliation proves impractical for all patients. Effective stratification considers both medication and patient factors, typically categorizing into high, moderate, and standard risk levels with corresponding reconciliation intensity. Medication factors commonly included in stratification include narrow therapeutic index, high-alert status, complex dosing requirements, and significant interaction potential. Patient factors typically include age extremes, organ dysfunction affecting medication clearance, communication barriers complicating history gathering, multiple comorbidities requiring complex regimens, and recent care transitions creating regimen fragmentation.

Patient population customization adapts reconciliation processes to specific clinical contexts rather than implementing identical procedures across diverse patient groups with varying reconciliation challenges. Pediatric customization includes age-appropriate interview techniques, specialized documentation capturing weight-based dosing and liquid medication concentrations, and enhanced caregiver involvement throughout the reconciliation process. Geriatric customization incorporates screening for potentially inappropriate medications, specific assessment of adherence capabilities, and evaluation of simplified regimen opportunities. Psychiatric setting customization addresses challenges including limited patient communication during acute episodes, verification difficulties with unreliable self-reporting, and complex psychotropic regimens with significant interaction potential. These customized approaches recognize that standardized reconciliation expecting identical process application across all contexts frequently fails to address population-specific challenges.

Urgency-based prioritization establishes appropriate sequence and timing expectations for reconciliation completion, recognizing that clinical circumstances significantly affect reconciliation urgency. Effective prioritization includes immediate reconciliation for emergent conditions where medication history directly influences urgent treatment decisions (e.g., acute coronary syndrome with potential home anticoagulant use), high-priority reconciliation for urgent but non-emergent conditions where medication information significantly influences initial management decisions, standard reconciliation for stable conditions where complete information gathering appropriately precedes treatment decisions, and deferred comprehensive reconciliation with interim essential information collection for unconscious or uncommunicative patients requiring initial stabilization before complete history development. This prioritization appropriately matches reconciliation timing to clinical needs rather than applying uniform timing expectations regardless of clinical context.

Resource allocation aligned with identified risk ensures that enhanced reconciliation practices receive sustainable support rather than implementation without appropriate resource provision. Best practices include staffing models with reconciliation workload explicitly incorporated into productivity expectations rather than added to existing responsibilities, technological support matched to reconciliation requirements rather than basic systems inadequate for complex reconciliation needs, dedicated physical spaces supporting uninterrupted reconciliation interviews in appropriate privacy, and specialized services addressing high-risk situations such as language interpretation, cognitive assessment support, and home medication verification. This risk-aligned resource provision prevents the common scenario of reconciliation expectations exceeding available resources, a mismatch frequently resulting in superficial compliance rather than meaningful safety improvement.

Process Reliability and Standardization

Forcing functions embed reconciliation completion into clinical workflows, preventing progression to subsequent activities until appropriate reconciliation steps occur. Effective implementation includes electronic health record configurations requiring reconciliation documentation before non-urgent order entry, automated verification of required reconciliation elements before accepting documentation as complete, medication order entry systems comparing new orders against documented home medications with discrepancy notification, and discharge workflow design requiring reconciliation completion before discharge order processing. These technological enforcement mechanisms supplement policy expectations with system-level requirements, ensuring consistent application regardless of individual practice patterns or workload pressures that might otherwise result in reconciliation shortcuts or omissions.

Standardized tools establish consistent reconciliation documentation across different providers, locations, and patient populations, enabling reliable information transfer throughout care transitions. Essential standardization includes uniform documentation formats capturing all necessary medication details, consistent terminology for reconciliation status and discrepancy categories, standardized verification level documentation indicating information reliability, and structured format for communicating reconciliation information during handoffs. Organizations with sophisticated reconciliation programs typically implement standardized electronic templates with required fields ensuring complete information capture, progressive disclosure design revealing relevant detail levels based on clinical need, and automated compilation creating consolidated views from multiple reconciliation points throughout patient care.

Quality assurance processes provide systematic verification that reconciliation meets established standards rather than relying on assumed quality without objective assessment. Effective approaches include concurrent review sampling evaluating reconciliation quality during patient care, retrospective analysis comparing reconciliation documentation against subsequently identified medication information to detect missed elements, direct observation of reconciliation practices assessing actual process execution beyond documentation review, and focused review of high-risk situations such as complex regimens or vulnerable populations where reconciliation errors carry greatest potential consequence. These verification activities support continuous improvement through identification of specific quality gaps rather than general performance assumptions.

Performance feedback systems create accountability while supporting individual and system-level improvement through objective data regarding reconciliation practices. Comprehensive feedback includes provider-specific metrics comparing individual performance against organizational benchmarks, department-level aggregation identifying systematic improvement opportunities, organization-wide trending demonstrating longitudinal performance changes, and when available, comparison against external standards establishing broader performance context. Effective feedback extends beyond simple completion metrics to include quality indicators such as discrepancy identification rates, verification level achievement, and correlation with medication safety outcomes. Regular review cadences establish expected performance discussions rather than occasional attention, while tiered reporting tailors information detail to specific audience needs from executive overview to individual performance coaching.

Integration with Patient Care and Safety Systems

Connection with broader medication safety programs establishes reconciliation as integral safety system component rather than isolated process, creating synergistic relationships with complementary safety initiatives. Effective integration includes incorporating reconciliation findings into adverse drug event investigations identifying system vulnerability patterns, utilizing medication safety committee oversight for reconciliation program evaluation, integrating reconciliation compliance into comprehensive medication safety metrics rather than separate measurement, and applying common improvement methodologies across reconciliation and other medication safety initiatives. This connected approach prevents reconciliation from becoming disconnected documentation exercise divorced from broader safety culture and improvement activities.

Patient engagement as reconciliation partners represents evolution beyond viewing patients as simple information sources to active participation in accuracy verification and decision-making. Progressive approaches include providing patients with reconciliation documentation for review and correction before finalization, establishing mechanisms for patients to report discrepancies they identify in medication documentation, involving patients in decisions regarding medication continuation or modification based on home experience information, and incorporating patient-reported adherence patterns into reconciliation to distinguish prescribed from actual regimens. This engagement recognizes patients as valuable reconciliation resources with unique knowledge about their medication experiences rather than passive recipients of reconciliation services.

Health information exchange connectivity addresses the fundamental reconciliation challenge of fragmented information across multiple care settings, establishing broader information access beyond individual organization boundaries. Effective connectivity includes bidirectional information sharing with community pharmacy systems, access to prescription fill data from pharmacy benefit managers, primary care medication list exchange capabilities, and when available, regional health information exchange participation providing consolidated medication history across multiple healthcare organizations. While technical and privacy challenges continue to limit comprehensive health information exchange implementation, organizations with mature reconciliation programs increasingly implement strategic connectivity with highest-value external information sources addressing the most significant reconciliation information gaps.

Continuous learning systems transform reconciliation from static process to evolving capability through systematic programmatic improvement based on performance experience. Essential components include regular review of reconciliation-related safety events identifying improvement opportunities, structured assessment of reconciliation practices during significant medication errors determining contribution to adverse outcomes, periodic literature review incorporating emerging evidence into local practices, and participation in collaborative improvement initiatives sharing experience across organizations. This learning orientation creates ongoing reconciliation program enhancement addressing evolving challenges rather than fixed implementation after initial development, establishing medication reconciliation as dynamic safety system rather than procedural requirement.

Things to Remember

- ☑ Admission reconciliation creates an accurate foundation for inpatient therapy through comprehensive information collection from multiple sources, systematic verification, and clear documentation connecting home medications to admission orders.
- ☑ Transfer reconciliation addresses internal transition vulnerabilities through active medication profile review, order set transitions preventing unintended duplications, structured handoff communication, and technology support.
- ☑ Discharge reconciliation provides critical verification before transitioning to self-management through comprehensive review, explicit documentation comparing pre-admission and discharge regimens, integrated prescription generation, and effective patient education.
- ☑ Best practices include dedicated personnel resources, interdisciplinary accountability, standardized documentation formats, risk stratification, and technology integration embedding reconciliation within workflow

systems.

- ☑ Reconciliation addresses the fundamental safety risk of information fragmentation during care transitions causing unintended therapy changes.
- ☑ Effective implementation requires both technical accuracy in medication lists and clinical judgment regarding therapeutic appropriateness of continuing, modifying, or discontinuing medications.

Multiple Choice Questions

1. Admission medication reconciliation creates an accurate foundation for inpatient therapy through:
   a) Reviewing only medications dispensed by the hospital pharmacy
   b) Comprehensive information collection from multiple sources with systematic verification
   c) Accepting patient self-report without additional verification
   d) Focusing exclusively on prescription medications without over-the-counter products
2. Transfer reconciliation addresses internal transition vulnerabilities through:
   a) Automatically continuing all previous medications without review
   b) Complete medication discontinuation with new ordering at each transition
   c) Active medication profile review during unit or service changes
   d) Limiting information transfer to controlled substances only

3. Discharge reconciliation provides critical verification before transitioning to self-management through:
   a) Providing standard educational materials without individualization
   b) Focusing exclusively on new medications without addressing pre-admission regimens
   c) Comprehensive review comparing pre-admission and discharge regimens
   d) Delegating all medication education to community pharmacies
4. Which of the following is NOT typically considered a best practice in medication reconciliation?
   a) Risk stratification directing enhanced efforts toward highest-risk situations
   b) Standardized documentation formats supporting consistent information capture
   c) Conducting reconciliation as a separate process disconnected from clinical decision-making
   d) Interdisciplinary accountability systems with clearly defined responsibilities
5. The primary purpose of medication reconciliation is to:
   a) Reduce medication costs through formulary substitutions
   b) Establish information accuracy throughout care transitions
   c) Eliminate the need for clinical judgment in prescribing decisions
   d) Transfer responsibility for medication management to patients

6. Risk factors warranting enhanced reconciliation processes include:
   a) Young adult patients with limited medication use
   b) Patients taking multiple high-risk medications with complex regimens
   c) Brief hospitalizations for minor procedures
   d) Patients with a single community pharmacy and provider
7. Effective discharge medication education should include:
   a) Technical information focused on pharmacological mechanisms
   b) Standardized information without adaptation to health literacy levels
   c) Purpose, administration instructions, side effects, and monitoring requirements
   d) Emphasis on rare adverse effects without prioritization of common concerns
8. The most accurate sources for medication reconciliation typically include:
   a) Family member recollection without verification
   b) Healthcare provider documentation without patient confirmation
   c) Multiple sources including patient interview, pharmacy records, and previous medical records
   d) Hospital formulary listings of commonly prescribed medications
9. Technology support for medication reconciliation:
   a) Eliminates the need for clinical judgment in

the reconciliation process
b) Functions effectively without integration into clinical workflows
c) Enables information synchronization between care areas reducing manual transcription
d) Works best as a standalone system separate from the electronic health record

10. Medication discrepancies discovered during reconciliation:
a) Should always be resolved by continuing the most recently prescribed therapy
b) Require clinical judgment to determine appropriate resolution based on patient needs
c) Are best addressed by defaulting to the highest dose of any conflicting information
d) Should be resolved exclusively by the primary admitting physician without consultation

Self-Assessment Questions

1. Critically analyze the process of admission medication reconciliation, including best practices, common challenges, and strategies to improve accuracy and efficiency.
2. Evaluate the unique considerations, challenges, and implementation strategies for medication reconciliation during internal patient transfers between different levels of care.
3. Analyze the discharge medication reconciliation process and its role in preventing adverse drug events during the transition from hospital to community settings.
4. Discuss the evidence supporting medication reconciliation as a safety intervention and its impact on patient outcomes, readmissions, and healthcare costs.
5. Evaluate the roles and responsibilities of different healthcare professionals in the medication reconciliation process and models for interprofessional collaboration.
6. Analyze how health information technology can support medication reconciliation processes, including both benefits and limitations of current systems.
7. Discuss strategies for engaging patients and families in the medication reconciliation process to improve accuracy and adherence.
8. Evaluate approaches to measuring the quality and effectiveness of medication reconciliation processes, including meaningful metrics and

performance indicators.

9. Analyze the unique challenges of medication reconciliation in vulnerable populations (elderly, low health literacy, multiple chronic conditions) and strategies to address these challenges.
10. Discuss how medication reconciliation processes should be adapted across different healthcare settings, including emergency departments, ambulatory care, and long-term care facilities.

Bibliography

1. Mueller SK, Sponsler KC, Kripalani S, Schnipper JL. Hospital-based medication reconciliation practices: a systematic review. Arch Intern Med. 2012;172(14):1057-69.
2. Kwan JL, Lo L, Sampson M, Shojania KG. Medication reconciliation during transitions of care as a patient safety strategy: a systematic review. Ann Intern Med. 2013;158(5 Pt 2):397-403.
3. Tam VC, Knowles SR, Cornish PL, Fine N, Marchesano R, Etchells EE. Frequency, type and clinical importance of medication history errors at admission to hospital: a systematic review. CMAJ. 2005;173(5):510-5.
4. Cornish PL, Knowles SR, Marchesano R, Tam V, Shadowitz S, Juurlink DN, et al. Unintended medication discrepancies at the time of hospital admission. Arch Intern Med. 2005;165(4):424-9.
5. Lehnbom EC, Stewart MJ, Manias E, Westbrook JI. Impact of medication reconciliation and review on clinical outcomes. Ann Pharmacother. 2014;48(10):1298-312.
6. Hron JD, Manzi S, Dionne R, Chiang VW, Brostoff M, Altavilla SA, et al. Electronic medication reconciliation and medication errors. Int J Qual Health Care. 2015;27(4):314-9.
7. Schnipper JL, Kirwin JL, Cotugno MC, Wahlstrom SA, Brown BA, Tarvin E, et al. Role of pharmacist counseling in preventing adverse drug events after hospitalization. Arch Intern Med. 2006;166(5):565-71.
8. World Health Organization. The High 5s Project - Standard Operating Protocol for Medication Reconciliation. Geneva: World Health Organization; 2014.
9. Mekonnen AB, McLachlan AJ, Brien JE. Pharmacy-led medication reconciliation programmes at hospital transitions: a systematic review and meta-analysis. J Clin Pharm Ther. 2016;41(2):128-44.
10. Institute for Healthcare Improvement. How-to Guide: Prevent Adverse Drug Events by Implementing Medication Reconciliation. Cambridge, MA: Institute for Healthcare Improvement; 2011.

CHAPTER 11

HIGH-ALERT MEDICATIONS

Abstract

High-alert medications present elevated harm risk when used incorrectly, requiring specialized safety systems beyond standard medication protocols. Identification and classification methodologies establish standardized recognition using evidence-based approaches including ISMP lists categorizing medications by risk profile, WHO classifications providing international standardization, and institutional customization addressing specific patient populations and services. Special handling requirements create multilayered protection through segregated storage preventing selection errors, restricted access limiting handling to qualified personnel, concentration standardization reducing calculation requirements, and distinctive labeling ensuring immediate recognition throughout the medication use process. Safety protocols establish consistent practices addressing unique risk points through restricted prescribing authorization, standardized order sets embedding safety parameters, independent verification requirements, and medication-specific protocols for anticoagulants, insulin, chemotherapy, and opioids reflecting their distinctive risk characteristics. Monitoring systems provide essential surveillance through systematic physiological parameter assessment, scheduled laboratory monitoring, patient-reported outcome tracking, and technology-assisted continuous monitoring, complemented by clearly defined response protocols, interdisciplinary intervention teams, and quality assurance.

Keywords: *Risk stratification, specialized protocols, verification requirements, concentrated oversight, parameter monitoring*

Learning Objectives

After completion of the chapter, the learners should be able to:

- Remember the criteria used to identify and classify high-alert medications.
- Understand how special handling requirements reduce the risk of errors with high-alert medications.
- Apply appropriate safety protocols to manage different categories of high-alert medications.
- Analyze monitoring systems for detecting potential adverse events with high-alert medications.
- Evaluate the effectiveness of various safeguards for different high-alert medication categories.
- Create comprehensive safety systems addressing the unique risks of specific high-alert medications

IDENTIFICATION AND CLASSIFICATION

High-alert medications pose elevated risks for patient harm when used incorrectly, necessitating systematic identification and classification to implement appropriate safety measures throughout the medication use process. These medications require exceptional attention due to their inherent risk characteristics, with standardized identification systems supporting consistent safety approaches across healthcare settings.

Definition and Risk Characteristics

High-alert medications are defined by their heightened potential to cause significant patient harm when used in error, distinguished from other medications where mistakes may cause harm but with less severity or frequency. This designation focuses specifically on the magnitude of potential harm rather than simply error frequency, recognizing that certain medications present disproportionate risk warranting enhanced safety precautions. The concept originated from sentinel event analyses revealing that a relatively small subset of medications was consistently implicated in serious or fatal medication errors, leading to formalized identification of these agents for targeted safety interventions.

Narrow therapeutic index represents a primary risk characteristic, with minimal separation between therapeutic and toxic doses creating limited safety margin for dosing errors. Medications in this category typically demonstrate less than a 2-fold difference between effective and harmful doses, meaning that even relatively small dosing errors can produce serious toxicity. Examples include warfarin, where modest overdosing can cause life-threatening hemorrhage; digoxin, where excessive dosing leads to potentially fatal arrhythmias; and aminoglycoside antibiotics, where narrow separation between therapeutic and nephrotoxic levels necessitates precise dosing and monitoring. This limited safety margin makes these medications particularly vulnerable to harm from calculation errors, documentation mistakes, or administration inaccuracies.

Rapid physiological impact constitutes another defining characteristic, with medications capable of producing immediate serious effects without opportunity for intervention before harm occurs. Neuromuscular blocking agents exemplify this category, causing respiratory paralysis within minutes of administration without adequate respiratory support. Similarly, vasopressors and vasoactive medications produce immediate hemodynamic effects that can rapidly become life-threatening with incorrect dosing. This rapid action contrasts with medications having more gradual effects where adverse consequences develop slowly enough for detection and intervention before severe harm occurs, allowing correction of potential errors before significant consequences materialize.

End-organ damage potential identifies medications capable of causing permanent or severe injury to critical organs, creating lasting harm beyond the medication's immediate effects. Chemotherapeutic agents illustrate this category, with potential for irreversible bone marrow suppression, cardiac damage, or neurotoxicity from overdosing. Anticoagulants present risk for intracranial or other major hemorrhage with permanent neurological sequelae or death. Contrast media can cause permanent renal injury in vulnerable patients. This potential for irreversible harm distinguishes these agents from medications where adverse effects, while potentially serious, typically resolve after discontinuation without permanent damage.

Specialized administration requirements characterize many high-alert medications, with complex preparation, delivery, or monitoring needs creating multiple error opportunities throughout the medication use process. Parenteral nutrition exemplifies this category, requiring precise electrolyte calculation, specialized preparation facilities, and careful monitoring during administration. Anesthesia induction agents involve complex weight-based calculations, rapid physiological effects requiring immediate monitoring capability, and specific administration techniques. These specialized requirements create vulnerability at multiple process points from preparation through administration, with errors at any stage potentially resulting in patient harm.

Table 11.1: High-Alert Medication Categories and Examples

Category	Risk Factors	Common Examples	Error Prevention
Anticoagulants	Narrow therapeutic range, bleeding risk	Warfarin, heparin, DOACs	Dosing accuracy, monitoring, drug interactions
Insulins	Variable dosing, hypoglycemia risk	All insulins, especially concentrated forms	Concentration verification, independent checks, timing
Opioids	Respiratory depression, sedation	Fentanyl, hydromorphone, methadone	Dose calculation, monitoring, naloxone access
Neuromuscular Blockers	Respiratory arrest if given inappropriately	Vecuronium, rocuronium, pancuronium	Segregated storage, warning labels, ventilation availability
Concentrated Electrolytes	Cardiac arrhythmias, death	Potassium chloride, hypertonic sodium chloride	Restricted access, dilution protocols, administration rate

Standardized Lists and Classification Systems

The Institute for Safe Medication Practices (ISMP) maintains the most widely recognized high-alert medication lists, providing evidence-based identification of medications requiring enhanced safety precautions. These lists derive from multiple data sources including adverse event reporting systems, published error reports, sentinel event analyses, and expert consensus panels. Separate lists address different healthcare settings, recognizing that medication risk profiles vary based on practice context, monitoring capabilities, and patient populations. The acute care list includes medications specific to hospital settings, the community/ambulatory list focuses on outpatient risks, and the long-term care list addresses nursing facility contexts. Regular updates incorporate emerging safety information and new medications, maintaining contemporary relevance as therapeutic options evolve.

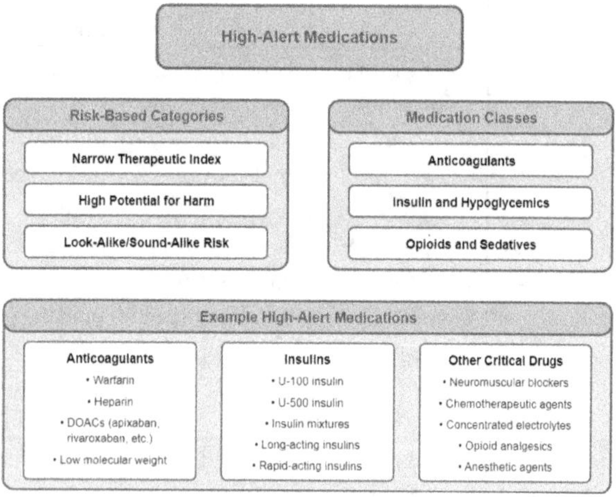

Figure 11.1: High-Alert Medication Classification

World Health Organization high-alert medication classification provides international standardization supporting global medication safety initiatives. This classification identifies "High-Alert Medications/High-Risk Medications" as designated substances requiring specialized handling, storage, prescribing, dispensing, administration, and monitoring processes due to elevated potential for patient harm. The WHO framework extends beyond simple medication listing to include implementation guidance for risk reduction strategies, with particular emphasis on resource-limited settings where advanced technological safety systems may be unavailable. This international standardization supports consistent safety approaches across diverse healthcare systems while accommodating local practice variations and resource constraints.

Class-based versus medication-specific identification represents a fundamental classification decision with significant implementation implications. Class-based approaches identify entire medication categories as high-alert based on shared risk characteristics, such as designating all anticoagulants rather than specific agents within this class. This approach provides comprehensive safety coverage including newly approved medications within established classes, but may direct safety resources toward lower-risk members of broadly defined categories. Medication-specific identification designates individual agents based on documented harm patterns, providing more targeted focus but potentially missing newly introduced high-risk medications without established error patterns. Most contemporary systems employ hybrid approaches, identifying both high-alert classes and specific high-risk medications within lower-risk classes.

Risk stratification within high-alert designation creates differentiated safety approaches proportional to specific medication risk profiles rather than applying identical precautions to all identified agents. Sophisticated classification systems typically establish multiple risk tiers with corresponding safety requirements based on harm potential, administration complexity, and available mitigation strategies. Highest-risk medications such as neuromuscular blocking agents, concentrated electrolytes, and chemotherapy typically receive maximum safeguards including extensive prescribing restrictions, multiple verification requirements, and specialized handling protocols. Moderate-risk agents may receive selected interventions focusing on their specific risk characteristics rather than comprehensive high-intensity precautions. This stratified approach enables appropriate resource allocation while maintaining safety emphasis proportional to actual risk.

Setting-Specific Considerations

Pediatric high-alert medication identification addresses the unique vulnerability of pediatric patients, where developmental pharmacology, weight-based dosing requirements, and limited communication capabilities create distinctive risk patterns. Pediatric-specific classification typically includes medications with narrow therapeutic index in children even when used safely in adults (e.g., chloral hydrate, phenytoin), agents requiring complex weight-based calculations with significant harm potential from computational errors (e.g., opioids, insulin), and medications with significantly different pediatric pharmacokinetics creating age-specific toxicity risks. Notable pediatric additions to standard adult high-alert lists include oral hypoglycemics (greater hypoglycemia risk in children), immunosuppressants (higher toxicity vulnerability), and certain oral liquid preparations where concentration confusion presents heightened risk for children.

Critical care environment classification acknowledges the unique medication risk profile in intensive care settings, where patient acuity, multiple continuous infusions, and rapid clinical changes create distinctive safety challenges. Critical care-specific high-alert designations typically emphasize vasoactive medications with immediate hemodynamic effects, sedatives and neuromuscular blocking agents affecting respiratory drive, concentrated electrolyte solutions, and complex titrated medications requiring frequent adjustment based on physiological parameters. The critical care context may actually reduce risk for certain high-alert medications through enhanced monitoring capabilities and specialized staff expertise, while simultaneously increasing risk for other agents due to complex administration requirements and rapidly changing patient conditions.

Ambulatory and home care contexts present unique high-alert medication considerations due to reduced professional oversight, variable patient self-management capabilities, and limited monitoring compared to inpatient settings. Classification for these environments typically emphasizes medications with serious consequences from adherence errors (e.g., immunosuppressants, anticoagulants), agents requiring complex self-administration techniques (e.g., injectable medications, inhaled therapies with specific technique requirements), and medications with significant cognitive impact affecting self-monitoring capability (e.g., opioids, hypnotics). Community-specific high-alert designations often include oral anticoagulants, insulin products designed for self-administration, oral chemotherapeutic agents, and medications requiring therapeutic drug monitoring that may be inconsistently performed in ambulatory settings.

Institutional customization of high-alert classifications

adapts standard systems to specific organizational risk profiles based on patient populations, services offered, and historical safety event patterns. Effective customization involves systematic evaluation of adverse drug events and near-misses to identify medications consistently involved in local safety issues, assessment of practice patterns identifying frequently used high-risk therapies justifying enhanced safeguards, and consideration of available safety resources to establish realistic implementation priorities. While maintaining core high-alert medications identified in standardized lists, customization may add organization-specific agents based on local experience or modify risk stratification to address institutional vulnerability patterns. This balanced approach maintains alignment with evidence-based standards while addressing unique organizational risk factors that may not appear in generalized classifications.

Identification Methodologies

Retrospective event analysis represents the traditional foundation for high-alert medication identification, examining documented harm events to identify medications consistently involved in serious adverse outcomes. This approach typically involves systematic review of incident reports, sentinel events, liability claims, and published case reports to identify medications causing disproportionate harm relative to utilization frequency. Advanced methodology includes assessment of harm magnitude and preventability for identified cases, distinguishing medications causing severe preventable harm warranting high-alert designation from those with unavoidable adverse effects despite appropriate use. The primary limitation of retrospective identification lies in its reactive nature, requiring harm occurrence before risk identification rather than proactive risk prevention.

Proactive risk assessment methodologies complement retrospective analysis by identifying potential high-alert medications before actual harm events occur. Failure Mode and Effects Analysis (FMEA) systematically evaluates medication use processes to identify potential failure points and their consequences, enabling high-alert designation based on potential harm rather than actual events. Socio-Technical Probabilistic Risk Assessment (ST-PRA) quantifies event probability and severity across complete medication use processes, supporting risk-based classification with structured estimation rather than awaiting event occurrence. These proactive approaches prove particularly valuable for newly introduced medications without established error patterns but with pharmacological characteristics suggesting significant harm potential.

Expert consensus processes incorporate specialized knowledge into high-alert identification when empirical data remains limited or inconsistent. Structured approaches including Delphi methodology or nominal group technique systematically gather expert judgment regarding medication risk profiles, create formal consensus through iterative evaluation, and document decision rationales supporting classification decisions. These processes typically involve multidisciplinary panels including pharmacists, physicians, nurses, medication safety specialists, and risk management professionals, ensuring diverse perspectives on medication risks across different practice contexts. While less rigorous than data-driven identification, well-designed consensus methodology provides valuable classification guidance when complete evidence remains unavailable.

Integration of pharmacological characteristics with

actual error potential establishes comprehensive high-alert identification addressing both intrinsic medication properties and practical usage patterns. This balanced approach recognizes that theoretical risk based solely on pharmacological profile may not translate into actual harm without corresponding error vulnerability in practical usage. Similarly, medications with frequent errors but limited harm potential may not warrant high-alert designation despite error prevalence. Effective integration considers factors including typical usage patterns, administration complexity, available safety systems, provider familiarity, and monitoring standards alongside pharmacological risk characteristics to establish appropriate classification reflecting both intrinsic risk and practical safety context.

SPECIAL HANDLING REQUIREMENTS

Special handling requirements for high-alert medications establish systematic safeguards throughout the medication use process, creating multiple layers of protection from procurement through administration and monitoring. These specialized procedures address the elevated harm potential of high-alert agents through deliberate process modifications that reduce error likelihood and enhance error detection before patient harm occurs.

Storage and Accessibility Controls

Segregated storage systems physically separate high-alert medications from routine inventory, creating distinct access patterns that highlight their special status while preventing selection errors. Effective implementations include dedicated storage sections within automated dispensing cabinets, separate refrigerator sections for high-alert refrigerated products, and distinct storage modules within carousel systems or robotics. Beyond simple separation, sophisticated approaches employ color-coding systems consistently identifying high-alert storage areas, physical barriers requiring conscious override to access high-risk medications, and graduated access restrictions with more stringent controls for highest-risk agents. These segregation strategies prevent accidental selection when seeking similarly named but lower-risk medications while creating consistent visual and workflow reminders of high-alert status.

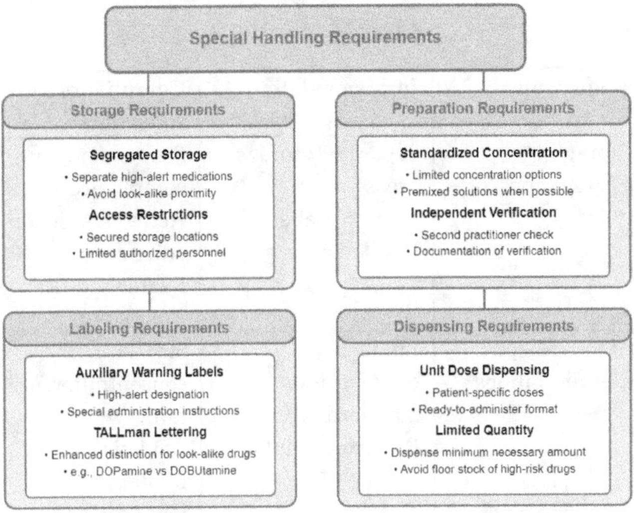

Figure 11.2: Special Handling Requirements for High-Alert Medications

Restricted access protocols establish formal limitations on personnel authorized to access high-alert medications, ensuring that only individuals with appropriate training and authorization handle these agents. Implementation approaches range from basic systems requiring supervisor approval or second-person verification before dispensing high-alert medications to sophisticated electronic controls including biometric identification, special access credentials, or dual authentication requirements for highest-risk agents. Access tracking systems maintain comprehensive records detailing who accessed specific high-alert medications, when access occurred, and quantities removed, creating audit trails supporting both security monitoring and usage pattern analysis. Progressive systems implement tiered access restrictions matching authorization levels to specific medication risk profiles rather than applying uniform controls to all high-alert agents.

Table 11.2: Special Handling Requirements for High-Alert Medications

Requirement	Implementation	Compliance Indicators
Storage Segregation	Separated storage areas Warning labels Limited access	Proper storage compliance Access restriction adherence Regular audit completion
Standardized Concentrations	Limited concentrations Standard order sets Premixed solutions	Standard concentration use rate Deviation frequency Error rates related to concentration
Independent Double-Checks	Defined check process Documentation requirements Critical check points	Double-check compliance rate Quality of verification process Error interception rate
Dispensing	Automated	Dispensing error

Controls	dispensing safeguards Pharmacy verification Special labeling	rates Override frequency Labeling compliance

Concentration and packaging standardization reduces error potential by eliminating unnecessary variation in high-alert medication presentations. This approach establishes standard concentrations for parenteral products, consistent package sizes and concentrations for oral medications, and uniform packaging within medication classes. For example, insulin standardization might establish regular insulin at one consistent concentration throughout an organization rather than stocking multiple concentration options, while opioid standardization could establish uniform packaging distinct from non-opioid analgesics. These standardization initiatives reduce cognitive burden during product selection and verification, eliminate calculation requirements that introduce error potential, and support familiarity through consistent presentation rather than requiring adaptation to multiple formulation options.

Look-alike risk mitigation addresses the specific hazard of high-alert medications being confused with lower-risk agents due to naming or packaging similarities. Strategies include storage separation preventing adjacency of similar-appearing products, auxiliary labeling with special high-alert designations, procurement decisions favoring distinct packaging when available, and when necessary, repackaging to create visual differentiation when products cannot be distinguished in manufacturer packaging. For sound-alike medications, communication standardization including read-back requirements, spelling verification during verbal orders, and naming conventions such as tall-man lettering create auditory distinction preventing confusion between similar-sounding high-alert and conventional medications. These differentiation strategies reduce selection errors that prove particularly dangerous when involving high-alert agents where incorrect selection carries substantial harm potential.

Preparation and Dispensing Safeguards

Pharmacy preparation centralization represents a fundamental safety strategy for high-alert medications, shifting preparation from patient care areas to pharmacy environments with specialized expertise, dedicated facilities, and enhanced verification procedures. This approach applies particularly to high-alert parenteral medications requiring compounding, calculations, or precise measurement where error potential increases with preparation complexity. Centralized preparation enables implementation of specialized verification procedures, environmental controls supporting accurate measurement, and standardized labeling systems not feasible in decentralized preparation models. For highest-risk preparations such as chemotherapy or pediatric high-alert medications, dedicated preparation areas with enhanced engineering controls and specialized staff assignments further reduce error potential through environmental optimization and focused expertise.

Compounding automation employs technology to enhance preparation accuracy for complex high-alert medications, reducing reliance on manual processes vulnerable to human error. Automated compounding devices for parenteral nutrition precisely measure multiple nutrient components while maintaining documentation of exact quantities used. Robotic chemotherapy systems provide accurate drug measurement while reducing staff exposure to hazardous agents. Gravimetric verification systems confirm prepared concentration through precise weight measurement rather than visual estimation. These technologies provide particular value for high-alert medications with complex preparation requirements, narrow therapeutic indices requiring precise concentration control, or severe consequences from preparation errors that traditional manual verification might not detect.

Standardized preparation protocols establish consistent methodologies for high-alert medication compounding, creating procedural reliability through elimination of unnecessary process variation. These protocols specify exact preparation sequences, approved diluents with specific volumes, standard concentrations aligning with administration devices, mixing procedures ensuring homogeneity, beyond-use dating with supporting stability data, and specific labeling requirements including auxiliary warnings. Protocol standardization reduces cognitive burden by eliminating unnecessary decision points during preparation, enables development of specialized expertise through consistent methodology, and supports verification through predictable preparation patterns rather than case-by-case judgment requiring deeper product knowledge.

Independent double-check systems provide verification of high-alert medication preparation accuracy before dispensing, creating an additional safety layer beyond standard pharmacy processes. Comprehensive verification includes calculation confirmation by a second individual without knowledge of the first calculation, independent component identification before preparation, process verification during critical preparation steps, and final product inspection against standardized criteria. Advanced double-check systems employ structured documentation capturing specific verification elements rather than simple co-signatures, utilize technology support such as barcode verification or photographic documentation of critical steps, and implement verification independence requirements preventing bias from known expectations. This redundant verification proves particularly valuable for high-alert medications with complex preparation requirements where single-point verification provides inadequate protection against consequential errors.

Labeling and Identification Systems

Distinctive labeling for high-alert medications creates immediate visual recognition of their special status throughout the medication use process, supporting appropriate handling from preparation through administration. Effective approaches include standardized auxiliary labels specifically indicating high-alert status, consistent color-coding systems applied to both storage locations and individual medication labels, and prominent warning symbols highlighting specific risk characteristics (e.g., paralytic agents, vesicants). Sophisticated labeling systems employ tiered approaches with distinctive indicators for different high-alert categories, standardized formats positioning critical information consistently across all high-alert products, and enhanced prominence for essential safety information such as concentration and maximum dose limits. This visual differentiation creates immediate recognition supporting heightened vigilance whenever high-alert medications enter the medication use process.

Concentration prominence addresses the specific risk of mathematical errors when high-alert medications require dose calculation based on concentration.

Enhanced labeling approaches include large-font concentration display, standardized concentration positioning on all high-alert labels, numerical and unit distinction preventing misreading (e.g., mg clearly differentiated from mcg), and for highest-risk medications, calculation assistance incorporated directly on labels. Specialized concentration displays for patient-specific preparations include both concentration and total content information (e.g., "50 mg/50 mL = 1 mg/mL; Total dose: 50 mg"), total volume and infusion rate guidance, and when appropriate, weight-based dosing information. This concentration emphasis reduces calculation errors that prove particularly dangerous with high-alert medications where mathematical mistakes can result in multiple-fold dosing errors.

Tall-man lettering implementation differentiates look-alike high-alert medication names through selective capitalization of distinguishing portions, reducing selection errors from name similarity. This approach follows FDA and ISMP conventions for specific medication pairs with documented confusion patterns, creating visual distinction between similar names. For example, HYDROmorphone and morphine distinction prevents potentially fatal confusion between opioids with significantly different potencies, while DOBUTamine and DOPamine differentiation prevents hemodynamic disasters from vasopressor confusion. Consistent implementation across all contexts including computer screens, medication labels, automated dispensing cabinet displays, and documentation creates reliable distinction throughout the medication use process rather than isolated application in limited contexts.

Standardized auxiliary information requirements establish consistent supplementary guidance beyond basic medication identification, addressing specific risks associated with high-alert medications. These requirements typically include mandatory warning labels for particularly dangerous agents (e.g., "Paralyzing Agent - Patient Must Be Ventilated"), route specificity preventing wrong-route administration (e.g., prominent "For Intrathecal Use Only" labeling), explicit rate restrictions for medications where administration speed directly affects safety, and specific storage requirements affecting medication stability and safety. For patient-specific preparations, standardized auxiliary information often includes patient identifiers, beyond-use dating with specific time limitations, and special handling requirements during administration. This standardized approach ensures critical safety information consistently accompanies high-alert medications rather than variable inclusion based on individual practitioner judgment.

Transportation and Delivery Controls

Specialized transport systems for high-alert medications establish secure transfer methods from preparation areas to administration locations, preventing both delivery errors and unauthorized access during transport. Physical approaches include dedicated sealed containers visually distinct from routine medication transport, tamper-evident packaging indicating potential interference during transport, and locking mechanisms for highest-risk agents requiring controlled access even during movement between locations. Procedural controls include restricted transport personnel authorization limiting handling to specifically trained individuals, direct hand-off requirements preventing unattended medication placement, and documentation creating transport audit trails from preparation to delivery. These specialized systems prove particularly important for high-alert medications where delivery to incorrect patients or unauthorized access during transport could result in significant harm.

Time-sensitive delivery protocols address the specific risks associated with high-alert medications requiring precise administration timing, preventing both premature delivery creating unauthorized access risk and delayed delivery potentially compromising patient care. These protocols typically include prioritization systems identifying high-alert medications requiring expedited transport, explicit timing guidance for medications with stability limitations after preparation, and specialized handling for temperature-sensitive high-alert products requiring controlled conditions during transport. Advanced approaches employ electronic tracking systems monitoring high-alert medication movement throughout facilities, automated alerts for delayed deliveries requiring intervention, and contingency routing supporting delivery despite normal transport system interruptions.

Pneumatic tube restrictions establish specific policies regarding high-alert medications unsuitable for automated transport systems due to physical characteristics, stability concerns, or security requirements. Typical restrictions include prohibitions against chemotherapeutic agent transport preventing contamination from container breakage, limitations on fragile high-alert preparations vulnerable to physical stress during transport, and restrictions on controlled substances or other high-risk agents requiring continuous secure custody. These restrictions prevent both medication damage potentially affecting therapeutic effectiveness and security compromises creating diversion opportunities during transport, acknowledging that convenience of automated transport must sometimes yield to safety considerations for highest-risk medications.

Verification at receipt creates additional safety protection by confirming high-alert medication accuracy at the transition between transport and administration environments. Comprehensive verification includes confirmation that the delivered medication matches the ordered therapy, validation of patient-specific preparation against current orders, verification that medication integrity remained intact during transport, and documentation establishing clear custody transfer from transport to administration personnel. Advanced verification systems employ technology support including barcode scanning confirming correct medication selection, photographic verification of medication appearance, and electronic documentation creating verification audit trails. This transition point verification proves particularly valuable for high-alert medications administered in critical care environments where multiple infusions and rapidly changing patient conditions create heightened risk for administration errors if incorrect medications arrive at the point of care.

SAFETY PROTOCOLS

Safety protocols for high-alert medications establish standardized processes addressing unique risk points throughout the medication use continuum, creating consistent safety practices that reduce reliance on individual vigilance or memory. These protocols transform general safety principles into specific operational procedures, establishing clear expectations for high-alert medication management across all practitioners and care settings.

Prescribing Requirements

Restricted prescriber authorization implements tiered prescribing privileges based on expertise, training, and credential verification, limiting high-alert medication ordering to qualified practitioners with demonstrated competence. Comprehensive systems establish medication-specific credentialing requirements rather than broad prescribing categories, recognizing that expertise with one high-alert class doesn't necessarily transfer to others. Implementation approaches include electronic order entry configurations limiting order capability based on verified credentials, formal privilege delineation within credentialing systems, and for highest-risk agents, specialty service consultation requirements before initiation. These restrictions ensure that high-alert medication therapy begins with knowledgeable prescribing decisions aligned with current evidence and patient-specific considerations rather than unfamiliar prescribers potentially unaware of critical risk factors.

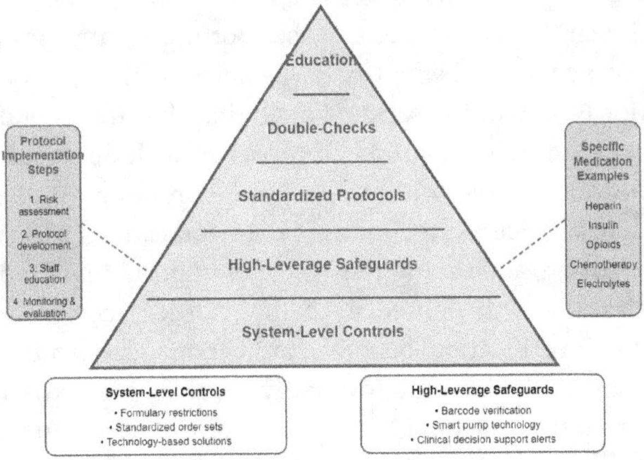

Figure 11.3 Safety Protocol for High-Alert Medications

Standardized order sets transform complex high-alert medication prescribing into structured formats with embedded safety features, reducing reliance on memory while incorporating evidence-based protocols. Effective order sets include weight-based dosing calculators for medications requiring patient-specific dose determination, clinically appropriate dose ranges preventing excessive dosing, required monitoring parameters ensuring appropriate surveillance during therapy, and standard administration instructions eliminating ambiguity. For high-alert medication classes with multiple agents, order sets often include decision support guiding appropriate agent selection based on clinical factors, standardized initial dosing replacing variable practitioner patterns, and tapering schedules when abrupt discontinuation presents risks. This standardization reduces unnecessary variation while embedding safety boundaries within the ordering process rather than relying on downstream detection of potentially inappropriate prescribing.

Indication documentation requirements establish mandatory documentation of therapeutic purpose for high-alert medications, supporting appropriate assessment of benefit-risk balance while enabling verification that the selected agent matches the intended purpose. Implementation approaches include required indication fields within electronic ordering systems, structured selection from approved indications for each medication, and for highest-risk agents, documentation of contraindication absence before order completion. Beyond verification benefits, indication documentation supports clinical monitoring by establishing expected therapeutic outcomes, enables appropriate duration decisions based on treatment purpose, and facilitates discontinuation when the original indication resolves. This explicit purpose documentation proves particularly valuable during care transitions, providing clear therapeutic intent information when new providers assume responsibility for ongoing high-alert medication management.

Independent prescription verification establishes systematic review of high-alert medication orders before implementation, providing expert evaluation of appropriateness independent from the original prescribing decision. Comprehensive verification includes assessment of indication appropriateness, dose evaluation against patient-specific factors (weight, organ function, interacting medications), review of required monitoring parameter specification, and verification of therapy duration appropriateness. Verification responsibility typically resides with clinical pharmacists possessing specialized medication expertise, though some organizations implement physician-to-physician verification for highest-risk agents such as chemotherapy. Implementation approaches range from prospective verification required before order activation to retrospective review within defined timeframes based on urgency and risk assessment, with critical interventions documented to support both individual case correction and system improvement through aggregate pattern analysis.

Administration Procedures

Time-out procedures before high-alert medication administration establish formal pause points for final verification, creating deliberate process interruption that prevents automatic continuation without appropriate safety checks. Comprehensive time-out protocols include verification of patient identity using multiple identifiers, confirmation of medication selection with required re-check of medication label against order, dose calculation verification using independent mathematical process, assessment of current patient status including parameters affecting medication appropriateness, and confirmation of required monitoring capability before administration. For highest-risk medications, structured checklists guide the time-out process, ensuring consistent verification of all critical elements regardless of administrator experience or environmental distractions. This deliberate process interruption proves particularly valuable for high-alert medications where administration represents the final opportunity for error interception before patient exposure.

Two-provider verification for administration creates human redundancy at the critical administration phase, requiring independent assessment by two qualified providers before high-alert medication reaches patients. Unlike simple co-signatures documenting presence, effective two-provider verification requires true independence where each provider performs verification without knowledge of the other's conclusion, structured documentation of specific elements verified by each provider, and clear delineation of verification responsibilities. Implementation approaches include physical presence of both providers during critical phases such as chemotherapy initiation, sequential verification with documentation before continuing administration steps, and for highest-risk agents such as epidural medications, full double-checks at each administration process stage from preparation through delivery.

Special administration techniques for specific high-alert categories address unique risks associated with particular medication classes or administration routes. Chemotherapy administration protocols include extravasation prevention measures, specialized venous access requirements, appropriate sequencing for multi-agent regimens, and emergency response preparation for hypersensitivity reactions.

Table 11.3: Safety Protocols for Specific High-Alert Medications

Medication	Risks	Required Safety Protocols
Insulin	Dosing errors, hypoglycemia	Units-only (no abbreviations) Independent dose verification Standardized concentration
Anticoagulants	Bleeding, drug interactions	Weight-based dosing protocols Monitoring parameters Reversal agent availability
Chemotherapy	Toxicity, dosing errors	Independent verification Body surface area calculation Cumulative dose tracking
Opioids	Respiratory depression, overdose	Conservative initial dosing Monitoring requirements Naloxone availability
Parenteral Nutrition	Electrolyte imbalances, infection	Standardized formulations Compatibility checks Administration protocols

Epidural medication protocols establish specialized connections preventing inadvertent intravenous administration, distinct labeling preventing confusion with parenteral medications, and positioning requirements maximizing intended effect while minimizing systemic absorption. Neuromuscular blocking agent protocols include ventilation capability verification, distinct administration timing separate from sedation, and specialized labeling with paralytic warnings. These medication-specific protocols address unique risks beyond general high-alert safeguards, tailoring protection to specific harm mechanisms associated with different medication categories.

Patient education and engagement strategies transform patients from passive recipients to active participants in high-alert medication safety, creating additional verification through informed recipient involvement. Comprehensive approaches include pre-administration education explaining medication purpose, expected effects, and significant risks; teaching specific warning signs requiring immediate notification; demonstrating appropriate administration techniques for self-administered high-alert medications; and establishing clear communication mechanisms for medication concerns. Advanced engagement strategies include providing patients with expected dose information supporting verification before administration, teaching family members monitoring parameters for high-risk effects, and implementing teach-back methodology confirming actual understanding rather than simply documenting information provision. This engagement proves particularly valuable for high-alert medications where patients often detect subtle adverse effects before they become apparent through clinical assessment.

Specific Medication Class Protocols

Anticoagulant safety protocols address the consistent involvement of these agents in serious medication errors, establishing comprehensive management systems addressing their unique risks. Core protocol elements include standardized dosing tools replacing variable calculation approaches, required baseline and ongoing coagulation monitoring before dose adjustments, structured dose modification algorithms based on laboratory results, and enhanced patient education regarding bleeding risk recognition. Advanced protocols implement anticoagulation management services providing specialized expertise, systematic transition management between different anticoagulants, periprocedural management guidance for interruption and resumption, and reversal agent availability ensuring immediate response capability for bleeding emergencies. These comprehensive approaches address the entire anticoagulant management process rather than isolated administration safeguards, recognizing that anticoagulant safety requires longitudinal management systems beyond point-of-care protections.

Insulin management systems establish specialized protocols for this high-alert medication consistently involved in significant medication errors across diverse healthcare settings. Effective systems include standardized concentration policies eliminating variable insulin dilutions, distinct storage separating insulin from other injectable medications, specialized order sets with safety boundaries preventing extreme dosing, and required blood glucose monitoring coordinated with administration timing. Advanced protocols implement glycemic management services providing specialized expertise for complex regimens, standard correction factor approaches replacing variable practitioner patterns, transitional management guidance between different insulin formulations, and hypoglycemia management protocols ensuring prompt response to adverse effects. These comprehensive systems address both preventable dosing errors and appropriate response systems when adverse effects occur, recognizing insulin's narrow therapeutic index requiring both error prevention and effective complication management.

Chemotherapy safety systems establish specialized protocols addressing both conventional safety concerns and unique risks associated with these high-alert medications including vesicant properties, narrow therapeutic indices, and complex scheduling requirements. Comprehensive approaches include diagnosis and protocol verification before initiation, body surface area calculation double-checks, cumulative dose tracking preventing toxicity from lifetime exposure, and specialized extravasation management protocols. Advanced systems implement computerized prescriber order entry designed specifically for chemotherapy with embedded maximum dose warnings, preparation verification using gravimetric analysis, specialized administration training requirements, and protocol adherence monitoring ensuring appropriate sequencing and timing across multiple cycles. These specialized systems recognize that chemotherapy safety requires domain-specific expertise beyond general medication safety principles, with protocols designed specifically for oncology practice rather than adaptations of general high-alert safeguards.

Opioid stewardship programs establish comprehensive management systems addressing the significant risks associated with these widely used high-alert analgesics. Effective programs include standardized order sets with appropriate dosing ranges based on opioid tolerance assessment, required co-prescribing of naloxone for high-risk patients, automated monitoring of sedation levels and respiratory status during therapy, and structured tapering protocols preventing withdrawal from abrupt discontinuation. Advanced approaches implement pain management consultation services for complex cases, prescription monitoring program integration identifying concerning usage patterns, multimodal analgesia protocols reducing opioid requirements, and opioid-specific patient education addressing both therapeutic expectations and safety concerns. These comprehensive programs address the complete opioid management process from initial prescribing through ongoing monitoring and appropriate discontinuation, recognizing that safety requires systematic approaches beyond isolated administration safeguards.

Emergency Situation Management

Override protocols establish controlled exception processes for urgent situations where standard high-alert medication safeguards could delay critical therapy, balancing safety with clinical urgency. Effective protocols include clear criteria defining qualifying emergency situations, explicit documentation requirements recording override rationale, designated approval authority for override decisions, and specific procedure modifications appropriate during emergencies while maintaining essential safety elements. Implementation approaches typically establish tiered override categories with corresponding requirements based on acuity level and medication risk, ensuring that life-saving medications remain accessible during emergencies while maintaining appropriate safeguards for medications without immediate mortality impact. Post-override review processes determines all exceptions for appropriateness, identifying both legitimate overrides meeting emergency criteria and potential inappropriate circumvention requiring intervention.

Reversal agent availability ensures immediate response capability for high-alert medication adverse effects, establishing systematic access to antidotes or antagonists for highest-risk agents. Comprehensive approaches include standard locations for reversal agents in all areas where corresponding high-alert medications are used, automated dispensing cabinet configuration ensuring reversal agent access without delays, regular inventory verification confirming continuous availability, and clear labeling supporting rapid identification during emergencies. Beyond physical availability, effective programs include systematic education ensuring provider familiarity with reversal indications and dosing, standardized protocols guiding appropriate reversal agent administration, and simulation training preparing providers for rapid response during actual emergencies. This reversal readiness recognizes that despite prevention efforts, adverse effects may still occur with high-alert medications, requiring immediate mitigation capability to limit harm severity.

Standardized emergency response systems establish consistent approaches to high-alert medication emergencies across all care settings, ensuring appropriate resources regardless of incident location. Core elements include standardized emergency notification systems alerting appropriate response teams, consistent emergency cart configurations with relevant reversal agents and resuscitation equipment, clearly defined team member responsibilities during responses, and documented algorithms guiding emergency management. Advanced systems implement simulation training specifically addressing high-alert medication emergencies, rapid response teams with specialized medication expertise, post-event debriefing processes identifying improvement opportunities, and regular protocol updates incorporating lessons from actual events. This systematic approach recognizes that emergency response effectiveness significantly influences harm magnitude when high-alert medication adverse events occur, with organized responses potentially limiting damage from initial medication events.

Documentation and reporting requirements establish clear expectations for recording emergency situations involving high-alert medications, supporting both immediate clinical care and subsequent system improvement. Comprehensive documentation includes detailed chronology of the event with specific timing of symptom onset and interventions, complete medication administration history including doses and administration times, specific patient response to both the medication and subsequent interventions, and laboratory or diagnostic studies obtained during the emergency. Reporting systems capture both adverse events and near-misses in structured formats supporting aggregate analysis, with specific classification identifying high-alert medication involvement to enable focused safety improvement. This documentation serves multiple purposes including clinical care continuity, educational value for similar future situations, quality improvement data supporting system enhancement, and when appropriate, regulatory reporting fulfilling external requirements.

MONITORING SYSTEMS

Monitoring systems for high-alert medications establish systematic surveillance throughout therapy, enabling early detection of adverse effects, efficacy assessment, and appropriate therapy adjustment based on patient response. These systems create essential feedback mechanisms verifying that medications with narrow therapeutic indices and significant toxicity potential remain within safe and effective parameters throughout treatment.

Parameter Selection and Protocols

Physiological parameter monitoring establishes systematic assessment of vital organ function affected by high-alert medications, enabling early detection of adverse effects before serious harm occurs. Comprehensive monitoring includes respiratory parameters for medications affecting ventilatory drive, cardiovascular measures for agents with hemodynamic effects, neurological assessment for medications affecting consciousness or neuromuscular function, and metabolic monitoring for agents affecting electrolyte balance or glucose regulation. Protocol development requires careful parameter selection matching specific medication effects, establishing appropriate assessment frequency balancing detection sensitivity against resource requirements, defining significant change thresholds warranting intervention, and specifying required actions when parameters exceed safety boundaries. These structured approaches transform general awareness of medication risks into specific monitoring expectations consistently applied regardless of individual provider vigilance.

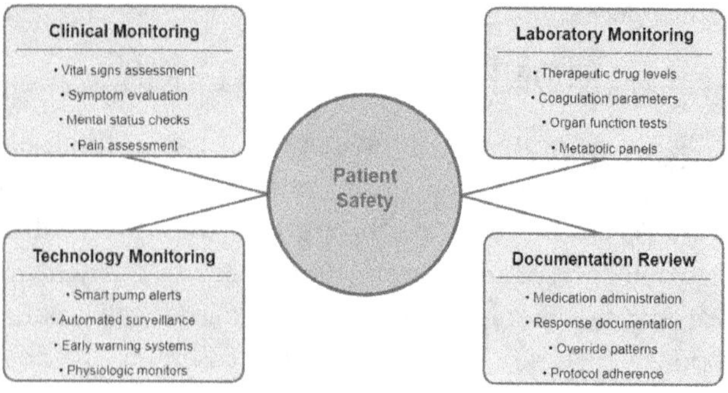

Figure 11.4: Monitoring System Framework for High-Alert Medications

Laboratory monitoring protocols establish systematic assessment of medication effects not readily apparent through clinical observation, providing objective measures of both therapeutic and toxic effects. Effective protocols specify required baseline testing establishing reference points for subsequent comparison, monitoring frequency appropriate to medication pharmacokinetics and risk profile, critical value thresholds requiring immediate intervention, and specific actions required for significant abnormalities. For medications with established therapeutic ranges such as vancomycin, aminoglycosides, or anticonvulsants, protocols typically include timing guidance for sample collection relative to administration, interpretation guidelines for results, and dosage adjustment algorithms based on measured levels. These structured approaches ensure consistent monitoring across different providers and care settings, preventing the common safety gap of appropriate medication initiation without subsequent monitoring to verify safety and effectiveness.

Patient-reported outcome monitoring establishes systematic assessment of subjective effects not captured through physiological measurements or laboratory testing, recognizing that patients often detect meaningful medication effects before they become objectively measurable. Structured approaches include standardized symptom assessment tools administered at defined intervals, specific questioning about known medication effects during routine assessment, threshold criteria for clinically significant symptoms warranting intervention, and documentation systems capturing response patterns across time. Advanced monitoring incorporates electronic symptom reporting between encounters, standardized severity scaling allowing trend identification, and systematic assessment of functional impact beyond simple symptom presence. This subjective monitoring proves particularly valuable for high-alert medications with effects on cognition, comfort, or function that significantly influence therapeutic benefit-risk balance but remain inadequately captured through objective measures alone.

Table 11.4: Monitoring Systems for High-Alert Medications

Monitoring Type	Assessment Parameters	Documentation Requirements
Clinical Monitoring	Vital signs Mental status Pain levels Specific symptoms	Monitoring flowsheets Assessment documentation Intervention documentation
Laboratory Monitoring	Therapeutic drug levels Organ function tests Electrolytes Specific markers	Result documentation Timing of tests Action taken on results
Technology-Based Monitoring	Smart pump alerts Physiologic monitors Automated surveillance	Alert responses Override reasons System checks
Adverse Event Monitoring	ADR detection Near-miss identification Trigger tool surveillance	Event reports Investigation documentation Action plans

Risk-stratified monitoring intensity establishes differentiated surveillance based on patient-specific factors affecting vulnerability to adverse effects, allocating monitoring resources according to actual risk profiles rather than uniform approaches for all patients. Effective stratification considers factors including age extremes affecting medication clearance, organ dysfunction influencing metabolism or elimination, genetic variations affecting medication response, interacting medications potentiating effects or toxicity, and baseline functional status affecting reserve capacity when adverse effects occur. Implementation typically establishes tiered monitoring protocols with increasing intensity for higher-risk situations, specific guidance for monitoring enhancement when risk factors emerge during therapy, and required documentation supporting monitoring decisions for highest-risk scenarios. This personalized approach recognizes that identical medication regimens present significantly different risk profiles in different patients, requiring monitoring customization rather than standardized approaches based solely on medication identity.

Technology-Assisted Monitoring

Continuous physiological monitoring systems provide uninterrupted surveillance of critical parameters affected by high-alert medications, enabling immediate detection of adverse effects without reliance on intermittent assessment. Systems commonly employed include continuous pulse oximetry detecting respiratory depression from opioids, electrocardiographic monitoring identifying arrhythmias or conduction abnormalities from cardiac medications, and hemodynamic monitoring capturing blood pressure changes from vasoactive agents. Advanced implementations include centralized monitoring stations with automated alerting for parameter deviations, alarm customization based on patient-specific baseline values rather than generic thresholds, and sophisticated pattern recognition identifying concerning trends before individual parameters reach critical values. These technological approaches address the fundamental limitation of intermittent manual assessment potentially missing critical changes between scheduled evaluations, particularly valuable during sleep periods or when patients cannot self-report developing symptoms.

Smart infusion pump technology creates continuous monitoring of medication administration parameters, ensuring that delivery remains within predefined safety limits throughout infusion. Core capabilities include drug libraries with predefined concentration options eliminating programming errors, soft limits generating warnings when doses exceed typical ranges, hard limits preventing administration of potentially lethal doses, and automated documentation of all programming changes and limit overrides. Advanced features include interoperability with electronic health records enabling automatic pump programming based on verified orders, weight-based dose calculation verification, secondary infusion coordination preventing delivery sequence errors, and integration with physiological monitoring systems enabling parameter-based infusion adjustment. These technologies create particular value for high-alert medications administered as continuous infusions, where manual programming errors or failure to adjust rates based on patient response represent significant risk points inadequately addressed through traditional process controls.

Clinical decision support systems provide automated surveillance of high-alert medication therapy, identifying potential safety issues through continuous electronic monitoring of medication orders, laboratory values, and patient parameters. Basic implementations include automated alerts for laboratory abnormalities related to medication effects, dosage warnings when orders exceed safety thresholds, and interaction notifications when new medications potentially affect existing high-alert therapy. Sophisticated systems implement surveillance algorithms integrating multiple data points to identify complex safety issues, predictive analytics identifying patients at elevated risk for adverse effects before occurrence, and symptom pattern recognition detecting medication toxicity signatures across seemingly unrelated clinical manifestations. These systems extend monitoring capability far beyond human surveillance capacity, continuously evaluating thousands of potential safety signals across entire patient populations to identify issues requiring human attention and intervention.

Telehealth monitoring extends high-alert medication surveillance beyond traditional healthcare environments, enabling professional oversight during home administration of agents previously restricted to supervised settings. Implementation approaches include video observation of self-administration techniques ensuring appropriate preparation and delivery, remote physiological monitoring transmitting critical parameters to healthcare teams, electronic symptom reporting with automated triage based on severity, and scheduled virtual assessment by specialized pharmacists or nurses. Advanced programs implement escalation protocols with tiered response based on finding severity, remote monitoring equipment specifically designed for home use without technical expertise requirements, and integration with emergency response systems for critical situations requiring immediate intervention. These approaches enable safe administration of high-alert medications in home environments previously considered too risky without direct professional supervision, increasing patient convenience while maintaining appropriate safety oversight.

Response Systems and Escalation

Alert parameter definition establishes objective thresholds for monitoring findings requiring clinical intervention, ensuring consistent response to potentially significant changes regardless of individual interpretation variability. Comprehensive definitions include numerical boundaries for quantitative parameters (laboratory values, vital signs, pain scores), descriptive criteria for qualitative assessments (mental status changes, functional limitations, subjective symptoms), and trend patterns requiring attention even when individual values remain within broad normal ranges. Effective implementation includes tiered alert levels distinguishing findings requiring immediate intervention from those warranting increased monitoring or scheduled reassessment, context-sensitive thresholds accounting for patient-specific factors affecting interpretation, and explicit documentation requirements when monitoring reveals significant deviations. These defined parameters transform general monitoring into actionable information with clear intervention triggers rather than subjective judgments about finding significance.

Escalation protocols establish standardized response pathways when monitoring identifies concerning findings, ensuring appropriate and timely intervention proportional to clinical significance. Structured protocols define specific actions required at each alert level, responsible personnel for different response components, appropriate timeframes for intervention completion, and required documentation of both findings and resulting actions. Implementation approaches include algorithm-based response guidance eliminating uncertainty about appropriate actions, automated notification systems alerting responsible providers about significant findings, backup notification pathways when primary responders prove unavailable, and verification systems confirming intervention completion within required timeframes. These formalized responses prevent the common safety gap where concerning findings receive appropriate documentation but delayed or inconsistent intervention, particularly valuable for high-alert medications where rapid response often significantly influences outcome severity.

Interdisciplinary response teams provide specialized expertise for complex high-alert medication issues identified through monitoring, supplying advanced management capabilities beyond primary team resources. These teams typically include clinical pharmacists with advanced pharmacotherapy knowledge, physicians with specific expertise in complicated medication management, and specially trained nurses experienced in complex medication response situations. Implementation models include dedicated response teams available through formal consultation for non-urgent situations, rapid response capabilities for emergent issues requiring immediate specialized intervention, and proactive rounding specifically reviewing high-risk medication regimens before problems develop. These specialized resources prove particularly valuable for unusual adverse effects requiring sophisticated management, complex pharmacokinetic issues necessitating advanced dosing adjustments, or multifaceted medication interactions requiring coordinated modification of multiple interacting therapies.

Trigger response documentation creates comprehensive records of monitoring findings, resulting interventions, and patient outcomes, supporting both immediate clinical care and retrospective quality improvement. Thorough documentation includes specific monitoring findings triggering intervention, assessment details clarifying clinical significance, interventions implemented with timing and responsible providers, subsequent monitoring confirming response appropriateness, and final resolution status of the identified issue. Beyond individual case management, aggregate documentation enables systematic analysis identifying common triggers requiring protocol refinement, intervention patterns suggesting education or resource needs, and outcome trends demonstrating system effectiveness. This documentation transforms individual clinical responses into organizational learning opportunities, using each monitoring-triggered intervention as data supporting continuous improvement of both monitoring parameters and response systems.

Quality Assurance and Improvement

Monitoring compliance assessment evaluates actual performance against established monitoring standards, identifying gaps between expected and actual surveillance of high-alert medications. Effective assessment includes regular chart review examining documentation of required monitoring parameters, timing verification confirming appropriate monitoring frequency, completeness evaluation ensuring all protocol elements receive attention, and intervention review verifying appropriate response to significant findings. Automated approaches increasingly supplement manual review through electronic health record reporting identifying missing documentation, laboratory system alerts for overdue monitoring tests, and electronic medication administration record analysis revealing gaps in required assessments. These compliance evaluations prevent the common quality gap where well-designed monitoring protocols exist on paper but receive inconsistent implementation in actual practice, particularly during high-workload periods when monitoring activities may receive lower priority than more visible care aspects.

Adverse event analysis specifically determines monitoring effectiveness during actual patient harm situations, evaluating whether existing surveillance detected developing problems appropriately and triggered timely intervention. Comprehensive analysis includes detailed event timeline reconstruction identifying earliest detectable indication of developing problems, comparison between actual monitoring performed and protocol requirements, assessment of appropriate monitoring interpretation when findings appeared, evaluation of response timeliness when significant results emerged, and identification of potential monitoring enhancements that might improve future detection. This focused examination extends beyond general adverse event review to specifically address monitoring system performance, recognizing that well-designed surveillance should identify developing problems before significant harm occurs when functioning as intended.

Monitoring parameter refinement establishes systematic processes for updating surveillance requirements based on emerging evidence, experience with actual events, and evolving medication usage patterns. Effective refinement includes regular literature review identifying new information about medication effects requiring monitoring adjustment, analysis of monitoring patterns revealing parameters consistently normal or consistently abnormal suggesting potential modification, evaluation of false positive alerts creating unnecessary interventions, and assessment of alert fatigue patterns indicating potential threshold adjustment requirements. Formal review processes typically involve interdisciplinary input ensuring both clinical relevance and practical feasibility, pilot testing of proposed changes before widespread implementation, and appropriate documentation supporting monitoring modifications. This continuous refinement prevents monitoring ossification where outdated parameters continue despite emerging evidence suggesting better alternatives, ensuring that surveillance remains aligned with current knowledge rather than historical patterns.

Monitoring technology optimization creates ongoing enhancement of electronic systems supporting high-alert medication surveillance, addressing both technical capabilities and human factors aspects affecting effectiveness. Implementation includes regular review of alert override patterns identifying potential threshold adjustments or format improvements, monitoring workflow analysis revealing integration opportunities enhancing efficiency, evaluation of false negative patterns where significant issues escaped electronic detection, and assessment of documentation burden potentially creating shortcuts compromising quality. Advanced approaches implement human factors engineering methodologies specifically examining monitoring system usability, incorporate frontline user feedback in system refinement, and conduct simulation testing of proposed changes before production implementation. This continuous optimization recognizes that initial technology implementation represents starting point rather than final solution, with ongoing refinement essential as both technology capabilities and clinical knowledge evolve over time.

Things to Remember

☑ High-alert medications require specialized safety systems due to elevated harm risk when used incorrectly, with standardized identification using evidence-based classification methodologies.

☑ Special handling includes segregated storage preventing selection errors, restricted access, concentration standardization reducing calculation requirements, and distinctive labeling ensuring recognition.

☑ Safety protocols establish consistent practices through restricted prescribing authorization, standardized order sets, independent verification requirements, and medication-specific protocols for high-risk categories.

☑ Monitoring systems provide essential surveillance through systematic physiological assessment, laboratory monitoring, patient-reported outcome tracking, and technology-assisted continuous monitoring.

☑ Response protocols with clearly defined parameters, interdisciplinary intervention teams, and escalation pathways ensure appropriate action when monitoring identifies concerning patterns.

☑ Quality assurance processes verifying monitoring effectiveness, compliance with specialized protocols, and appropriate response to identified issues complete comprehensive high-alert medication management.

Multiple Choice Questions

1. High-alert medications are primarily identified based on:

   a) Medication cost and reimbursement considerations

   b) Elevated harm risk when used incorrectly

   c) Frequency of prescription within the organization

   d) Complexity of administration techniques

2. Which organization provides widely recognized high-alert medication lists that serve as the foundation for many institutional programs?

   a) Centers for Disease Control and Prevention (CDC)

   b) American Medical Association (AMA)

   c) Institute for Safe Medication Practices (ISMP)

   d) World Health Organization (WHO)

3. Special handling requirements for high-alert medications might include:

   a) Storage with similar-looking medications to improve efficiency

   b) Standardized concentrations and limited variety of strengths

   c) Verbal orders as the preferred ordering method

   d) Calculation of doses without verification tools

4. Safety protocols for high-alert medications typically include:

   a) Independent verification focused only on controlled substances

b) Standardized order sets embedding safety parameters

c) Simplified administration techniques without double-checks

d) Limited documentation requirements to save time

5. Which of the following is NOT typically classified as a high-alert medication?

   a) Insulin

   b) Anticoagulants

   c) Neuromuscular blocking agents

   d) First-generation cephalosporins

6. Monitoring systems for high-alert medications should include:

   a) Assessment limited to the primary intended effect of the medication

   b) Documentation only when abnormal findings are present

   c) Systematic physiological parameter assessment based on medication risks

   d) Identical monitoring parameters regardless of specific medication

7. Concentration standardization for high-alert medications:

   a) Is unnecessary with computerized calculations

   b) Reduces calculation requirements and potential errors

   c) Should be avoided to ensure dose flexibility

   d) Is primarily important for oral but not parenteral medications

8. Which approach to high-alert medication safety provides the highest level of protection

according to the hierarchy of effectiveness?
a) Warning labels identifying high-alert status
b) Policies requiring double-checking
c) Staff education about high-alert medications
d) Forcing functions preventing dangerous combinations

9. Distinctive labeling for high-alert medications:
a) Should be identical across all medication categories
b) Is unnecessary with electronic medication records
c) Ensures immediate recognition throughout the medication use process
d) Works best when subtle and understated

10. Medication-specific protocols for anticoagulants would typically include:
a) Standard dosing without laboratory monitoring
b) Administration by any available staff member
c) Standardized reversal protocols and monitoring parameters
d) Limited documentation of therapeutic response

Self-Assessment Questions

1. Analyze the criteria and methods used to identify and classify high-alert medications, evaluating evidence-based approaches to prioritization and risk assessment.
2. Critically evaluate special handling requirements for high-alert medications across different healthcare settings, including storage, preparation, dispensing, and administration safeguards.
3. Discuss comprehensive safety protocols for three different classes of high-alert medications, analyzing their effectiveness in preventing serious medication errors.
4. Evaluate monitoring systems for high-alert medications, including parameters, frequency, documentation, and response protocols for adverse events.
5. Analyze the unique risks and safety considerations associated with anticoagulants, discussing comprehensive approaches to reduce harm from these high-alert medications.
6. Discuss the challenges and strategies in implementing double-check procedures for high-alert medications, including considerations for effectiveness and workflow integration.
7. Evaluate the role of technology in improving high-alert medication safety, including smart pumps, automated dispensing, and clinical

decision support systems.

8. Analyze the educational needs of healthcare professionals regarding high-alert medications and effective strategies for knowledge dissemination and competency assessment.
9. Discuss standardization approaches for high-alert medications, including concentrations, dosing units, administration rates, and labeling, with evidence for their impact on safety.
10. Evaluate the ethical considerations in managing high-alert medications, including resource allocation, access restrictions, and balancing safety with clinical necessity

Bibliography

1. Institute for Safe Medication Practices. ISMP List of High-Alert Medications in Acute Care Settings. Horsham, PA: Institute for Safe Medication Practices; 2018.
2. Cohen MR, Smetzer JL, Tuohy NR, Kilo CM. High-alert medications: safeguarding against errors. In: Cohen MR, editor. Medication Errors. 2nd ed. Washington, DC: American Pharmacists Association; 2010. p. 317-411.
3. Federico F. The Five Rights of Medication Administration. Cambridge, MA: Institute for Healthcare Improvement; 2015.
4. Sakowski J, Newman JM, Dozier K. Severity of medication administration errors detected by a bar-code medication administration system. Am J Health Syst Pharm. 2008;65(17):1661-6.
5. Grissinger M. Your high-alert medication list is relatively useless without associated risk-reduction strategies. P T. 2016;41(10):598-600.
6. World Health Organization. Control of Concentrated Electrolyte Solutions. Patient Safety Solutions. 2007;1(5):1-3.
7. Paparella S. High-alert medications: shared accountability for risk identification and error prevention. J Emerg Nurs. 2010;36(5):476-8.
8. The Joint Commission. Sentinel Event Alert 11: High-alert medications and patient safety. Sentinel Event Alert. 1999 Nov 19.
9. Phillips J, Beam S, Brinker A, Holquist C, Honig P, Lee LY, et al. Retrospective analysis of mortalities associated with medication errors. Am J Health Syst Pharm. 2001;58(19):1835-41.
10. Manias E, Williams A, Liew D. Interventions to reduce medication errors in adult intensive care: a systematic review. Br J Clin Pharmacol. 2012;74(3):411-23.

CHAPTER 12

SAFETY PROGRAMS

Abstract

Safety programs establish systematic approaches to medication error prevention through structured systems supporting consistent practices across organizations. Program development begins with comprehensive needs assessment identifying specific vulnerabilities, proceeds through stakeholder engagement building essential support, continues with governance structure creation establishing clear authority, and culminates with standardized processes ensuring consistent application. Resource allocation transforms conceptual designs to operational reality through financial budgeting with return-on-investment analysis, human resource models establishing appropriate staffing, technology assessment supporting system selection, and educational resource development enabling knowledge transfer. Staff training creates necessary capabilities through baseline knowledge establishment, role-specific competency development, diverse methodologies including simulation and case-based learning, and reinforcement strategies maintaining skills beyond initial education. Evaluation methods provide accountability through balanced metrics addressing outcomes, processes and structural elements; systematic data collection with appropriate statistical analysis; regular review cadences ensuring consistent attention; and transparent reporting creating visibility throughout the organization.

Keywords: *Program infrastructure, Resource requirements, Competency development, Performance metrics, Continuous evaluation*

Learning Objectives

After completion of the chapter, the learners should be able to:

- Remember the essential components of medication safety program development.
- Understand how resource allocation supports effective implementation of safety initiatives.
- Apply appropriate staff training methodologies to develop medication safety competencies.
- Analyze evaluation methods to determine the effectiveness of safety programs.
- Evaluate the impact of program structure on medication safety outcomes.
- Create a comprehensive medication safety program addressing organizational needs.

PROGRAM DEVELOPMENT

Safety program development establishes systematic approaches to medication safety improvement, creating organized systems that transform safety principles into operational practices. Effective development processes build sustainable programs addressing organizational needs while incorporating evidence-based practices and regulatory requirements.

Needs Assessment and Gap Analysis

Comprehensive evaluation of existing safety systems provides essential foundation for program development, identifying both strengths to leverage and vulnerabilities requiring attention. This process typically includes analysis of historical medication safety events revealing recurring patterns, review of near-miss reports highlighting prevention opportunities, assessment of current safety practices against established standards, and comparison with industry benchmarks identifying performance gaps. Advanced methodologies incorporate structured self-assessment tools such as the ISMP Medication Safety Self-Assessment, safety culture surveys measuring staff perceptions and attitudes, simulation exercises testing system responses to safety challenges, and proactive risk assessments identifying potential failure points before actual events occur.

Gap prioritization establishes strategic focus for program development, ensuring that limited resources address highest-impact opportunities rather than dispersing effort across all identified needs. Effective prioritization methodologies consider multiple dimensions including potential harm severity, event probability, affected population size, available evidence supporting specific interventions, implementation feasibility, and alignment with organizational priorities. Structured approaches employ formal prioritization matrices incorporating weighted scoring across these dimensions, creating objective comparison between diverse improvement opportunities. This prioritization transforms potentially overwhelming gap inventories into manageable implementation sequences, preventing program stagnation from attempting simultaneously to address all identified needs.

Stakeholder engagement throughout development creates programs reflecting diverse perspectives while building essential support for implementation. Comprehensive engagement includes involvement of frontline staff experiencing daily medication processes, patients and families bringing unique safety perspectives, organizational leadership providing resources and authority, quality departments contributing methodology expertise, and information technology personnel supporting technical aspects of safety systems. Effective engagement methodologies range from formal committee structures with designated representation to focused workgroups addressing specific program elements, supplemented by broader feedback mechanisms ensuring that perspectives beyond formal participants receive consideration. This inclusive approach creates both stronger programs incorporating multiple viewpoints and essential implementation support from stakeholders who participated in development.

Regulatory compliance integration ensures that safety programs address mandatory requirements while maintaining focus on patient safety rather than mere regulatory satisfaction. Comprehensive integration reviews requirements from multiple authorities including federal regulations, state pharmacy laws, accreditation standards, professional organization guidelines, and payer quality programs. Effective approaches align required elements with broader safety goals, incorporating regulatory requirements within comprehensive programs rather than establishing separate compliance-focused initiatives disconnected from overall safety strategy. This integration prevents the common scenario where parallel systems address similar safety concerns through different mechanisms due to artificial separation between regulatory compliance and quality improvement, creating unnecessary duplication while potentially missing valuable synergies.

Program Structure

Vision and mission development establishes foundational purpose and direction for medication safety programs, creating shared understanding of ultimate goals and organizational commitment. Effective vision statements articulate aspirational end-states (e.g., "Zero preventable medication harm through systems supporting safe practice") while mission statements define operational purpose (e.g., "Develop, implement, and continuously improve medication systems that prevent errors and minimize harm"). These statements provide essential context for specific program elements, ensuring that tactical initiatives connect to strategic safety goals. Beyond content, development process significantly influences impact, with inclusive creation involving diverse stakeholders creating broader ownership than executive-dictated statements disconnected from frontline experience.

Governance structure design establishes decision-making systems, accountability mechanisms, and authority relationships supporting program implementation and ongoing operations. Effective structures typically include executive-level oversight committees providing strategic direction and resource authorization, operational committees managing implementation and daily functions, and working groups addressing specific program elements requiring specialized expertise. Clear delineation of responsibilities, decision authorities, reporting relationships, and performance expectations creates functional governance rather than merely formal structures. Program maturity often influences appropriate governance, with early development typically requiring stronger central coordination while mature programs may benefit from more distributed responsibility supporting local innovation within established systems.

Integration with quality infrastructure prevents medication safety isolation by establishing clear connections with broader quality and safety systems. Effective integration includes alignment with organizational quality committees creating bidirectional information flow, coordination with enterprise risk management addressing liability implications of medication safety, connection with regulatory compliance ensuring consistent approach to external requirements, and cohesion with patient safety programs beyond medication-specific concerns. This integration prevents medication safety from becoming disconnected silo with unique methodologies, inconsistent approaches, and resource competition against other quality priorities. Successful integration maintains medication safety visibility and specialized focus while leveraging broader quality resources and methodologies.

Standardized processes and tools establish consistent approaches to common safety activities, creating reliability and efficiency through elimination of unnecessary variation. Core standardization typically addresses adverse event investigation with consistent methodology and documentation, intervention implementation with standardized project management approaches, safety data collection using uniform definitions and methods, and program communication employing consistent formats and channels. Well-designed standardization establishes sufficient structure ensuring consistency while allowing appropriate flexibility for context-specific adaptation. This standardization prevents the inefficiency and variable quality resulting from continuously reinventing approaches to recurring safety activities, creating efficiency through consistent methodology while enabling meaningful comparison across different program components.

Implementation Planning

Phased implementation strategies establish realistic deployment sequences preventing overwhelming change while maintaining momentum toward comprehensive program development. Effective approaches typically begin with foundation elements creating essential infrastructure, proceed through high-priority interventions addressing greatest risks, continue with broader system enhancements expanding safety coverage, and culminate with advanced elements optimizing mature programs. Detailed planning addresses dependencies ensuring that necessary precursors precede dependent elements, resource limitations preventing simultaneous initiatives exceeding organizational capacity, and appropriate sequencing building early success supporting subsequent changes. This phased approach prevents both analysis paralysis from attempting perfect initial design and implementation failure from excessive simultaneous change overwhelming organizational capacity.

Project management methodology application brings structured discipline to implementation, ensuring that planned initiatives translate into operational reality through systematic execution processes. Comprehensive application includes clear project definition with specific scope boundaries, detailed work breakdown structures identifying component tasks, realistic timelines with milestone tracking, resource allocation with clear responsibility assignments, risk assessment identifying potential barriers, and regular status reporting maintaining accountability. Advanced implementation employs dedicated project management personnel for complex initiatives, standardized documentation ensuring consistent approach across multiple projects, and portfolio management balancing resource allocation across competing priorities. This disciplined approach prevents the common pattern where excellent program designs fail to achieve practical implementation due to inadequate execution processes.

Communication planning establishes strategic approaches for information sharing throughout program development and implementation, ensuring that all stakeholders maintain appropriate awareness while preventing information overload. Effective planning addresses multiple dimensions including audience identification with specific information needs, message development tailored to different stakeholder perspectives, channel selection matching communication goals and recipient preferences, and timing coordination ensuring appropriate information flow throughout implementation phases. Advanced approaches develop standardized communication templates ensuring consistent format and content, establish regular cadences creating predictable information flow, and implement feedback mechanisms confirming message receipt and understanding. This structured communication prevents both information gaps leaving key stakeholders unaware of important developments and excessive communication creating message fatigue and attention dilution.

Resistance management strategies proactively address the inevitable challenges to significant safety program changes, transforming potential opposition into constructive engagement. Comprehensive approaches begin with stakeholder analysis identifying groups likely affected by planned changes, proceed through impact assessment understanding specific concerns, continue with engagement strategies addressing identified issues, and establish ongoing feedback mechanisms detecting emerging resistance. Specific techniques include early involvement of potential resisters in program design, transparent communication about change rationale and expected benefits, pilot implementation demonstrating value before broader deployment, opinion leader engagement creating peer influence supporting adoption, and success celebration reinforcing value realization. This proactive management prevents the common scenario where technically sound safety programs fail to achieve intended benefits due to workforce resistance undermining effective implementation.

Table 12.1: Medication Safety Program Development

Development Phase	**Activities**	**Success Indicators**
Assessment	Gap analysis Safety culture survey Risk prioritization	Comprehensive risk profile Prioritized gap list Baseline measurements
Planning	Goal establishment Initiative selection Timeline development	Specific objectives Resource requirements Implementation timeline
Implementation	Pilot testing Policy development Education rollout	Milestone completion Adoption metrics Process measures
Sustainability	Monitoring systems Performance feedback Continuous improvement	Sustained compliance Outcome improvements Process integration

Documentation and Policies

Program charter development creates formal authorization and structural definition, establishing legitimate organizational foundation for medication safety activities. Comprehensive charters include purpose statements articulating program goals, scope definitions establishing boundaries and responsibilities, authority descriptions clarifying decision rights, membership specifications for governance bodies, operating procedures for routine activities, and resource commitments supporting program functions. Beyond content, approval process significantly influences program standing, with executive endorsement establishing clear organizational priority. This formal documentation transforms medication safety from informal initiative to authorized organizational function, creating sustainability beyond individual champions while establishing clear legitimacy for program activities.

Policy and procedure development translates program systems into operational guidance, creating clear expectations for safety practices throughout the medication use system. Effective development includes identification of critical processes requiring standardization, evidence review establishing best practice foundations, stakeholder input ensuring operational feasibility, clear writing in actionable language, appropriate approval reflecting organizational governance, and systematic implementation including education and competency verification. Beyond individual documents, comprehensive policy systems establish hierarchical structures with clear relationships between high-level policies, detailed procedures, and department-specific work instructions. This operational guidance transforms general safety principles into specific practice expectations, creating consistency across departments, shifts, and individual practitioners.

Role and responsibility documentation establishes clear accountability for medication safety functions, preventing critical activities from falling between organizational boundaries while avoiding unnecessary duplication. Detailed documentation specifies responsible parties for core functions including adverse event investigation, intervention implementation, data analysis, regulatory reporting, staff education, and technology safety evaluation. Effective approaches ensure appropriate alignment between responsibility, authority, and capability, preventing accountability assignments without corresponding decision rights or necessary resources. Beyond specific safety team roles, comprehensive documentation addresses medication safety responsibilities for all disciplines involved in medication use, creating shared responsibility culture rather than delegating safety solely to designated specialists.

Version control and document management systems ensure that current standards remain readily accessible while maintaining historical documentation for reference and regulatory purposes. Effective systems include standardized formatting creating consistent document appearance, systematic review cycles ensuring content currency, approval workflows maintaining appropriate governance, distribution mechanisms delivering updates to affected staff, access controls protecting sensitive information, and archival procedures preserving historical versions. Advanced approaches implement electronic document management systems supporting automated workflows, version tracking, access monitoring, and integration with training records. This systematic management prevents the common safety risk where multiple versions circulate simultaneously, creating confusion about current standards while potentially perpetuating outdated practices contrary to current safety evidence.

RESOURCE ALLOCATION

Resource allocation transforms safety program designs from conceptual systems to operational reality through strategic distribution of financial, human, and technological resources supporting implementation and sustained operations. Effective allocation balances competing priorities while ensuring that critical safety functions receive necessary support for successful execution.

Financial Resources

Budget development establishes financial foundations for medication safety programs, translating programmatic needs into specific resource requirements supporting implementation and ongoing operations. Comprehensive development includes detailed cost estimation for personnel requirements, technology investments, education programs, consulting services, and operational expenses; anticipation of both implementation and sustaining costs across multiple budget cycles; consideration of potential offsets from adverse event reduction, efficiency improvements, and reduced liability exposure; and alignment with organizational budget processes ensuring appropriate timing and format. Beyond technical components, effective budget development includes strategic positioning emphasizing safety investment benefits rather than merely expense requests, comparison with industry benchmarks establishing appropriate funding levels, and contingency planning addressing potential resource constraints.

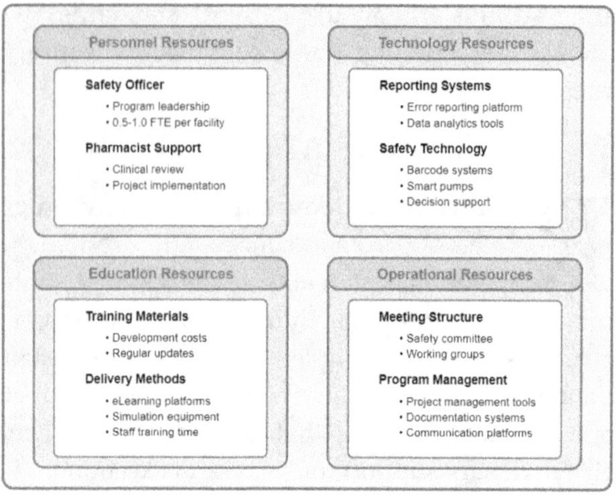

Figure 12.1 Resource Allocation Model for Medication Safety

Return on investment analysis supports resource allocation decisions through systematic evaluation of expected benefits relative to required investments, creating objective comparison between competing priorities. Comprehensive analysis includes quantification of direct financial benefits from adverse event reduction (reduced treatment costs, shortened lengths of stay, decreased readmissions), indirect benefits from improved operational efficiency, and avoidance costs from reduced liability exposure; comparison with implementation and operational costs over appropriate timeframes; calculation of standard financial metrics including return on investment percentage, payback period, and net present value; and sensitivity analysis testing how result variations affect conclusions. This analysis supports both initial program funding decisions and ongoing resource allocation adjustments, transforming safety investments from perceived cost centers to strategically justified initiatives with demonstrable financial benefits beyond direct patient safety improvements.

Grant and external funding opportunities expand available resources beyond internal organizational budgets, potentially accelerating program development while reducing direct financial impact. Effective strategies include systematic monitoring of funding opportunities from government agencies, private foundations, professional organizations, and industry partners; development of compelling proposals aligned with funder priorities while addressing organizational needs; cultivation of potential funding relationships before specific opportunities arise; and creation of appropriate infrastructure managing grant requirements including reporting, compliance, and sustainability planning. Successful approaches recognize external funding as program acceleration rather than fundamental support, maintaining core operational funding through internal mechanisms while utilizing external resources for enhancements, expansions, or specialized initiatives requiring additional investment beyond baseline operations.

Cost-sharing models distribute financial responsibilities across departments benefiting from medication safety improvements, preventing concentration of expenses within safety departments while actual benefits accrue elsewhere. Implementation approaches include charge-back mechanisms allocating direct safety staff costs to supported departments, shared funding models for technology investments benefiting multiple areas, departmental contributions to central safety budgets proportional to size or risk exposure, and performance-based models where departments realizing greatest safety improvements receive corresponding budget enhancements. These models transform medication safety from isolated cost center to distributed responsibility with shared financial commitment, creating broader organizational investment while aligning financial incentives with safety improvement rather than maintaining traditional budget silos disconnected from improvement outcomes.

Human Resources

Staffing models establish personnel systems supporting medication safety functions, creating appropriate capacity for program development, implementation, and ongoing operations. Comprehensive models address multiple dimensions including overall staffing ratios (typically expressed as dedicated safety full-time equivalents per organizational size metrics), skill mix between professional disciplines (pharmacists, nurses, physicians, quality specialists), role distribution between central and distributed functions, and appropriate reporting relationships ensuring necessary authority. Model development considers factors including organizational complexity, technology sophistication, regulatory environment, historical safety performance, and patient population risk characteristics. Effective models balance centralized expertise providing specialized knowledge with distributed personnel supporting local implementation, creating appropriate coverage while maximizing impact from limited dedicated resources.

Medication safety specialist development creates essential expertise beyond general clinical knowledge, establishing specialized capability for advanced safety functions requiring specific competencies. Development pathways include formal certification programs such as Certified Professional in-Patient Safety (CPPS), specialized fellowship or residency training focusing on medication safety, mentored practice under experienced safety professionals, and progressive responsibility expansion building practical expertise through supervised experience. Beyond individual development, organizational approaches include dedicated budget allocation for advanced training, career ladder structures recognizing and rewarding progressive expertise development, and succession planning ensuring program continuity despite individual transitions. This specialized development recognizes that effective medication safety requires specific knowledge and skills beyond general clinical practice, justifying dedicated investment in personnel development rather than assuming that clinical expertise automatically creates safety expertise.

Table 12.2: Resource Allocation for Medication Safety Programs

Resource Type	Essential Components	ROI Measures
Personnel	Safety officer Dedicated pharmacists Unit champions	Error reduction per FTE Intervention value Avoided costs
Technology	Clinical decision support Reporting systems Analytics tools	Error reduction rates Time savings Prevented harm costs
Educational	Training materials Simulation resources Knowledge assessment tools	Knowledge improvement Behavior change Error reduction
Physical	Safety zones Workspace design Storage systems	Error reduction Workflow efficiency Staff satisfaction

Committee structure and participation establishes

formal mechanisms for broader workforce engagement beyond dedicated safety personnel, extending program reach while incorporating diverse perspectives into safety activities. Effective structures typically include medication safety committees with multidisciplinary representation overseeing program direction, specialized workgroups addressing specific improvement initiatives, unit-based safety teams implementing local adaptations, and appropriate connections with organizational quality and governance committees. Participation expectations balance representation breadth ensuring diverse perspectives against practical size limitations affecting meeting effectiveness, with common approaches including core membership for essential perspectives supplemented by ad hoc participation for specific topics requiring additional expertise. This structured engagement extends safety program human resources far beyond dedicated personnel, creating force multiplication through distributed participation while building broader organizational safety culture through expanded involvement.

Leadership engagement strategies secure essential executive support converting strategic priorities into operational resources, ensuring that medication safety receives appropriate organizational attention and investment. Effective approaches include regular safety data presentation in leadership forums, executive participation in adverse event review processes, leadership rounding focusing specifically on medication safety concerns, direct reporting relationships between safety leadership and executive positions, and integration of safety metrics into leadership performance evaluation. Advanced strategies involve executives in safety program activities beyond passive reporting review, creating direct experience with medication processes rather than abstracted data review disconnected from operational reality. This engagement transforms safety from isolated technical function to strategic priority with corresponding resource allocation, establishing necessary foundation for successful program implementation beyond conceptual support without practical resource commitment.

Technology Resources

Technology assessment and selection creates systematic evaluation of potential safety technologies, ensuring appropriate investment in systems offering greatest safety improvement potential. Comprehensive assessment includes structured needs analysis identifying specific safety vulnerabilities potentially addressed through technology, market evaluation of available solutions, capability comparison against requirements, total cost of ownership calculation including implementation and ongoing operational expenses, and organizational readiness evaluation for successful adoption. Effective selection processes involve multidisciplinary teams including safety specialists, end users, information technology personnel, and financial representatives, creating balanced evaluation beyond vendor presentations or technical specifications alone. This systematic approach prevents both technology acquisition without clear safety purpose and missed opportunities where beneficial technologies remain unimplemented due to inadequate evaluation processes or misalignment with actual safety needs.

Implementation resource planning establishes realistic support requirements for technology deployment, addressing the substantial resources necessary beyond initial acquisition costs. Detailed planning includes staffing requirements for implementation teams, training resources for end-user education, technical support capacity during transition periods, project management personnel coordinating complex implementations, and operational adjustments accommodating productivity impacts during implementation phases. Effective planning considers timing coordination between multiple initiatives preventing simultaneous demands exceeding capacity, sequencing establishing logical progression building on previous implementations, and resource smoothing preventing extreme peaks and valleys in support requirements. This comprehensive planning prevents the common scenario where technically sound safety technologies fail to achieve intended benefits due to inadequate implementation support, creating disappointing results despite significant acquisition investments.

Integration with existing technology creates cohesive systems rather than isolated safety applications, establishing information flow supporting comprehensive safety functions across technological boundaries. Key integration priorities typically include connections between electronic health records and safety reporting systems enabling automated data extraction, linkages between smart infusion pumps and medication administration records creating closed-loop documentation, interfaces between pharmacy systems and clinical decision support ensuring consistent information presentation, and data warehouse connections supporting aggregate safety analytics across multiple source systems. Effective integration planning considers both technical interface requirements and workflow implications, creating seamless user experiences rather than fragmented interactions across multiple systems. This connected approach prevents safety technology islands operating independently from core clinical systems, addressing the patient safety risks created when critical information remains trapped within technological silos inaccessible at key decision points.

Technology support and maintenance ensures sustained functionality beyond initial implementation, recognizing that safety benefits require ongoing technical support rather than one-time deployment. Comprehensive support includes dedicated personnel for system administration and routine maintenance, regular update schedules keeping systems current with vendor enhancements and security requirements, systematic testing processes validating continued functionality after changes, performance monitoring identifying emerging issues before critical failures, and established support pathways addressing user questions and technical problems. Resource allocation specifically designates ongoing operational funding rather than solely implementation capital, preventing the common pattern where initially successful safety technologies gradually deteriorate without sustained support. This continued investment maintains technology safety benefits throughout system lifecycles rather than experiencing progressive degradation undermining initial improvement gains.

Educational Resources

Training program development establishes systematic approaches to safety knowledge and skill development, creating workforce capability supporting effective program implementation and operation. Comprehensive development includes needs assessment identifying specific knowledge gaps, curriculum design addressing identified needs with appropriate learning objectives, teaching methodology selection matching content requirements, faculty development ensuring quality instruction, and evaluation planning measuring both learning outcomes and behavioral application. Effective programs employ adult learning principles emphasizing practical application rather than merely theoretical knowledge, case-based methodologies connecting safety principles to actual practice scenarios, and multimodal approaches addressing diverse learning preferences. This structured development transforms general safety awareness into specific competencies supporting actual practice change, bridging the common gap between conceptual understanding and operational application.

Simulation and skills laboratory resources provide protected learning environments for safety practice development, enabling experience with high-risk situations without patient safety consequences. Effective simulation programs include dedicated physical spaces designed for realistic practice, appropriate equipment supporting authentic experience, trained facilitators guiding learning processes, and debriefing methodologies transforming experience into structured learning. Applications particularly valuable for medication safety include high-alert medication administration scenarios, emergency response to medication adverse events, communication practices during critical situations, and team coordination during complex medication processes. These experiential learning opportunities create practical skill development beyond didactic education alone, addressing the reality that many safety practices require procedural competence and teamwork capabilities rather than merely conceptual understanding.

Just-in-time learning resources support immediate knowledge access during actual work processes, addressing the limitations of traditional education removed from practice contexts. Implementation approaches include point-of-care references embedded within workflow systems, quick-reference guides located at medication preparation stations, mobile applications providing immediate medication information access, and mentor availability for real-time consultation during complex situations. Design considerations include information organization supporting rapid retrieval, content conciseness providing essential guidance without excessive detail, and format optimization for actual work environment constraints. These resources acknowledge the impossibility of retaining all necessary safety information through traditional education alone, creating supportive knowledge environments extending learning beyond formal training sessions into daily practice where actual safety decisions occur.

Staff release time allocation provides essential workforce availability for safety education participation, addressing the reality that training without attendance opportunity creates theoretical programs without practical impact. Effective allocation includes dedicated education time within regular scheduling, coverage arrangements maintaining operations during training sessions, appropriate distribution across shifts and departments ensuring comprehensive participation rather than convenient attendance, and accountability mechanisms ensuring actual utilization for intended purposes. Budgetary approaches include specific funding designated for education time rather than expecting departments to absorb costs within existing operational budgets, creating financial support for participation rather than education competing against immediate productivity demands. This deliberate allocation transforms safety education from theoretical availability to practical reality, addressing the common gap between developed programs and actual workforce participation.

STAFF TRAINING

Staff training establishes the knowledge, skills, and attitudes necessary for effective medication safety practices, creating workforce capability that translates safety programs from conceptual designs to operational reality. Comprehensive training addresses both technical competencies and safety culture development, recognizing that successful implementation requires both specific practice capabilities and supportive belief systems.

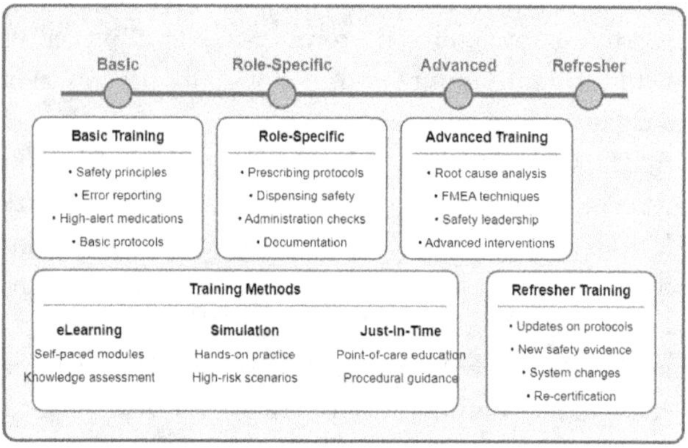

Figure 12.2: Medication Safety Staff Training

Core Competency Development

Baseline safety knowledge establishes fundamental understanding required by all staff involved in medication processes, creating common foundation supporting specific role-based competencies. Core content typically includes basic medication safety principles, common error mechanisms and prevention strategies, organizational reporting systems and procedures, just culture concepts supporting appropriate accountability, and specific high-alert medication risks relevant across disciplines. Effective approaches establish tiered knowledge expectations with universal baseline requirements complemented by role-specific knowledge appropriate to different positions, ensuring relevant content without unnecessary detail beyond specific responsibilities. This foundational knowledge creates shared understanding supporting interdisciplinary communication, appropriate risk recognition, and coordinated safety efforts across diverse roles rather than fragmented perspectives lacking common conceptual framework.

Table 12.3: Staff Training Models for Medication Safety

Training Approach	Best Applications	Implementation Methods
Foundational Training	New staff orientation, basic concepts	eLearning modules Competency validation Knowledge assessment
Role-Specific Training	Specialized functions, high-risk tasks	Simulation training Hands-on workshops Skills validation
Just-in-Time Training	New processes, urgent safety issues	Point-of-care instruction Quick reference guides Safety huddles
Team-Based Training	Interprofessional processes, handoffs	Interprofessional simulation Team exercises Communication tools

Role-specific competency identification establishes clear expectations for safety practices within specific positions, translating general safety principles into concrete behavioral requirements. Comprehensive identification includes systematic review of position responsibilities identifying safety-critical functions, risk assessment of potential failure points within role-specific activities, evidence review establishing best practices for identified risks, and translation into observable behaviors supporting clear performance expectations. Development typically involves collaboration between safety specialists contributing theoretical knowledge and frontline staff providing practical expertise, creating competency definitions reflecting both evidence-based practices and operational realities. This specific delineation transforms general safety awareness into concrete performance expectations, bridging the gap between conceptual safety principles and actual work practices necessary for error prevention.

Competency verification processes establish objective assessment of safety knowledge and skills, ensuring that educational efforts translate into actual capability rather than merely documented attendance. Effective verification includes knowledge assessment through testing or structured discussion, skills evaluation through direct observation or simulation performance, and behavioral assessment through workplace observation during actual practice. Advanced approaches implement competency verification schedules appropriate to criticality and complexity, with high-risk activities requiring more frequent reassessment than stable, lower-risk functions. Documentation systems maintain comprehensive records supporting both individual development planning and regulatory compliance, creating evidence trails beyond simple class rosters. This verification transforms safety training from activity completion to demonstrated capability, addressing the common gap between educational participation and actual practice competence.

Remediation and improvement planning establishes structured approaches when competency verification identifies performance gaps, creating supportive pathways to capability development rather than merely punitive consequences. Comprehensive planning includes root cause analysis identifying specific deficit sources (knowledge gaps, skill limitations, system barriers), individualized improvement plans addressing identified causes, resource identification supporting development activities, timeline establishment with milestone checkpoints, and reassessment processes confirming gap closure. Effective approaches emphasize improvement support rather than punitive orientation, recognizing that most competency gaps reflect system limitations in training, resources, or expectations rather than individual negligence or intentional noncompliance. This constructive approach addresses safety competency development as continuous improvement process rather than binary judgment, creating learning culture supporting ongoing development rather than fear-driven compliance focus.

Training Methodologies

Simulation-based training creates experiential learning opportunities for safety-critical activities, enabling practice with high-risk situations in protected environments before actual patient care application. Implementation ranges from simple role-playing exercises requiring minimal resources to sophisticated high-fidelity simulations with realistic environments and equipment. Applications particularly valuable for medication safety include high-alert medication preparation and administration, adverse event response and management, critical communication during safety events, and interdisciplinary coordination during complex medication processes. Effective design includes realistic scenario development reflecting actual practice challenges, appropriate fidelity matching learning objectives, skilled facilitation guiding experience without excessive intervention, and structured debriefing transforming experience into conceptual learning. This experiential approach addresses the limitations of didactic education for procedural and teamwork skills, creating practical capability development beyond theoretical knowledge.

Case-based learning employs actual safety events as educational foundation, connecting abstract safety principles to concrete situations while creating emotional engagement supporting retention and application. Comprehensive implementation includes case selection representing important safety concepts, appropriate de-identification protecting privacy while maintaining essential elements, structured discussion guides focusing attention on key learning points, and application activities translating case insights into practice changes. Effective facilitation balances psychological safety allowing honest discussion against accountability for improvement, avoiding both blame orientation undermining open conversation and consequence minimization diminishing improvement motivation. This methodology transforms safety events from isolated incidents to organizational learning opportunities, creating valuable educational resources from otherwise costly experiences while demonstrating commitment to transparency and improvement rather than concealment.

Team-based training approaches acknowledge the

interdisciplinary nature of medication safety, developing collaborative capabilities across professional boundaries rather than isolated role-specific skills. Implementation includes multidisciplinary participation in training sessions, scenario design incorporating multiple role perspectives, explicit attention to communication and coordination skills, and facilitation techniques addressing professional hierarchy issues potentially impeding open communication. Specific methodologies demonstrating effectiveness include TeamSTEPPS providing structured communication tools and coordination strategies, crew resource management adapting aviation team concepts to healthcare, and interprofessional simulation developing practical collaboration experience. This team focus addresses the reality that medication safety primarily fails at interface points between disciplines rather than within isolated professional activities, creating collaborative capability essential for comprehensive safety systems transcending individual vigilance.

Academic detailing and peer coaching establish individualized learning through direct workplace interaction, addressing the limitations of classroom education separated from actual practice environments. Implementation includes identification of credible peer coaches or academic detailers with both subject expertise and teaching capability, training in effective coaching techniques, protected time allocation for coaching activities, and documentation systems tracking interventions and outcomes. Effective approaches emphasize collaborative problem-solving rather than directive instruction, adaptation to individual learning needs and styles, connection with actual work challenges rather than theoretical scenarios, and progressive skill development through ongoing relationships rather than isolated interactions. This methodology creates sustainable behavior change through workplace-embedded learning, addressing the common gap between classroom knowledge and actual practice application in complex clinical environments.

Training Program

Scheduling and accessibility strategies ensure that developed training programs reach intended audiences, addressing the common gap between educational availability and actual workforce participation. Effective strategies include multiple session scheduling across various times accommodating different shifts and work patterns, recording options for staff unable to attend live sessions, unit-based delivery bringing education to work locations rather than requiring travel to central training facilities, and protected time allocation ensuring participation opportunity without compromising patient care or requiring off-duty attendance. Advanced approaches include capacity planning matching educational frequency with workforce size and turnover, coordination between competing educational requirements preventing scheduling conflicts, and prioritization systems ensuring critical safety training receives appropriate emphasis among multiple learning requirements. This deliberate accessibility planning transforms training programs from theoretical availability to actual workforce participation, addressing the reality that even excellent educational content proves ineffective without successful delivery to intended audiences.

Trainer development ensures that educational quality matches content importance, recognizing that effective safety education requires specific teaching skills beyond subject matter expertise alone. Comprehensive development includes instructor selection based on both content knowledge and teaching aptitude, formal training in adult education principles and methods, practice opportunities with feedback supporting skill development, and ongoing coaching addressing identified improvement opportunities. Advanced approaches implement trainer certification processes ensuring consistent quality standards, peer observation providing developmental feedback, and communities of practice supporting continued growth through shared experience. This investment acknowledges that educator capability significantly influences learning outcomes, justifying specific resource allocation for trainer development rather than assuming that subject expertise automatically creates teaching effectiveness for critical safety content.

Documentation systems establish comprehensive records of safety training activities, supporting both individual development tracking and organizational compliance with regulatory requirements. Effective systems include participant tracking with attendance verification, content documentation preserving specific topics covered, competency assessment records beyond mere participation documentation, and longitudinal tracking enabling analysis of training patterns and needs. Implementation considerations include integration with broader learning management systems preventing duplicate documentation requirements, accessibility for both individual participants and managers needing subordinate information, appropriate privacy protections for performance-related data, and reporting capabilities supporting both individual and aggregate analysis. This systematic documentation transforms training from isolated educational events to managed development processes, creating continuity across multiple learning experiences while maintaining necessary records for regulatory compliance and performance management.

Reinforcement and sustainment strategies address the natural degradation of knowledge and skills over time, maintaining safety capabilities between formal training intervals through systematic reinforcement activities. Implementation approaches include regular safety huddles reviewing key concepts and recent events, periodic skills refreshers addressing critical but infrequently used capabilities, safety newsletters or electronic communications reinforcing important principles, and leader rounding with intentional safety knowledge assessment and reinforcement. Effective strategies recognize the forgetting curve phenomenon where information retention decreases predictably without reinforcement, implementing systematic sustainment activities proportional to information criticality and usage frequency. This ongoing reinforcement transforms safety training from episodic events to continuous learning processes, addressing the reality that even excellent initial training proves insufficient without systematic maintenance activities supporting retention and application.

Specialized Training

High-alert medication training establishes enhanced knowledge and skills for medications presenting elevated harm risk, ensuring capability commensurate with potential consequences of errors. Comprehensive programs address specific high-alert classes with dedicated modules beyond general medication safety training, including detailed pharmacology affecting safe use, common error patterns with prevention strategies, required safety protocols and verification procedures, monitoring parameters with appropriate response thresholds, and reversal or rescue measures for adverse events. Implementation typically employs tiered approaches with universal awareness training for all staff complemented by detailed competency development for personnel directly involved in high-alert medication processes. Verification standards generally exceed those for routine medications, with more frequent reassessment, higher performance thresholds, and more rigorous documentation requirements. This specialized training acknowledges that medications with severe harm potential warrant elevated learning investment beyond standard approaches appropriate for lower-risk agents.

New technology training supports safe implementation of medication-related technologies, addressing the safety risks created when sophisticated systems receive inadequate user preparation. Effective approaches begin with needs assessment identifying specific knowledge and skill requirements for safe operation, proceed through curriculum development addressing both technical functions and safety implications, continue with hands-on practice in simulated environments before live implementation, and conclude with workplace support during initial usage periods. Advanced methodologies include role-specific training targeting different user needs, competency verification before independent system use, identification of super-users providing peer support, and post-implementation assessment identifying emerging learning needs after initial experience. This comprehensive preparation prevents the common scenario where safety technologies fail to deliver intended benefits due to inadequate user capability, transforming potential safety enhancements into actual practice improvements through appropriate user development.

New staff orientation establishes safety foundation for personnel entering the organization, creating immediate integration into existing safety systems rather than delayed enculturation through experience alone. Comprehensive orientation includes organization-specific safety event reporting procedures, particular high-alert medications emphasized within the setting, local safety technology operation, specific protocols and procedures beyond general professional knowledge, and communication channels for safety concerns or questions. Effective delivery balances information volume against absorption capacity, typically implementing phased approaches addressing immediate necessities before comprehensive coverage, connecting general safety principles with specific organizational applications, and providing ongoing support resources recognizing impossible complete retention from initial sessions. This deliberate orientation acknowledges that new personnel present elevated safety risk regardless of previous experience, requiring specific safety acculturation beyond general professional competence or previous organizational patterns.

Leadership safety training develops specialized capabilities for personnel with management responsibility, addressing their unique role in safety culture development and system management. Content typically includes safety leadership behaviors influencing frontline practices, just culture principles guiding appropriate accountability, safety event review facilitation skills, improvement methodology for system enhancement, resource allocation supporting safety initiatives, and performance management approaches addressing safety behavior. Implementation considerations include appropriate timing relative to leadership assumption, connection with broader leadership development rather than isolated safety training, practical application opportunities embedded within actual responsibilities, and peer networking supporting continued development through shared experience. This specialized development acknowledges that leadership significantly influences organizational safety performance beyond technical system design, creating capability for the critical cultural and managerial functions that transform theoretical safety programs into operational realities affecting daily practice.

EVALUATION METHODS

Evaluation methods establish systematic assessment of medication safety program effectiveness, providing objective determination of actual impact rather than assumed benefits from implementation activities alone. Comprehensive evaluation creates accountability for results while identifying improvement opportunities, supporting appropriate resource allocation based on demonstrated outcomes rather than theoretical expectations.

Metrics and Measurement Systems

Outcome metrics assess actual safety results achieved through program interventions, measuring direct patient impact rather than merely implementation activities or intermediate processes. Core outcome measures typically include adverse drug event rates capturing actual patient harm, severity-categorized medication error frequencies, preventable medication-related readmissions, and when available, medication-related mortality. Advanced measurement employs risk-adjusted methodologies accounting for patient population differences affecting expected event rates, uses multidimensional harm scales rather than binary presence/absence classification, and implements detection methodologies beyond voluntary reporting such as trigger tool reviews identifying events through clinical markers. These outcome assessments provide ultimate evaluation of program effectiveness, determining whether safety activities translate into actual patient benefit beyond process compliance or implementation completion.

Process metrics evaluate adherence to safety practices expected to reduce harm, providing earlier feedback than outcome measures while maintaining clearer connection to specific interventions. Common process measurements include compliance rates with established safety protocols, technology utilization metrics such as barcode scanning percentages or clinical decision support response patterns, safety documentation completeness, and high-alert medication verification process adherence. Effective implementation typically establishes clear operational definitions ensuring measurement consistency, employs sampling methodologies balancing comprehensive assessment against resource requirements, and implements risk-stratified approaches concentrating measurement resources on highest-impact processes. These assessments provide valuable intermediate evaluation before outcome changes become apparent, enabling rapid intervention when expected safety practices show compliance gaps rather than waiting for adverse outcomes to reveal process failures.

Structural metrics assess safety system components and resources, evaluating fundamental program elements supporting process reliability and outcome improvement. Typical structural measures include safety staffing ratios relative to organizational size, technology implementation percentages, policy and procedure completeness against established standards, safety committee functioning based on attendance and action completion, and training program enrollment capturing workforce participation in safety education. Effective measurement approaches consider both presence and quality of structural elements, moving beyond binary existence verification to functionality assessment determining whether structures operate as designed. These foundational assessments determine whether basic safety program components exist and function appropriately, providing essential context for process and outcome evaluation by establishing whether fundamental safety infrastructure supports expected practices and results.

Table 12.4: Evaluation Methods for Medication Safety Programs

Evaluation Type	Data Collection Methods	Reporting Approach
Process Evaluation	Direct observation Documentation audit System reports	Process control charts Compliance dashboards Implementation tracking
Outcome Assessment	Incident reports Chart review Trigger tools	Pre/post comparison Trend analysis Benchmarking
Return on Investment	Financial analysis Comparative outcomes Utilization data	Cost-benefit analysis Value demonstration Resource justification
Program Impact	Safety surveys Staff interviews Program assessment	Comprehensive evaluation Program development Strategic planning

Balanced scorecard approaches integrate multiple metric types into comprehensive evaluation systems, acknowledging that single-dimension assessment provides incomplete perspective on complex safety programs. Implementation typically includes selection of complementary metrics across outcome, process, and structural domains; establishment of appropriate weighting reflecting organizational priorities; development of visual display formats supporting meaningful interpretation; and regular review cycles with defined response expectations for different performance patterns. Advanced approaches incorporate leading indicators predicting future performance, lagging indicators confirming historical results, internal metrics tracking organizational progress against baseline, and external comparisons establishing performance context against broader standards. This multidimensional evaluation prevents narrow focus on isolated metrics that might create misleading impressions of overall program effectiveness, establishing comprehensive assessment supporting balanced improvement rather than distorted emphasis on limited measurement aspects.

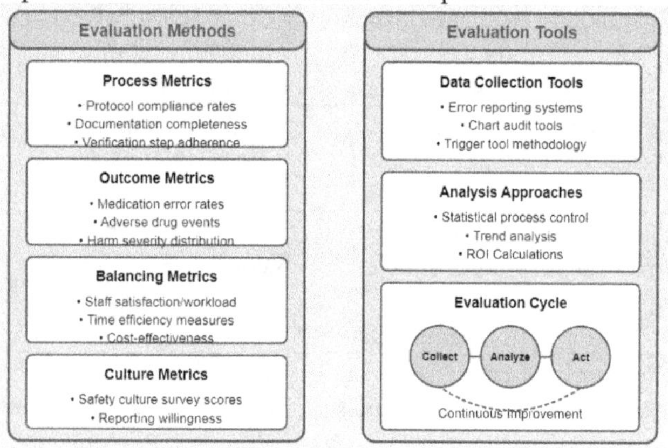

Figure 12.3 Medication Safety Program Evaluation

Data Collection and Analysis

Data source identification establishes information foundations for safety evaluation, determining both possibilities and limitations for program assessment. Comprehensive identification catalogs available sources including electronic health record data, incident reporting systems, pharmacy dispensing records, automated dispensing cabinet transactions, smart infusion pump logs, claims and liability information, and patient satisfaction or experience surveys. Effective assessment includes detailed understanding of each source's strengths and limitations, including capture comprehensiveness, data quality characteristics, accessibility for analysis purposes, historical availability for trending, integration capabilities with other sources, and potential biases affecting interpretation. This systematic inventory prevents both missed evaluation opportunities where valuable data remains unutilized and misguided assessment based on incomplete understanding of data limitations, creating realistic evaluation plans matched to actual information availability rather than theoretical measurement ideals beyond practical implementation.

Statistical methodology application brings analytical rigor to safety data interpretation, distinguishing meaningful patterns from random variation that might prompt inappropriate conclusions or actions. Basic applications include calculation of rates with appropriate denominators enabling meaningful comparison, trend analysis identifying significant changes over time, and comparative assessment determining performance relative to relevant benchmarks. More sophisticated approaches implement statistical process control methods distinguishing special cause variation requiring investigation from common cause variation representing expected system performance fluctuation, risk adjustment techniques accounting for population differences affecting expected event rates, and multivariate analysis identifying complex relationships between system factors and safety outcomes. This methodological rigor prevents both overreaction to normal performance variation and underresponse to significant safety signals, supporting appropriate improvement resource allocation based on valid statistical interpretation rather than anecdotal impression.

Qualitative assessment complements quantitative measures with contextual understanding, addressing the reality that numbers alone often inadequately capture complex safety dynamics. Implementation approaches include structured focus groups exploring safety perceptions and experiences, observational studies directly assessing safety practice implementation in clinical environments, safety culture surveys measuring beliefs and attitudes affecting behavior, and narrative analysis from event descriptions identifying themes beyond quantitative categorization. Effective qualitative assessment employs systematic methodologies ensuring analytical rigor beyond anecdotal impression, including representative sampling strategies, standardized data collection protocols, multiple analyst review reducing individual interpretation bias, and formal thematic analysis identifying consistent patterns across information sources. This complementary assessment adds essential context to quantitative findings, explaining why observed patterns occur rather than merely documenting their existence.

Data integration and visualization creates meaningful presentation from complex safety information, transforming raw data into actionable intelligence supporting program evaluation and improvement. Comprehensive approaches include data warehouse development aggregating information across multiple source systems, standardized definitions and taxonomies enabling meaningful combination, automated extraction and transformation processes maintaining current information, and appropriate data governance ensuring quality and security. Effective visualization employs principles including clear purpose definition for each display, appropriate format selection matching information characteristics and audience needs, visual hierarchy emphasizing most important elements, contextual information supporting interpretation, and interactive capabilities enabling exploration beyond static presentation. This translation from raw data to meaningful display prevents the common scenario where valuable safety information exists but remains underutilized due to accessibility or comprehension barriers, creating usable intelligence supporting both evaluation and improvement rather than mere data collection without practical application.

Performance Review Processes

Regular review cadences establish systematic evaluation timing, ensuring consistent attention to safety performance rather than sporadic assessment driven by events or external requirements. Effective cadence structures typically implement multiple review cycles with different frequencies and focuses: daily reviews addressing immediate safety concerns, weekly assessments monitoring short-term performance patterns, monthly evaluations tracking progress against improvement goals, quarterly reviews assessing broader performance trends, and annual comprehensive program evaluations. Implementation considerations include alignment with organizational meeting structures preventing duplicate reviews, appropriate participation ensuring necessary expertise and authority, standardized agenda creating review consistency, and clear responsibility assignment for identified actions. This deliberate timing creates reliable assessment rather than haphazard evaluation, establishing safety program accountability through predictable review expectations rather than intermittent attention lacking sustained focus.

Board and leadership review processes establish executive-level safety accountability, creating appropriate governance oversight beyond operational management. Effective processes include regular safety performance presentation in board meetings, structured reporting systems highlighting main metrics and significant events, clear explanation connecting technical information to governance implications, and explicit action expectations establishing accountability for identified issues. Implementation considerations include appropriate information synthesis preventing excessive detail obscuring important patterns, comparative data providing performance context, presentation formats accessible to non-clinical audiences, and connection between safety performance and strategic organizational priorities. This governance-level review establishes medication safety as board responsibility rather than delegated technical function, creating appropriate accountability at highest organizational levels for this fundamental quality and risk management domain.

Peer review and external assessment provide objective evaluation beyond internal perspective, addressing potential limitations from organizational blind spots or cultural normalization of problematic practices. Implementation approaches include participation in collaborative benchmarking programs comparing performance against similar organizations, external consultant review providing expert assessment against industry standards, accreditation surveys evaluating against established regulatory requirements, and peer exchange programs where similar organizations review each other's safety systems. Effective external assessment balances standardized evaluation against organization-specific context, employs reviewers with appropriate expertise and credibility, establishes non-punitive systems encouraging transparent sharing, and creates actionable recommendations rather than merely general observations. This external perspective complements internal evaluation with fresh viewpoints and broader comparative context, identifying improvement opportunities potentially overlooked within organizational boundaries while validating successful approaches against external standards.

Action planning processes translate evaluation findings into performance improvement, connecting assessment to actual practice change rather than merely documenting current state. Comprehensive planning includes root cause analysis for identified deficiencies, intervention development addressing fundamental causes rather than symptoms, responsibility assignment creating clear accountability for implementation, timeline establishment with milestone tracking, resource allocation supporting necessary actions, and follow-up mechanisms verifying effective implementation. Effective processes implement priority setting ensuring focus on highest-impact opportunities, feasibility assessment preventing unrealistic planning, collaborative development involving affected stakeholders, and appropriate approval ensuring necessary authority for significant changes. This deliberate connection between evaluation and action prevents the common quality gap where assessment becomes isolated documentation exercise without corresponding improvement, establishing complete evaluation cycles where findings drive actual safety enhancement rather than merely recording current performance.

Transparent Reporting and Communication

Internal performance communication establishes appropriate information sharing throughout the organization, creating awareness supporting both accountability and improvement beyond designated safety personnel. Effective approaches include tiered reporting matching information detail to audience needs and responsibilities, standardized formats creating consistent presentation across reporting cycles, balanced presentation acknowledging both successes and improvement opportunities, and clear connection between performance data and expected actions. Implementation considerations include appropriate distribution timing coordinated with improvement activities, accessibility ensuring information reaches intended audiences, understandable presentation avoiding technical jargon limiting comprehension, and feedback mechanisms confirming effective communication rather than merely information transmission. This transparency transforms safety performance from isolated quality department knowledge to organizational awareness, creating shared understanding supporting improvement beyond formal safety roles.

External reporting strategies address appropriate transparency with stakeholders outside the organization, balancing meaningful disclosure against potential misinterpretation or liability concerns. Considerations include regulatory reporting requirements establishing mandatory disclosures, voluntary transparency initiatives demonstrating organizational commitment to accountability, patient communication regarding specific safety events or identified risks, and community reporting establishing public trust through appropriate disclosure. Effective approaches implement standardized reporting formats enabling meaningful comparison, provide contextual information supporting appropriate interpretation, establish review processes ensuring accuracy before external release, and develop communication strategies addressing potential reactions to disclosed information. This external transparency acknowledges broader stakeholder interest in safety performance beyond organizational boundaries, establishing appropriate accountability while managing potential misunderstanding risks inherent in complex safety information.

Patient and family communication establishes appropriate safety information sharing with those directly affected by medication processes, acknowledging their legitimate interest in performance affecting their care. Implementation approaches include inclusion of safety metrics in patient-facing quality materials, specific communication about safety initiatives affecting patient experience, appropriate disclosure following adverse events, and engagement mechanisms gathering patient perspectives on safety priorities and concerns. Effective communication employs plain language accessible to non-medical audiences, honest presentation acknowledging both strengths and improvement opportunities, balanced information supporting informed decision-making without creating unnecessary anxiety, and appropriate privacy protection while maintaining meaningful transparency. This patient-centered communication recognizes that those receiving care represent primary stakeholders in safety performance, establishing appropriate information sharing supporting both informed choice and collaborative safety partnership.

Improvement story dissemination creates narrative understanding beyond metric presentation, using specific safety enhancement examples to illustrate broader program effectiveness and approach. Implementation includes identification of compelling improvement examples demonstrating main program elements, structured documentation capturing both process and outcomes, appropriate anonymization protecting involved individuals while maintaining essential elements, and strategic sharing through multiple channels including newsletters, organizational meetings, orientation programs, and external publications when appropriate. Effective approaches balance quantitative results with human impact illustration, acknowledge challenges alongside successes creating authentic rather than sanitized narratives, and connect specific improvements to broader safety principles supporting generalization beyond individual examples. This narrative approach complements metric-based evaluation with concrete illustrations making abstract safety concepts tangible, creating memorable understanding beyond statistical presentation while demonstrating practical program impact through specific examples rather than general assertions.

Things to Remember

- ☑ Program development begins with comprehensive needs assessment, proceeds through stakeholder engagement, continues with governance structure creation, and culminates with standardized processes ensuring consistent application.
- ☑ Resource allocation includes financial budgeting with return-on-investment analysis, human resource models establishing appropriate staffing, technology assessment, and educational resource development.
- ☑ Staff training creates necessary capabilities through baseline knowledge establishment, role-specific competency development, diverse methodologies including simulation, and reinforcement strategies maintaining skills.
- ☑ Evaluation methods provide accountability through balanced metrics addressing outcomes, processes and structural elements; systematic data collection; regular review; and transparent reporting.
- ☑ Successful safety programs require executive sponsorship providing necessary authority and resources beyond technical design excellence.
- ☑ Integration with broader organizational quality initiatives prevents isolated safety efforts disconnected from related improvement activities.

Multiple Choice Questions

1. Safety program development typically begins with:
   a) Implementing technological solutions
   b) Comprehensive needs assessment identifying specific vulnerabilities
   c) Staff disciplinary procedures for error prevention
   d) Regulatory compliance documentation
2. Effective governance structure for safety programs includes:
   a) Responsibility assigned exclusively to pharmacy departments
   b) Clear authority and reporting relationships with executive involvement
   c) Minimal committee structure to reduce administrative burden
   d) Focus on regulatory reporting without clinical integration
3. Resource allocation for safety programs should include:
   a) Equal distribution across all potential safety initiatives
   b) Focus exclusively on technology acquisition
   c) Financial budgeting with return-on-investment analysis
   d) Minimal staffing to reduce operational costs
4. Staff training for medication safety programs ideally incorporates:
   a) One-time orientation without ongoing reinforcement
   b) Identical content for all roles and departments

c) Diverse methodologies including simulation and case-based learning
d) Theoretical concepts without practical application

5. Evaluation methods for safety programs should:
   a) Focus exclusively on outcome measures like adverse event rates
   b) Include balanced metrics addressing outcomes, processes, and structural elements
   c) Prioritize staff satisfaction over safety outcomes
   d) Minimize data collection to reduce burden
6. Which approach to program development best supports sustainability?
   a) Implementing multiple simultaneous initiatives without prioritization
   b) Focusing exclusively on technology without workflow consideration
   c) Stakeholder engagement building essential support throughout development
   d) Rapid implementation without pilot testing or evaluation
7. Human resource models for safety programs should establish:
   a) Minimal dedicated staffing to reduce costs
   b) Appropriate staffing based on organization size and program scope
   c) Responsibility exclusively within quality departments without clinical involvement
   d) Centralized structure without unit-based representatives

8. Effective safety program communication strategies include:
   a) Limited information sharing to prevent potential liability
   b) Technical language demonstrating program sophistication
   c) Transparent reporting creating visibility throughout the organization
   d) Focus on negative outcomes to motivate improvement
9. Integration with broader organizational quality initiatives:
   a) Is unnecessary as safety programs function best in isolation
   b) Prevents fragmented approaches addressing similar issues through different methodologies
   c) Should be avoided to maintain program independence
   d) Is primarily important for marketing purposes
10. Staff competency development for medication safety:
    a) Is best achieved through written materials alone
    b) Should focus exclusively on pharmacists and physicians
    c) Requires baseline knowledge establishment and role-specific skill development
    d) Is complete after initial orientation without ongoing assessment

Self-Assessment Questions

1. Analyze the main elements of a comprehensive medication safety program development process, from initial assessment through implementation and evaluation.
2. Evaluate strategies for effective resource allocation in medication safety programs, including budgeting, staffing, technology investments, and return on investment analysis.
3. Critically analyze approaches to staff training in medication safety, including learning methods, content development, competency assessment, and maintenance of knowledge.
4. Discuss methods for evaluating medication safety programs, including selection of metrics, data collection strategies, analysis techniques, and translation into program improvements.
5. Analyze how organizational culture influences the effectiveness of medication safety programs and strategies for cultivating a supportive safety culture.
6. Evaluate the governance structures necessary for successful medication safety programs, including leadership roles, committee functions, and reporting relationships.
7. Discuss the integration of medication safety programs with other organizational initiatives such as quality improvement, risk management, and regulatory compliance.
8. Analyze strategies for sustaining medication

safety programs over time, addressing challenges of program fatigue, leadership changes, and competing priorities.

9. Evaluate approaches to medication safety program implementation across different healthcare settings (acute care, ambulatory, long-term care) and the unique considerations for each.
10. Discuss the role of external partnerships (professional organizations, collaboratives, vendors) in enhancing medication safety programs and facilitating knowledge sharing.

Bibliography

1. Wachter RM, Pronovost PJ. Balancing "no blame" with accountability in patient safety. N Engl J Med. 2009;361(14):1401-6.
2. Agency for Healthcare Research and Quality. A Framework for Safety Across the Care Continuum. Rockville, MD: AHRQ; 2016.
3. Weick KE, Sutcliffe KM. Managing the Unexpected: Resilient Performance in an Age of Uncertainty. 2nd ed. San Francisco: Jossey-Bass; 2007.
4. Singer SJ, Vogus TJ. Reducing hospital errors: interventions that build safety culture. Annu Rev Public Health. 2013;34:373-96.
5. Smetzer JL, Cohen MR. Lessons from the Denver medication error/criminal negligence case: look beyond blaming individuals. Hosp Pharm. 1998;33(6):640-57.
6. Nieva VF, Sorra J. Safety culture assessment: a tool for improving patient safety in healthcare organizations. Qual Saf Health Care. 2003;12 Suppl 2:ii17-23.
7. Schneider PJ, Pedersen CA, Montanya KR, Curran CR, Harpe SE, Bohenek W, et al. Improving the safety of medication administration using an interactive CD-ROM program. Am J Health Syst Pharm. 2006;63(1):59-64.
8. Reason JT. Managing the Risks of Organizational Accidents. Aldershot: Ashgate; 1997.
9. Pronovost P, Needham D, Berenholtz S, Sinopoli D, Chu H, Cosgrove S, et al. An intervention to decrease catheter-related bloodstream infections in the ICU. N Engl J Med. 2006;355(26):2725-32.
10. Kaplan HC, Brady PW, Dritz MC, Hooper DK, Linam WM, Froehle CM, et al. The influence of context on quality improvement success in health care: a systematic review of the literature. Milbank Q. 2010;88(4):500-59.

CHAPTER 13

EMERGENCY PREPAREDNESS

Abstract

Emergency preparedness establishes medication safety continuity during disruptions through proactive planning for situations threatening normal operations. Crisis management systems include early warning systems enabling timely identification, standardized incident command structures establishing clear authority, tiered decision-making processes matching response to emergency severity, and documentation systems maintaining accountability despite modified operations. Medication safety during emergencies employs adapted approaches including tiered safety systems implementing appropriate modifications based on crisis severity, simplified high-alert protocols maintaining essential safeguards, alternative distribution models addressing infrastructure disruptions, and enhanced monitoring compensating for reduced preventive systems. Contingency planning creates proactive readiness through vulnerability assessment identifying system weaknesses, scenario development establishing concrete planning contexts, alternative care site preparation, and workforce continuity strategies ensuring personnel availability despite community-wide disruptions. Disaster response addresses catastrophic situations through crisis standards of care implementation acknowledging necessary practice modifications, medication triage systems allocating limited supplies based on clinical priority, strategic national stockpile access procedures, and specialized approaches for vulnerable populations including chronic disease patients.

Keywords: *Crisis adaptation, Contingency preparedness, Supply management, Triage, Vulnerability assessment*

Learning Objectives

After completion of the chapter, the learners should be able to:

- Remember the key components of crisis management systems for medication safety.
- Understand how medication safety practices must adapt during emergency situations.
- Apply appropriate contingency planning methods to maintain medication safety during disruptions.
- Analyze the unique medication safety challenges presented by different emergency scenarios.
- Evaluate the effectiveness of disaster response strategies in preserving essential medication safety functions.
- Create comprehensive emergency medication management plans addressing different crisis scenarios.

CRISIS MANAGEMENT

Crisis management establishes systematic approaches to maintaining medication safety during acute events that disrupt normal operations, creating structured response capabilities that protect patients despite challenging circumstances. Comprehensive crisis management integrates preparation, response, and recovery activities into cohesive systems supporting medication safety throughout emergency situations.

Crisis Recognition and Classification

Early warning systems enable timely crisis identification, allowing proactive response before situations escalate to unmanageable levels. Effective systems monitor multiple indicators including supply chain disruptions affecting medication availability, infrastructure vulnerabilities threatening operational capacity, staffing fluctuations potentially compromising safety functions, and external threats with operational implications. Implementation approaches include automated surveillance of critical parameters, established notification thresholds triggering assessment, and clear escalation pathways when concerning patterns emerge. Advanced systems incorporate predictive analytics identifying potential crises before actual manifestation, environmental scanning detecting emerging threats, and integration with regional or national alert networks providing broader situational awareness. These proactive identification capabilities transform crisis management from reactive response to anticipatory preparation, enabling controlled activation of emergency protocols rather than chaotic reaction to fully developed crises.

Standardized classification systems establish consistent categorization of emergency situations, supporting appropriate response matched to crisis characteristics rather than inconsistent reaction based on individual interpretation. Comprehensive systems address multiple dimensions including crisis scope (localized versus system-wide), duration expectations (transient versus sustained), impact severity (inconvenience versus existential threat), and available response time (immediate versus developing). Implementation typically employs tiered classification with corresponding response levels, specific criteria defining different categories, and clear authority designation for classification decisions. Well-designed systems balance sufficient differentiation enabling appropriately calibrated responses against excessive complexity potentially creating confusion during high-stress situations. This standardized approach prevents both overreaction consuming unnecessary resources and under-response leaving critical needs unaddressed, aligning response intensity with actual situation requirements.

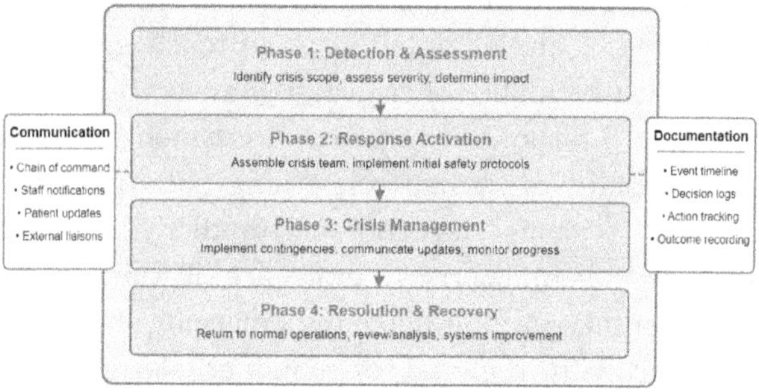

Figure 13.1 Crisis Management for Medication-Related Emergencies

Activation protocols establish clear procedures for crisis response initiation, preventing both delayed implementation when necessary and premature activation causing needless disruption. Effective protocols specify decision authority at different crisis levels, required assessment before activation, notification requirements when protocols engage, documentation expectations for activation decisions, and deactivation criteria determining when normal operations resume. Implementation considerations include appropriate balance between hierarchical authority ensuring coordination and distributed capability allowing rapid response when designated leaders prove unavailable, decision support tools guiding activation judgments during stressful circumstances, and communication templates ensuring comprehensive notification despite crisis pressure. These structured processes transform crisis response from improvised reaction to systematized activation, ensuring that response mechanisms engage appropriately based on established criteria rather than variable individual decisions under pressure.

Situational assessment methodologies establish structured approaches to ongoing crisis evaluation, creating accurate understanding supporting appropriate response adjustments as conditions evolve. Implementation includes initial rapid assessment establishing baseline situation parameters, ongoing monitoring tracking condition changes, structured update processes ensuring information currency, and comprehensive reassessment at defined intervals testing whether initial assumptions remain valid. Effective methodologies employ standardized systems ensuring consistent evaluation dimensions, multiple information sources preventing narrow perspective, verification processes confirming critical information before significant decisions, and explicit attention to evolving medication safety implications throughout the crisis. These assessment capabilities prevent response stagnation based on initial understanding despite changing circumstances, creating adaptive management matched to actual conditions rather than fixed reaction regardless of situation evolution.

Command Structures and Decision Processes

Incident command systems establish unified management structures during crises, creating clear authority relationships, responsibility assignments, and communication channels despite disrupted normal operations. Comprehensive implementation includes designated command positions with defined responsibilities, succession planning ensuring leadership continuity despite individual unavailability, structured reporting relationships creating clear information flow, and scalable systems adapting to different crisis magnitudes. Medication-specific elements within these structures typically include pharmacy representation in command groups, designated medication safety leadership roles, clear authority regarding formulary modifications or substitution decisions, and defined relationships with supply chain management addressing medication availability. These formal structures transform crisis response from chaotic individual actions to coordinated organizational functions, establishing clear decision pathways and accountability despite operational disruption.

Decision-making systems provide structured approaches to medication-related judgments during crises, supporting sound choices despite time pressure, limited information, and heightened stress. Effective systems include triage systems prioritizing critical medication needs over less essential functions, benefit-risk assessment tools supporting modified standards appropriate to crisis circumstances, ethical systems guiding resource allocation during scarcity, and documentation requirements maintaining accountability despite emergency conditions. Implementation typically includes pre-established decision criteria reducing cognitive burden during crises, designated authority for different decision types, consultation requirements for highest-risk modifications, and review processes validating critical decisions when circumstances permit. These systems acknowledge that crisis conditions necessitate different decision approaches than normal operations, providing structured support for difficult choices rather than expecting routine processes to function effectively during emergencies.

Table 13.1: Crisis Management for Medication-Related Emergencies

Crisis Type	Critical Considerations	Communication Protocols
Medication Shortage	Critical medication prioritization Alternative therapy identification Usage restrictions	Provider notifications Restriction protocols Patient communication
Serious Medication Error	Patient stabilization Secondary risk prevention Immediate notification	Chain of command Documentation requirements Disclosure process
Technology Failure	Downtime procedures Manual safeguards Recovery processes	Downtime notification Work process changes Recovery updates
Contamination Event	Product quarantine Patient identification Alternative supplies	Alert protocols Tracking processes Regulatory reporting

Communication systems establish reliable information exchange during crises despite potential infrastructure disruption, ensuring that critical medication safety information reaches appropriate recipients despite challenging conditions. Comprehensive systems include multiple redundant communication pathways preventing single-point failures, standardized formats ensuring consistent information transmission regardless of channel, verification processes confirming critical message receipt, and structured update cadences maintaining information currency. Medication-specific implementations typically include priority designations ensuring critical safety information receives transmission precedence, specialized formats for complex medication information, verification requirements for high-risk medication instructions, and closed-loop communication for critical therapy changes. These systems acknowledge that communication represents a primary vulnerability during crises, implementing specific safeguards ensuring that essential medication information continues flowing despite general communication challenges.

Authority delegation and empowerment strategies establish appropriate decision capability throughout the organization during crises, enabling timely action despite potential isolation from normal authority structures. Effective strategies include pre-defined delegation parameters identifying decisions authorized at different organizational levels during emergencies, clear documentation of temporary authority extensions, appropriate limitations maintaining necessary safety boundaries despite expanded authorization, and post-crisis review validating decisions made under emergency authority. Medication-specific implementations typically address dispensing authority modifications, formulary deviation permissions, documentation requirement adjustments, and verification practice alterations appropriate to crisis circumstances. This deliberate empowerment transforms crisis response from paralysis awaiting unavailable approval to appropriate action within established parameters, acknowledging that effective emergency management requires distributed decision capability beyond normal hierarchical structures.

Communication and Coordination

Internal communication strategies establish reliable information exchange within the organization during crises, ensuring that essential medication safety information reaches appropriate recipients despite challenging conditions. Effective strategies include tiered notification systems matching information detail to recipient needs and responsibilities, multiple redundant channels preventing single-point communication failures, standardized formats creating consistent information structure regardless of channel, and regular update cadences maintaining information currency. Implementation typically employs pre-developed templates addressing common crisis communication needs, designated communication roles ensuring consistent responsibility despite staff changes, and closed-loop verification for critical safety information. These structured approaches prevent the common crisis communication failures of information overload overwhelming critical details, inconsistent messaging creating confusion, and critical gaps leaving essential functions without necessary guidance.

External stakeholder communication addresses information exchange with parties outside the organization, ensuring appropriate awareness of crisis impacts on medication management capabilities and requirements. Main stakeholders typically include referring providers requiring awareness of modified medication management capabilities, health system partners involved in patient transfer or resource sharing, regulatory agencies requiring notification of standard practice modifications, and community resources potentially supporting medication access during disruptions. Effective communication includes clear description of operational impacts affecting external parties, specific guidance regarding modified procedures during the crisis, realistic timeframe expectations for resolution, and designated contact points for questions or coordination needs. This external transparency prevents misalignment between organizational capabilities and external expectations, establishing realistic understanding supporting appropriate adaptation rather than continued normal expectations despite crisis limitations.

Interdepartmental coordination mechanisms establish collaborative function across organizational boundaries during crises, addressing the heightened importance of seamless cooperation when normal operations face disruption. Implementation approaches include cross-functional response teams bringing diverse expertise to crisis management, liaison positions facilitating information exchange between departments, joint planning processes ensuring aligned response actions, and unified command structures establishing clear authority across departmental boundaries. Medication-specific coordination typically focuses on critical interfaces including pharmacy-nursing collaboration ensuring appropriate administration despite supply challenges, pharmacy-medical staff communication regarding therapeutic alternatives during shortages, and pharmacy-supply chain coordination addressing inventory management during distribution disruptions. These mechanisms acknowledge that departmental boundaries often become crisis vulnerability points where normal interaction patterns break down, implementing specific coordination safeguards maintaining essential relationships despite emergency pressures.

Regional and network collaboration establishes systematic cooperation beyond organizational boundaries, leveraging broader resources and capabilities during crises exceeding individual facility capacity. Effective collaboration includes resource-sharing agreements establishing parameters for medication exchange during shortages, patient transfer protocols ensuring appropriate therapy continuation during movements, shared information systems supporting coordinated response across multiple facilities, and joint training activities building cross-organizational relationships before crises occur. Implementation typically involves formal agreements established during normal operations, designated coordination roles activated during emergencies, standardized communication protocols ensuring efficient information exchange, and regular capability updates maintaining awareness of partner resources. This extended coordination acknowledges that significant crises typically affect multiple organizations simultaneously, requiring collaborative approaches beyond individual response capabilities.

Documentation and After-Action Review

Modified documentation requirements establish appropriate record-keeping expectations during crises, balancing essential safety documentation against practical limitations when normal processes exceed emergency capabilities. Effective modifications include identification of critical documentation elements requiring maintenance regardless of circumstances, streamlined formats reducing documentation burden during crisis operations, alternative recording methods when primary systems become unavailable, and prioritization systems focusing limited documentation resources on highest-risk medications and situations. Implementation typically involves pre-established emergency documentation protocols defining minimum requirements, templates supporting efficient recording despite challenging conditions, clear authority for documentation requirement modification, and procedures for information integration when normal systems resume. These adapted approaches acknowledge that standard documentation expectations may prove impossible during significant disruptions while maintaining essential records supporting safe medication management despite emergency conditions.

Real-time documentation of crisis decisions creates accountability and continuity despite modified operations, establishing clear records of situation assessments, considered alternatives, selected actions, and implementation results. Comprehensive documentation includes chronological decision logs capturing main judgments with rationales, policy modification records detailing temporary changes with justifications, resource allocation decisions with prioritization criteria, and authority delegation documentation clarifying modified responsibility assignments. Implementation typically employs dedicated documentation roles ensuring consistent recording despite operational pressures, standardized formats supporting efficient capture of essential information, and regular review processes validating documentation adequacy throughout the crisis. This concurrent recording transforms crisis management from retrospectively reconstructed activities to contemporaneously documented actions, creating both operational continuity as personnel change and appropriate accountability for decisions made under emergency conditions.

After-action review processes establish structured analysis following crisis resolution, transforming experience into organizational learning that improves future emergency response. Effective processes include comprehensive event timeline reconstruction documenting both actions and outcomes, multidisciplinary participation ensuring diverse perspectives on performance assessment, structured evaluation systems ensuring consistent analysis dimensions, and specific attention to medication safety performance throughout the crisis. Implementation typically involves designated responsibility for review coordination, protected time allocation ensuring thorough assessment despite recovery pressures, and appropriate psychological safety supporting honest evaluation without blame orientation. The most valuable reviews balance recognition of successful elements worth reinforcement with identification of improvement opportunities addressing observed limitations, creating balanced assessment rather than either exclusively critical or defensive evaluation.

Improvement implementation mechanisms translate after-action insights into actual preparedness enhancements, connecting review findings to specific operational changes before future emergencies occur. Effective mechanisms include formal improvement plans with specific action items, responsibility assignments creating clear accountability for implementation, timeline establishment with milestone tracking, resource allocation supporting necessary enhancements, and follow-up processes verifying effective completion. Implementation considerations include priority setting focusing on highest-impact improvements, feasibility assessment ensuring realistic planning, cross-functional involvement when changes affect multiple departments, and appropriate authorization when modifications require significant resource commitment or policy changes. These systematic approaches prevent the common gap between insightful after-action analysis and actual operational improvement, ensuring that identified enhancement opportunities translate into concrete preparedness changes rather than merely documented observations without practical application.

MEDICATION SAFETY DURING EMERGENCIES

Medication safety during emergencies requires specialized approaches addressing the unique challenges created when normal operations face disruption, establishing modified practices that maintain essential safety protections despite resource limitations, infrastructure challenges, and extraordinary pressures. These adapted methodologies acknowledge that standard practices may prove impossible during crises while establishing alternative approaches preserving fundamental safety principles despite emergency conditions.

Modified Procedures and Standards

Tiered safety systems establish differentiated practices based on emergency severity, implementing appropriate modifications matched to actual conditions rather than binary choices between normal standards and complete suspension. Comprehensive approaches typically define multiple response levels with corresponding practice modifications: Level 1 maintaining near-normal practices with minor adjustments, Level 2 implementing moderate modifications while preserving essential safety elements, Level 3 employing significant adaptations focusing exclusively on critical protections, and Level 4 representing catastrophic conditions requiring minimal viable practices.

Table 13.2: Medication Safety Strategies During Emergencies

Emergency Type	Safety Risks	Mitigation Strategies
Natural Disasters	Supply disruption Storage compromise Documentation challenges	Emergency formulary Storage contingencies Paper backup systems
Mass Casualty	High volume pressure Staffing limitations Protocol deviations	Simplified protocols Role expansion preparation Triage-based priorities
Utility Failures	Refrigeration loss Electronic system failure Communication barriers	Temperature monitoring Downtime procedures Backup communication
Infectious Disease	Isolation challenges PPE interference Staff limitation	Dedicated medication areas Modified verification processes Remote verification options

Medication-specific implementations address verification requirements, documentation expectations, dispensing procedures, and administration practices appropriate to different emergency intensities. This graduated approach prevents both rigid adherence to normal standards that may prove impossible during serious disruptions and unnecessary abandonment of essential safeguards during manageable situations requiring only limited adaptation.

Independent double-check modifications address the reality that normal verification practices may exceed available resources during emergencies while maintaining essential verification for highest-risk medications and situations. Effective modifications include risk-stratified approaches concentrating limited verification resources on most critical medications, procedure simplification maintaining core safety elements with streamlined processes, alternative verification mechanisms when standard approaches become unavailable, and clear authority for practice modification appropriate to emergency conditions. Implementation typically involves pre-defined protocols specifying which medications require maintained verification regardless of circumstances, streamlined procedures designed specifically for emergency conditions, and documentation expectations appropriate to modified practices. These adapted approaches acknowledge verification as both essential safety element and potential resource constraint during emergencies, establishing appropriate balance between safety preservation and operational feasibility.

Documentation requirement adjustments establish realistic record-keeping expectations during emergencies, focusing limited resources on essential safety information while temporarily suspending less critical elements. Comprehensive adjustments identify core documentation components required regardless of circumstances (essential patient information, actual medication administration, critical monitoring results), elements that may receive simplified recording during moderate emergencies (detailed timing information, routine assessment parameters, non-critical interventions), and components that may be temporarily suspended during severe disruptions (routine documentation supporting billing or regulatory requirements without direct safety implications). Implementation includes clear authority designation for requirement modification, specific guidance regarding minimum expectations at different emergency levels, and appropriate processes for information reconstruction when normal operations resume. These adjusted expectations acknowledge that complete normal documentation may prove impossible during significant disruptions while maintaining essential records supporting safe medication management.

Emergency Type	Key Safety Risks	Safety Strategies
Natural Disasters (Hurricanes, Floods, Earthquakes)	• Supply chain disruption • Power/refrigeration loss • Electronic system failures	• Emergency medication caches • Backup power for storage • Paper documentation systems
Mass Casualty Events (Terrorism, Major Accidents)	• High patient volume • Need for rapid response • Staffing limitations	• Mass casualty protocols • Prepackaged emergency kits • Simplified verification process
Pandemic/Epidemic (Infectious Disease Outbreaks)	• Medication shortages • Isolation barriers • Staff illness/reduction	• Conservation protocols • Remote verification systems • Extended BUD protocols
Infrastructure Failures (Power Outages, IT System Failures)	• EHR/CPOE unavailability • Refrigeration loss • Communication barriers	• Downtime procedures • Generator backup • Alternate communication plans

Figure 13.2: Medication Safety for Different Emergency Types

Automated safeguard modifications address potential technology limitations during emergencies, establishing alternative safety mechanisms when electronic systems face disruption. Effective approaches include downtime procedures maintaining essential safety checks during system unavailability, manual workarounds replacing automated verification processes, paper-based alternatives for electronic documentation, and modified override protocols appropriate to emergency conditions. Implementation typically involves pre-established procedures designed specifically for technology disruption scenarios, regular practice during non-emergency conditions ensuring staff familiarity, designated technology assessment roles during crises, and clear authority for safeguard modification decisions. These alternative approaches acknowledge the potential vulnerability created by technology dependence during emergencies while establishing appropriate backup mechanisms maintaining fundamental safety protections despite system limitations.

Resource Allocation and Conservation

Medication prioritization systems establish systematic approaches to allocating limited medication supplies during shortages, ensuring that available resources address highest-priority needs through objective allocation processes. Comprehensive systems typically employ multiple classification dimensions including therapeutic category (life-sustaining, urgent, important but deferrable, optional), patient acuity (critical, unstable, stable), availability of therapeutic alternatives, and conservation potential through dose adjustment or duration limitation. Implementation involves multidisciplinary committees establishing prioritization criteria before crises occur, clear decision authority during actual shortages, transparent processes communicating allocation rationales, and regular reassessment as conditions evolve. These structured approaches prevent both inequitable distribution based on non-clinical factors and inconsistent allocation from variable individual judgments, establishing fair resource distribution based on clinical need and potential benefit despite supply limitations.

Therapeutic substitution protocols establish pre-approved alternative medication options for critical therapies, enabling rapid adaptation when primary agents become unavailable without requiring case-by-case approval processes exceeding emergency decision capabilities. Effective protocols include comprehensive alternative listings for essential medication classes, clinical guidance regarding dosage conversion between agents, monitoring recommendations appropriate to alternative medications, and implementation considerations addressing practical conversion processes. Development typically involves pharmacy and therapeutics committee review establishing clinically appropriate alternatives, informatics support creating order set modifications facilitating rapid conversion, and educational resources supporting clinical staff unfamiliar with alternative agents. These pre-established alternatives prevent both treatment interruptions while awaiting substitution decisions and inappropriate alternatives selected without adequate clinical review, maintaining therapeutic continuity despite supply disruptions.

Dose conservation strategies establish medication-sparing approaches during supply limitations, extending available inventory through modified utilization practices without compromising essential therapy. Implementation approaches include dose optimization ensuring appropriate utilization without excess, duration limitation restricting therapy to clinically necessary periods, formulation changes conserving limited supplies (e.g., conversion from intravenous to oral therapy when clinically appropriate), batching of prepared medications minimizing waste from partial container utilization, and beyond-use dating extension based on stability data rather than routine practice. Development involves pharmacist leadership identifying appropriate conservation opportunities, medical staff collaboration establishing clinical appropriateness, and nursing input regarding practical implementation feasibility. These systematic approaches prevent both premature exhaustion of critical supplies and unnecessary restriction of appropriate therapy, optimizing limited resources through clinically sound conservation rather than arbitrary restriction.

Specialized distribution models establish modified medication delivery systems during emergencies, adapting normal distribution practices to crisis conditions while maintaining essential control and accountability. Implementations include centralized dispensing consolidating limited pharmacy staff resources, mobile pharmacy operations bringing medication access to relocated patient care areas, batch delivery systems replacing individual medication distribution, and modified charge capture processes maintaining essential financial functions with simplified mechanisms. Operational considerations include security provisions preventing diversion despite modified controls, storage requirement maintenance for temperature-sensitive medications, verification processes appropriate to alternative distribution models, and tracking systems ensuring accountability despite altered dispensing patterns. These adapted approaches acknowledge that normal distribution models may prove unsustainable during significant operational disruption while establishing viable alternatives maintaining essential medication availability and basic safety controls despite emergency conditions.

High-Alert Medication Management

Simplified high-alert protocols maintain essential safety elements for dangerous medications despite emergency conditions, preserving critical protections while adapting to resource limitations and operational constraints. Effective approaches include streamlined verification procedures maintaining independent checks with simplified documentation, concentrated oversight focusing limited resources on most hazardous medications, modified preparation procedures maintaining safety with adapted processes, and enhanced monitoring compensating for reduced preventive safeguards. Implementation typically involves pre-defined emergency protocols specifying minimum requirements regardless of crisis conditions, clear authority for protocol modification appropriate to circumstances, and specific guidance regarding adaptation priorities when complete protocol maintenance proves impossible. These emergency-specific approaches acknowledge both the continued risk presented by high-alert medications during crises and the potential impracticality of full standard protocols, establishing appropriate balance between safety preservation and operational feasibility under challenging conditions.

Concentrated oversight models focus limited supervisory resources on highest-risk medication processes during emergencies, ensuring appropriate safety monitoring despite personnel limitations and competing priorities. Implementation approaches include designated safety personnel with specific high-alert monitoring responsibility, scheduled safety rounds focusing specifically on high-risk medication areas, targeted verification processes concentrating on critical medications, and remote supervision capabilities supporting oversight despite physical access limitations. Operational considerations include clear role definition distinguishing safety oversight from operational responsibilities, appropriate authority ensuring effective intervention when issues identified, and communication pathways establishing reliable information flow despite emergency conditions. These focused approaches acknowledge the impossibility of maintaining normal comprehensive oversight during significant disruptions while establishing essential monitoring for most critical medication processes with highest potential harm.

Modified storage approaches maintain appropriate security and segregation for high-alert medications despite potential infrastructure disruption, preserving fundamental safety protections while adapting to emergency conditions. Effective adaptations include alternative secure storage locations when primary areas become unavailable, temporary storage units meeting essential requirements when permanent solutions prove inaccessible, manual tracking systems replacing electronic controls during technology disruptions, and enhanced physical security compensating for automated system limitations. Implementation considerations include pre-identified alternative locations meeting basic requirements, portable secure storage units available for rapid deployment, and clear authority for storage modification decisions appropriate to emergency conditions. These contingency approaches acknowledge potential infrastructure vulnerability during emergencies while establishing viable alternatives maintaining essential medication security and segregation despite facility or technology disruptions.

Enhanced monitoring compensates for potentially reduced preventive safeguards during emergencies, increasing surveillance of patient response when normal pre-administration protections face limitation. Implementation approaches include increased assessment frequency detecting adverse effects earlier, focused monitoring protocols concentrating on highest-risk medications, simplified assessment tools facilitating consistent evaluation despite resource constraints, and prioritized laboratory testing ensuring essential monitoring despite capacity limitations. Operational considerations include clearly defined monitoring parameters establishing minimum expectations regardless of emergency conditions, responsibility designation ensuring consistent accountability despite staffing challenges, and documentation requirements appropriate to crisis circumstances. This intensified surveillance acknowledges the potential increased error risk during emergencies when normal preventive systems face constraints, establishing compensatory detection mechanisms identifying adverse effects promptly when prevention capabilities may be compromised.

Communication and Handoff Challenges

Simplified handoff tools maintain essential information transfer during emergencies despite time pressure, cognitive overload, and potential staffing disruptions challenging normal handoff processes. Effective tools include focused formats concentrating on critical medication information, standardized structures ensuring consistent coverage despite variable personnel, visual cues highlighting highest-risk therapies requiring special attention, and abbreviated documentation balancing completeness against practical constraints. Implementation typically involves pre-developed emergency handoff templates designed specifically for crisis conditions, prioritized content identifying essential elements requiring transmission regardless of circumstances, and minimal documentation requirements supporting practical completion despite challenging conditions. These adapted approaches acknowledge that comprehensive normal handoffs may prove unsustainable during significant disruptions while establishing viable alternatives maintaining essential safety communication despite emergency limitations.

Cross-training and role flexibility support continuity despite staffing disruptions during emergencies, enabling essential medication functions despite potentially unavailable specialists. Implementation approaches include targeted cross-training focused on critical medication tasks, simplified procedures designed for execution by broader staff groups during emergencies, clear guidance materials supporting unfamiliar role performance, and appropriate supervision ensuring patient safety when personnel operate beyond normal responsibilities. Development considerations include identification of essential functions requiring continuity regardless of specialist availability, realistic assessment of capabilities transferable to broader staff groups, simplified protocols suitable for execution with limited training, and appropriate scope limitations preventing high-risk activities exceeding basic cross-training. This enhanced workforce flexibility acknowledges potential specialist unavailability during significant emergencies while establishing appropriate alternative capability maintaining essential medication functions despite staffing limitations.

Visual management systems enhance communication during emergencies when normal information transfer may face challenges, creating easily recognized indicators supporting appropriate medication management despite potentially limited verbal or electronic communication. Effective implementations include color-coding systems identifying different medication categories or status conditions, standardized symbols communicating main information without detailed text, visible indicators showing critical therapy timing or requirements, and simplified visual patient profiles highlighting essential medication information. Development considerations include intuitive design requiring minimal explanation, consistency across all emergency locations, appropriate prominence ensuring visibility during chaotic conditions, and sufficient differentiation preventing confusion between similar indicators. These visual approaches acknowledge communication vulnerability during crises while establishing alternative information transfer mechanisms supporting appropriate medication management despite potential verbal or electronic communication limitations.

Family engagement strategies maintain critical medication information continuity despite potential electronic record disruption during emergencies, leveraging patient and family knowledge as valuable information source when normal documentation proves unavailable. Effective approaches include structured medication history interviews eliciting specific information about current therapies, medication listing tools supporting comprehensive documentation of reported medications, verification processes confirming critical information accuracy, and appropriate integration with available electronic information establishing complete profiles. Implementation considerations include interview guides supporting consistent information collection, documentation tools capturing essential details, verification approaches appropriate to emergency conditions, and clear processes for resolving discrepancies between reported and documented medications. This engagement acknowledges both the potential vulnerability of electronic medication records during emergencies and the valuable information resource represented by patients and families, establishing appropriate processes leveraging this knowledge during crisis situations.

CONTINGENCY PLANNING

Contingency planning establishes systematic preparation for potential emergencies before they occur, creating proactive readiness rather than reactive response to disruptions affecting medication management. Comprehensive planning addresses diverse potential scenarios, developing specific response capabilities matched to different emergency types while creating flexible adaptability for unanticipated situations.

Risk Assessment and Scenario Development

Vulnerability assessment identifies potential weaknesses in medication systems that could compromise safety during emergencies, enabling targeted preparation addressing specific risk points before actual disruptions occur. Comprehensive assessment evaluates multiple dimensions including infrastructure vulnerabilities (power dependence, water requirements, physical security), technology fragility (downtime risks, backup limitations, recovery timeframes), supply chain weaknesses (single-source dependencies, inventory limitations, distribution vulnerabilities), and workforce constraints (specialized skill requirements, minimum staffing needs, geographic concentration). Effective methodologies employ structured evaluation tools ensuring consistent assessment across different system components, multidisciplinary participation bringing diverse perspectives to vulnerability identification, and regular reassessment capturing changes in system characteristics or external threat environments. This proactive identification transforms general emergency preparation into targeted readiness addressing specific organizational vulnerabilities, focusing resources on highest-risk areas rather than generic preparation inadequately matched to actual risk profiles.

Table 13.3: Medication-Related Contingency Planning Elements

Contingency Element	Planning Requirements	Documentation Needs
Emergency Supply Chain	Alternative suppliers Stockpile management Transportation backup	Supplier contacts Inventory requirements Acquisition protocols
Backup Procedures	Manual processes Alternative workflows Verification adaptations	Downtime procedures Paper forms Authority matrices
Staff Planning	Cross-training Role expansion protocols Remote work capabilities	Emergency credentialing Just-in-time training Staff recall procedures
Recovery Processes	Data reconciliation Return to normal operations Post-event review	Recovery checklists Verification processes After-action templates

Scenario development creates specific emergency situations for planning purposes, establishing concrete contexts for contingency development rather than abstract preparation inadequately connected to potential realities. Effective development includes both high-probability scenarios based on historical experience or known vulnerabilities and high-consequence possibilities representing rare but catastrophic situations, creating comprehensive preparation spanning different emergency types and severities. Specific scenarios valuable for medication-focused planning include prolonged power outages affecting refrigeration and electronic systems, supply chain disruptions creating critical medication shortages, staffing crises from disease outbreaks or mass casualty events, facility damage requiring partial or complete evacuation, and technology failures affecting ordering, dispensing, and documentation systems. This specific context transforms general emergency concepts into concrete situations supporting detailed planning, enabling realistic preparation addressing practical challenges rather than theoretical readiness disconnected from operational realities.

Criticality analysis establishes priority systems for contingency planning, identifying medication functions requiring maintenance regardless of circumstances versus those accepting temporary suspension during emergencies. Comprehensive analysis evaluates factors including direct life safety implications, adverse effect potential from therapy interruption, availability of alternative approaches, recovery complexity if suspended, and interdependence with other critical functions. Implementation typically creates tiered classification with corresponding continuity requirements: Level 1 functions requiring continuous maintenance without interruption, Level 2 functions accepting brief disruption with rapid recovery, Level 3 functions tolerating extended interruption with eventual restoration, and Level 4 functions suitable for suspension throughout emergencies with post-crisis recovery. This prioritization prevents both inadequate protection for truly critical functions and wasted resources maintaining non-essential capabilities during crises, establishing appropriate continuity requirements matched to actual operational importance rather than attempting uniform protection across all medication functions regardless of criticality.

Impact and probability mapping creates visual representation of different emergency scenarios, supporting resource allocation decisions through clear illustration of both likelihood and consequence severity. Effective mapping employs matrix structures positioning scenarios based on occurrence probability (from remote to virtually certain) and potential impact (from minor inconvenience to catastrophic disruption), creating quadrant classification guiding different preparation approaches. High-probability, high-impact scenarios typically receive most intensive preparation with detailed plans and specific resource allocation; low-probability, high-impact situations warrant specialized preparation despite infrequent occurrence; high-probability, low-impact events generally require streamlined response procedures without extensive resource commitment; and low-probability, low-impact possibilities may receive basic monitoring without detailed preparation. This visual representation transforms complex risk relationships into clear decision guidance, supporting appropriate resource allocation proportional to both likelihood and consequence rather than preparing equally for all possibilities regardless of probability or impact.

Essential Resources and Capabilities

Inventory management strategies establish appropriate medication stockpiles for emergency situations, creating on-hand supplies supporting continued operations despite potential distribution disruptions. Effective strategies balance multiple considerations including storage costs for rarely used inventory, expiration management preventing waste from unused stockpiles, storage space limitations constraining physical inventory, and cashflow implications of increased on-hand supplies. Implementation approaches include identification of critical medications requiring enhanced inventory based on therapeutic importance and supply vulnerability, par level adjustments increasing standard stock for essential items, rotation systems preventing expiration of emergency supplies, and regional collaboration spreading stockpile costs across multiple organizations. Advanced approaches implement dynamic inventory models adjusting holdings based on current threat assessments, supplier reliability history, and seasonal risk factors. This deliberate stockpiling transforms potential medication unavailability from crisis-time scramble to pre-planned mitigation, establishing appropriate reserves matched to organizational needs and risk profiles.

Backup system development creates alternative capabilities for critical medication functions, establishing operational redundancy when primary systems face disruption. Comprehensive development includes paper-based alternatives for electronic ordering and documentation systems, manual processes replacing automated dispensing functions, alternative communication channels when primary methods become unavailable, reserve power sources for critical medication storage and preparation equipment, and backup data systems maintaining essential information despite primary system failure. Implementation considerations include appropriate resource allocation proportional to system criticality, regular testing ensuring actual functionality rather than theoretical capability, usability design supporting effective operation during high-stress situations, and appropriate maintenance ensuring readiness despite infrequent utilization. These redundant capabilities transform potential single-point failures into manageable disruptions, maintaining essential medication functions through alternative mechanisms rather than accepting complete capability loss when primary systems fail.

Alternative care site planning establishes medication management capabilities outside normal care locations, creating operational readiness for situations requiring facility evacuation or extraordinary patient surge exceeding normal capacity. Effective planning includes medication supply arrangements for alternate sites, storage capability meeting security and environmental requirements, preparation space supporting continued compounding activities, essential reference information accessibility, and necessary equipment for safe medication administration. Implementation typically involves pre-positioned supply caches at designated alternate locations, mobile pharmacy units capable of rapid deployment, agreements with partner facilities for space utilization during emergencies, and standardized setup procedures supporting rapid operational capability establishment. These preplanned alternatives transform potential location disruption from improvised reaction to systematic relocation, maintaining essential medication capabilities despite facility unavailability through pre-established alternative arrangements.

Workforce continuity planning ensures adequate

personnel availability during emergencies despite potential staff unavailability from disaster effects, transportation disruptions, or competing personal obligations during community-wide events. Comprehensive planning includes minimum staffing models identifying essential positions requiring coverage regardless of circumstances, cross-training programs developing versatile capabilities across broader staff groups, designated emergency roles potentially differing from normal responsibilities, and mutual aid agreements with partner organizations supporting personnel sharing during crises. Implementation considerations include appropriate expectation setting regarding emergency responsibilities, practical support addressing personal preparedness enabling work availability, compensation policies appropriate to extraordinary circumstances, and family support arrangements removing conflicts between professional and personal responsibilities during community-wide events. This deliberate personnel planning transforms potential workforce shortage from crisis-time gap to pre-addressed consideration, establishing appropriate staffing continuity through systematic preparation rather than assumption of normal availability during abnormal circumstances.

Standard Operating Procedures and Protocols

Emergency-specific protocols establish detailed guidance for medication management during different disruption scenarios, creating predetermined approaches for common emergency situations requiring modified practices. Comprehensive development includes specific protocols for situations including power outages affecting medication refrigeration and electronic systems, water service disruption impacting sterile preparation capabilities, supply chain interruptions creating critical shortages, information system failures affecting ordering and documentation, and evacuation scenarios requiring patient transfers with appropriate medication continuity. Effective protocols specify activation criteria establishing when emergency procedures apply, detailed operational guidance regarding modified practices, decision authority identifying who may authorize procedure implementation, and termination parameters determining when normal operations resume. These predetermined procedures transform emergency response from improvised reaction to guided implementation, replacing crisis-time procedure development with execution of established protocols matched to specific emergency types.

Decision tools support systematic judgment during emergency situations despite stress, time pressure, and limited information typically challenging decision quality during crises. Effective tools include structured systems guiding high-consequence decisions such as therapeutic substitution during critical shortages, triage algorithms directing limited medication resources to patients with greatest potential benefit, checklists ensuring comprehensive consideration of relevant factors despite cognitive limitations during emergencies, and documentation templates capturing essential decision elements supporting both implementation and post-crisis review. Development considerations include appropriate balance between guidance structure and necessary flexibility for unanticipated situations, usability under stress conditions, accessibility during infrastructure disruptions, and sufficient simplicity supporting practical utilization despite emergency pressures. These decision supports transform complex emergency judgments from vulnerable individual determinations to structured processes with appropriate guidance, maintaining decision quality despite challenging conditions through predetermined systems specifically designed for crisis application.

Standard operating procedures for recovery establish systematic approaches to normal operations restoration, creating predetermined pathways from emergency functions to routine practices following disruption resolution. Comprehensive procedures address multiple recovery dimensions including inventory restoration following emergency stockpile utilization, documentation reconciliation integrating emergency records with normal systems, technology transition from manual processes back to electronic systems, therapeutic standardization returning from emergency alternatives to preferred agents, and quality verification ensuring appropriate safety restoration despite transition disruption. Implementation considerations include phased approaches preventing simultaneous change overwhelming adaptation capabilities, clear transition authority establishing when specific functions resume normal operations, appropriate verification ensuring full capability restoration before emergency procedure termination, and systematic assessment identifying potential improvement opportunities for future emergency response. These recovery procedures transform crisis resolution from haphazard normalization to systematic restoration, establishing appropriate transition supporting both operational continuity and safety maintenance throughout the recovery process.

Regulatory compliance considerations establish appropriate balance between normal standards and practical emergency limitations, creating predetermined approaches to compliance management during situations where full adherence proves impossible. Effective approaches include identification of regulatory requirements suitable for modification during emergencies, pre-established communication channels with regulatory authorities supporting timely notification of necessary adaptations, documentation systems capturing modified practices with appropriate justification, and progressive restoration planning returning to full compliance through systematic transition. Implementation typically involves proactive regulatory engagement before emergencies occur, development of specific compliance management plans for foreseeable disruptions, designated responsibility for regulatory communication during crises, and appropriate record-keeping supporting post-emergency review. These predetermined approaches transform potential compliance conflicts from crisis-time complications to pre-addressed considerations, establishing appropriate regulatory management through systematic planning rather than improvised navigation of competing requirements during actual emergencies.

Testing and Continuous Improvement

Simulation exercises test emergency plans under controlled conditions, validating capability while developing staff experience before actual crises occur. Comprehensive exercise programs include tabletop simulations discussing theoretical response to presented scenarios, functional exercises testing specific capabilities without full activation, and full-scale drills implementing complete emergency operations in realistic conditions. Medication-specific exercises valuable for preparedness assessment include dispensing capability during electronic system failure, preparation continuity despite infrastructure disruption, distribution functionality with transportation limitations, and therapeutic decision-making during simulated shortages. Effective implementation includes realistic scenario development reflecting actual organizational vulnerabilities, multidisciplinary participation representing all affected functions, objective evaluation identifying performance gaps, and structured debriefing transforming exercise experience into specific improvement actions. These controlled practice opportunities transform theoretical plans into validated capabilities, building both system verification and personnel experience before facing actual emergency conditions.

Regular plan reviews maintain contingency readiness despite changing conditions, ensuring that prepared responses remain aligned with current operational realities and emerging threats. Comprehensive review processes address multiple dimensions including organizational changes affecting planned response capabilities, facility modifications altering evacuation requirements or alternative care options, technology evolution creating different vulnerability patterns, staffing changes affecting identified roles and responsibilities, and external threat environment developments presenting new challenges requiring preparation. Implementation typically includes scheduled reviews at defined intervals, event-triggered reassessment following significant organizational changes, multidisciplinary participation ensuring diverse perspective consideration, and systematic update processes maintaining plan currency. These regular evaluations transform emergency planning from static documents to evolving guidance, maintaining actual response capability through continuous adaptation rather than allowing prepared approaches to gradually disconnect from operational reality through unaddressed change.

Lessons learned integration establishes systematic

improvement based on actual emergency experiences, transforming real events into enhanced future capability through structured analysis and implementation. Effective integration includes comprehensive after-action review identifying both successful elements worth reinforcement and improvement opportunities addressing observed limitations, root cause analysis determining fundamental performance factors rather than superficial observations, specific improvement recommendations with practical implementation guidance, and formal action planning creating accountability for enhancement implementation. Implementation considerations include appropriate timing balancing prompt review capturing fresh observations against sufficient distance allowing objective assessment, inclusive participation ensuring diverse perspective consideration, psychological safety supporting honest evaluation without blame orientation, and resource allocation enabling actual improvement beyond mere recommendation documentation. This structured learning transforms emergency experiences from isolated events to continuous improvement opportunities, building enhanced capability through systematic adaptation based on actual performance rather than maintaining unchanged approaches despite identified limitations.

External evaluation provides objective assessment from knowledgeable outside perspective, identifying potential vulnerabilities or improvement opportunities that may remain unrecognized within organizational boundaries. Implementation approaches include regulatory authority review evaluating compliance with emergency preparedness requirements, accreditation organization assessment examining contingency planning against established standards, peer organization exchange providing comparative perspective from similar institutions, and specialized consultant evaluation bringing industry-wide experience to organizational assessment. Effective utilization includes appropriate preparation ensuring productive assessment rather than superficial review, transparent information sharing enabling thorough evaluation, non-defensive reception of identified opportunities, and systematic implementation planning addressing valuable recommendations. This external perspective complements internal assessment with fresh viewpoints and broader comparative context, identifying improvement opportunities potentially overlooked within organizational boundaries while validating successful approaches against external standards and practices.

DISASTER RESPONSE

Disaster response establishes systematic approaches to maintaining medication safety during large-scale events exceeding normal emergency management capabilities, addressing the unique challenges created by catastrophic situations requiring extraordinary measures beyond standard contingency preparations. These specialized responses acknowledge the fundamental differences between manageable emergencies and true disasters, implementing appropriate adaptations supporting medication safety despite potentially severe resource limitations and infrastructure disruptions.

Triage and Resource Allocation

Crisis standards of care implementation establishes formalized transition to modified practice expectations during disasters, acknowledging when resource limitations prevent normal operations while creating ethical systems for altered standards appropriate to catastrophic circumstances. Comprehensive implementation includes formal declaration processes establishing when crisis standards apply, specific guidance regarding modified practices appropriate to disaster conditions, ethical systems supporting difficult resource allocation decisions, and documentation requirements maintaining accountability despite emergency conditions. Medication-specific elements typically address modified dispensing practices during severe shortages, simplified verification procedures when normal double-checks prove impossible, adjusted documentation requirements balancing accountability against practical limitations, and altered administration practices appropriate to disaster conditions. This formal transition transforms disaster response from failed attempt at normal operations to appropriate adaptation matched to actual conditions, establishing realistic expectations and ethical systems supporting necessary modifications rather than leaving practitioners caught between impossible standards and undefined alternatives.

Medication triage systems establish systematic approaches to allocating limited supplies during disasters, creating objective systems supporting difficult distribution decisions when demand exceeds availability. Effective systems include categorization systems classifying medications based on factors including life-sustaining necessity, immediate versus deferrable need, availability of therapeutic alternatives, and patient condition affecting potential benefit; decision processes establishing who makes allocation judgments when needed; documentation requirements capturing both decisions and supporting rationale; and appeals mechanisms addressing disagreements while maintaining necessary decisiveness.

Table 13.4: Disaster Response Considerations for Medication Management

Response Phase	Medication Management Priorities	Quality Assurance
Immediate Response	Critical medication availability Emergency protocols activation Triage-based distribution	Real-time error tracking Protocol compliance checks Critical incident review
Ongoing Operations	Supply management Modified workflows Documentation continuity	Daily safety huddles Abbreviated audits Modified safety checks
Extended Response	Conservation strategies Alternative therapy protocols Staff rotation planning	Adapted monitoring protocols Focused safety reviews Pattern analysis
Recovery	Return to standard processes Documentation reconciliation System restoration validation	Process restoration verification Post-event analysis Improvement planning

Implementation typically involves multidisciplinary development establishing clinically appropriate criteria, ethics committee input ensuring alignment with organizational values, leadership approval providing necessary authority, and staff education creating understanding before actual implementation necessity.

These systematic approaches transform potential allocation chaos from subjective individual judgments to structured processes with transparent criteria, supporting both practical distribution decisions and ethical practice despite severe resource constraints.

Modified dispensing models establish alternative medication distribution approaches during disasters, adapting normal practices to extraordinary circumstances while maintaining essential safety and accountability. Implementation approaches include centralized dispensing consolidating limited pharmacy staff and inventory, mobile pharmacy operations bringing medication access to displaced populations, nurse-managed systems with appropriate pharmacist oversight when normal pharmacy operations prove impossible, and community distribution mechanisms for chronic medications when healthcare facilities become overwhelmed. Operational considerations include security provisions preventing diversion despite modified controls, verification processes appropriate to alternative dispensing models, documentation systems matching practical limitations while maintaining basic accountability, and appropriate regulatory communication regarding necessary practice modifications. These alternative approaches acknowledge that normal dispensing models may prove unsustainable during disasters while establishing viable alternatives maintaining essential medication access despite catastrophic disruption.

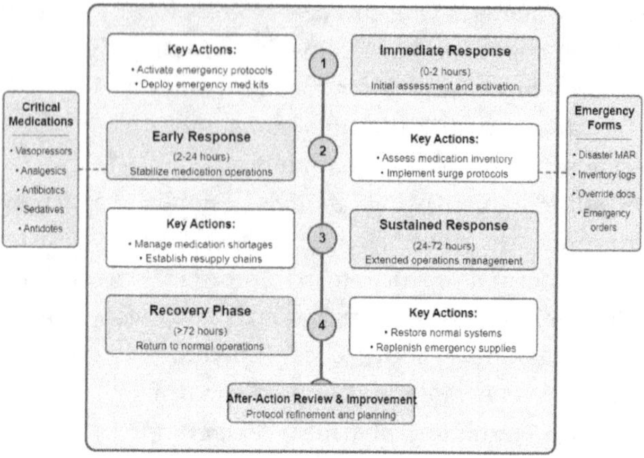

Figure 13.3 Disaster Response Medication Management

Ethical systems guide difficult decisions during disasters when resource limitations prevent meeting all needs, establishing principled approaches to unavoidable choices rather than leaving practitioners without moral guidance during devastating circumstances. Comprehensive systems address foundational principles including justice in resource distribution, proportionality matching intervention intensity to potential benefit, transparency regarding decision criteria, respect for human dignity despite resource constraints, and procedural fairness ensuring consistent process application. Medication-specific applications include allocation principles during critical shortages, prioritization systems when normal therapy for all proves impossible, modified risk acceptance appropriate to disaster circumstances, and documentation expectations maintaining accountability despite practical limitations. These ethical structures transform potentially arbitrary or inconsistent disaster decisions to principled choices with moral foundation, supporting both practical action and practitioner moral integrity despite circumstances forcing difficult choices between competing needs exceeding available resources.

Emergency Supply Management

Strategic national stockpile access establishes procedures for obtaining federally maintained emergency medication supplies during disasters exceeding local resource capabilities, creating predetermined pathways to supplemental inventory when normal supply chains prove inadequate. Comprehensive procedures include request processes specifying required information and appropriate authorization, receiving procedures establishing secure acceptance capability, distribution systems allocating received supplies based on predetermined prioritization, inventory management maintaining accountability despite emergency conditions, and documentation requirements supporting post-event reconciliation. Implementation considerations include pre-event relationship development with relevant authorities, staff familiarity with request procedures before actual needs arise, appropriate storage capability for potentially substantial supply quantities, and distribution planning addressing both internal organizational needs and potential community-wide responsibilities. These established procedures transform national stockpile access from unfamiliar crisis-time navigation to predetermined pathways with clear processes, enabling appropriate supplemental resource utilization through systematic preparation rather than improvised attempts during actual disasters.

Alternative supply sources establish additional inventory access beyond standard channels, creating diverse options when primary suppliers face disruption during widespread disasters. Effective development includes identification of alternative pharmaceutical wholesalers beyond primary vendors, direct manufacturer relationships providing contingency access when distribution networks fail, partner healthcare organization agreements enabling resource sharing during regional events, and non-traditional source relationships such as veterinary supply chains offering limited alternatives for certain medications. Implementation considerations include appropriate contractual arrangements establishing emergency access rights, quality assurance procedures verifying product integrity from non-routine sources, and regulatory compliance ensuring appropriate licensure and authorization despite modified procurement approaches. These diversified supply relationships transform potential single-point distribution failure into manageable disruption with alternatives, maintaining essential medication availability through multiple access pathways rather than complete dependency on potentially vulnerable primary suppliers during widespread disasters affecting normal distribution networks.

Medication cache deployment establishes rapid inventory distribution capability during disasters, creating predetermined medication packages supporting immediate response before more sophisticated supply management becomes operational. Effective implementation includes strategically positioned caches at potential disaster response locations, standardized contents based on anticipated emergency needs, regular inventory review ensuring continued usability, appropriate security preventing unauthorized access, and deployment protocols establishing release authority and documentation requirements. Content development typically focuses on emergency medications with predictable disaster demand including analgesics, antibiotics, tetanus prophylaxis, emergency cardiac medications, respiratory agents, and basic chronic disease maintenance therapies. These prepared packages transform initial disaster response from delayed scramble awaiting supply organization to immediate capability with prepositioned inventory, providing essential medications during critical early response periods before traditional supply chains can be established or restored.

Extemporaneous compounding capacity establishes capability to create necessary medications when manufactured products become unavailable during disasters, providing alternative preparation approaches when standard supplies face disruption. Comprehensive development includes expertise maintenance in fundamental compounding techniques, reference resource accessibility providing formulation information during infrastructure disruption, essential equipment and supply stockpiling supporting basic preparation capability, quality control procedures appropriate to emergency conditions, and appropriate regulatory communication regarding necessary practice modifications. Implementation considerations include realistic capability assessment preventing overestimation of practical production capacity, prioritization systems focusing limited resources on most critical preparations, appropriate labeling ensuring product identification despite emergency conditions, and documentation supporting post-disaster review. This alternative production capability transforms potential therapy interruption during manufactured product unavailability to continued treatment through local preparation, maintaining essential medication access through adaptable production capabilities rather than complete dependency on potentially disrupted commercial manufacturing and distribution during widespread disasters.

Continuity of Care for Vulnerable Populations

Chronic disease management strategies establish approaches to maintaining essential ongoing therapy during disasters, addressing the particular vulnerability of patients requiring continuous medication for condition control. Effective strategies include medication identification systems highlighting highest-priority chronic therapies where interruption creates greatest harm, extended prescription initiatives providing additional supply before anticipated disasters, patient education regarding personal emergency medication management, and abbreviated history collection tools capturing essential chronic therapy information when full records prove unavailable. Implementation typically involves interdisciplinary development identifying critical maintenance medications, information system reports generating vulnerable patient lists for proactive outreach, and community partnerships supporting continued access despite healthcare facility disruption. These systematic approaches transform chronic disease patients from particularly vulnerable disaster populations to specifically addressed priorities with predetermined management strategies, maintaining essential therapy continuity through deliberate planning rather than accepting potentially dangerous treatment interruptions during system disruption.

Special population planning addresses unique medication needs of vulnerable groups during disasters, establishing specific approaches for populations requiring specialized pharmaceutical management. Comprehensive planning typically addresses pediatric considerations including age-appropriate formulations and weight-based dosing capabilities; geriatric needs such as medication reconciliation for complex regimens and cognitive limitation accommodations; pregnancy requirements including teratogenic risk avoidance and condition-specific therapies; and patients with functional needs requiring specialized administration approaches or medication forms. Implementation involves interdisciplinary development identifying population-specific requirements, specialized stockpiling ensuring appropriate formulation availability, targeted education preparing staff for unique needs, and community partnerships identifying vulnerable individuals requiring specific outreach. These focused approaches transform special populations from overlooked disaster victims to specifically considered groups with predetermined support strategies, addressing unique medication requirements through intentional planning rather than discovering unmet needs during actual response.

Medication reconciliation adaptation establishes modified approaches to therapy continuity during disasters, addressing the challenges of maintaining appropriate medication management when normal information sources and verification processes face disruption. Effective adaptation includes abbreviated reconciliation tools focusing on most critical information, alternative verification sources when traditional records prove unavailable, modified documentation requirements balancing completeness against practical limitations, and decision support for therapeutic substitution when identical medication continuation proves impossible. Implementation considerations include realistic expectation setting regarding possible reconciliation quality during severe disruption, priority establishment ensuring most critical medications receive greatest attention, and appropriate accountability documentation supporting post-disaster review. These modified approaches acknowledge that comprehensive normal reconciliation may prove impossible during catastrophic circumstances while establishing appropriate alternatives maintaining essential therapy continuity despite information limitations and resource constraints.

Home-bound patient support establishes medication delivery capability during disasters when normal access mechanisms face disruption, addressing the vulnerability of individuals unable to reach distribution points due to mobility limitations, transportation disruption, or safety concerns. Implementation approaches include mobile dispensing operations bringing medications directly to isolated populations, community health worker programs conducting home visits with basic medication supplies, telecommunication triage identifying highest-priority delivery needs, and coordination with emergency services providing transportation when pharmaceutical delivery proves unfeasible. Operational considerations include security provisions during distribution in potentially unstable environments, verification procedures confirming appropriate recipient identification despite limited documentation, inventory management ensuring accountable distribution despite field conditions, and appropriate prioritization focusing limited resources on most critical needs. These outreach capabilities transform home-bound individuals from forgotten disaster victims to specifically addressed populations with dedicated support strategies, maintaining essential medication access through deliberate outreach rather than accepting potential therapy interruption during circumstances preventing normal healthcare facility access.

Recovery and System Restoration

Phased restoration planning establishes systematic approaches to normal operations resumption following disasters, creating predetermined pathways from emergency functions to routine practices that maintain safety throughout the transition. Comprehensive planning includes recovery sequence determination based on clinical priority and dependency relationships, resource allocation supporting progressive restoration, verification procedures confirming appropriate functionality before reliance, and contingency provisions addressing potential setbacks during the recovery process. Medication-specific elements typically address inventory replenishment following emergency depletion, technology restoration when electronic systems resume availability, staffing normalization as emergency deployment concludes, therapeutic standardization returning from disaster alternatives to preferred agents, and quality system reinstatement ensuring appropriate safety restoration. These structured approaches transform disaster recovery from chaotic normalization attempts to systematic restoration processes, establishing appropriate transition supporting both operational resumption and safety maintenance throughout the recovery continuum.

Documentation reconciliation establishes information continuity between disaster operations and normal systems, addressing the potential gaps created when emergency conditions necessitate modified recording practices or alternative documentation methods. Effective reconciliation includes systematic collection of emergency records created during disaster conditions, methodical integration into permanent systems maintaining information continuity, gap identification when critical information remains unavailable, and appropriate notation regarding emergency circumstances affecting normal documentation standards. Implementation considerations include realistic expectations regarding possible reconciliation completeness after catastrophic disruption, prioritization focusing limited resources on most critical information integration, appropriate regulatory communication regarding documentation modifications, and quality verification ensuring that reconciled information accurately reflects actual therapy despite transition between recording systems. This systematic information management transforms potential post-disaster documentation chaos to structured information continuity, maintaining essential treatment records despite transitions between emergency and normal operating conditions.

After-action analysis establishes structured evaluation of disaster medication management performance, transforming response experience into specific improvement opportunities enhancing future capability. Comprehensive analysis includes detailed chronology reconstruction documenting main events and decisions, objective performance assessment identifying both successful elements and improvement opportunities, root cause analysis determining fundamental factors rather than superficial observations, and specific recommendation development with practical implementation guidance. Medication-specific evaluation typically addresses inventory adequacy for actual disaster needs, distribution effectiveness reaching vulnerable populations, therapeutic decision quality during resource limitations, documentation sufficiency supporting post-disaster continuity, and staff performance under emergency conditions. These systematic assessments transform disaster response from isolated experience to organizational learning opportunity, creating valuable insight supporting specific preparedness enhancement rather than leaving important lessons uncaptured as operations normalize.

Staff support and recovery addresses the

psychological impact of disaster response on healthcare personnel, recognizing that effective system restoration requires attention to human factors beyond technical operations. Comprehensive support includes critical incident stress management during and immediately following disaster operations, structured debriefing opportunities processing difficult experiences, continued psychological support addressing delayed stress reactions, workload management preventing exhaustion during extended recovery operations, and appropriate recognition acknowledging extraordinary service during challenging circumstances. Implementation considerations include leadership emphasis establishing psychological support as organizational priority rather than optional consideration, confidential access encouraging utilization without stigma concerns, practical accessibility integrated with work schedules, and continued availability recognizing that stress reactions often emerge during recovery rather than immediate response. This deliberate attention transforms staff from operational resources to valued individuals requiring support, maintaining long-term capability through appropriate recovery assistance rather than risking delayed burnout compromising sustained restoration capacity after initial disaster response concludes.

Things to Remember

- ☑ Crisis management systems include early warning systems, standardized incident command structures, tiered decision-making processes matching response to emergency severity, and documentation maintaining accountability.
- ☑ Medication safety during emergencies employs adapted approaches including tiered safety

systems implementing appropriate modifications, simplified high-alert protocols, alternative distribution models, and enhanced monitoring.

- ☑ Contingency planning creates proactive readiness through vulnerability assessment, scenario development, alternative care site preparation, and workforce continuity strategies ensuring personnel availability.
- ☑ Disaster response addresses catastrophic situations through crisis standards of care implementation, medication triage systems allocating limited supplies, strategic national stockpile access, and specialized approaches for vulnerable populations.
- ☑ Effective emergency planning addresses both anticipated scenarios based on risk assessment and adaptive capacity for unanticipated situations requiring flexible response.
- ☑ Regular testing through simulations, tabletop exercises, and limited-scale drills verifies plan effectiveness before actual emergencies occur

Multiple Choice Questions

1. Crisis management systems for medication safety include:
   a) Elimination of all safety protocols during emergencies
   b) Standardized incident command structures establishing clear authority
   c) Centralization of all medication decisions with a single individual
   d) Identical approaches regardless of emergency severity
2. Medication safety during emergencies employs:

a) Abandonment of all safety procedures to increase efficiency
b) Tiered safety systems implementing appropriate modifications based on crisis severity
c) Identical procedures as normal operations regardless of circumstances
d) Focus exclusively on controlled substances without consideration of other medications

3. Alternative distribution models during infrastructure disruptions might include:
a) Eliminating documentation of medication administration
b) Batched dispensing with adjusted verification processes
c) Removing pharmacist review from the medication process
d) Allowing unrestricted access to all medication supplies

4. Contingency planning creates proactive readiness through:
a) Focus exclusively on natural disasters without considering other emergencies
b) Generalized approaches without specific scenario planning
c) Vulnerability assessment identifying system weaknesses
d) Planning conducted by emergency management without clinical input

5. Crisis standards of care implementation addresses:
a) Normal operation standards without modification

b) Necessary practice modifications acknowledging emergency constraints
c) Elimination of all standards during emergencies
d) Focus exclusively on documentation rather than clinical practice

6. Medication triage systems during disasters:
a) Always ensure normal medication availability without modification
b) Allocate limited supplies based on clinical priority
c) Focus exclusively on acute medications without consideration of chronic therapies
d) Operate without predefined criteria for decision-making

7. Strategic national stockpile considerations include:
a) Unlimited medication availability making local planning unnecessary
b) Immediate access without activation procedures
c) Understanding access procedures, timeline, and integration with local systems
d) Focus exclusively on controlled substances and antibiotics

8. Early warning systems for medication-related emergencies:
a) Are unnecessary with robust response capabilities
b) Should focus exclusively on external disasters
c) Enable timely identification and proactive response

d) Function best without integration with broader emergency management

9. Workforce continuity strategies ensuring personnel availability might include:
   a) Expectation that all staff will be available regardless of circumstances
   b) Cross-training, emergency credentialing, and staffing adjustments
   c) Reliance exclusively on existing staff without external support mechanisms
   d) Focus on physicians without consideration of other essential personnel
10. Effective emergency planning addresses:
   a) Only the most likely scenarios based on historical experience
   b) Response without consideration of recovery processes
   c) Both anticipated scenarios and adaptive capacity for unanticipated situations
   d) Technology failures without consideration of staffing challenges

Self-Assessment Questions

1. Critically analyze the components of an effective crisis management plan for medication-related emergencies, including roles, communication, decision-making, and response protocols.
2. Evaluate strategies to maintain medication safety during different types of emergencies (natural disasters, pandemics, infrastructure failures), including considerations for prioritization and resource allocation.
3. Analyze comprehensive contingency planning approaches for medication management during emergencies, addressing supply chain disruptions, staffing shortages, and system failures.
4. Discuss the main elements of an effective medication-focused disaster response protocol, including immediate actions, sustained operations, and recovery phases.
5. Evaluate the unique medication safety challenges during mass casualty incidents and strategies to maintain safe practices under extreme pressure.
6. Analyze approaches to maintaining the cold chain and other special storage requirements during emergencies where infrastructure may be compromised.
7. Discuss strategies for cross-training healthcare professionals to ensure medication safety competencies during emergency situations

when typical roles may be disrupted.

8. Evaluate the role of community partnerships (other healthcare facilities, suppliers, government agencies) in enhancing emergency preparedness for medication management.
9. Analyze how medication stockpiling and alternative supply systems should be developed, maintained, and deployed during emergencies.
10. Discuss how organizations should conduct post-emergency reviews of medication management performance and integrate lessons learned into future preparedness plans

Bibliography

1. Institute of Medicine. Crisis Standards of Care: A Systems Framework for Catastrophic Disaster Response. Washington, DC: National Academies Press; 2012.
2. Hick JL, Hanfling D, Burstein JL, DeAtley C, Barbisch D, Bogdan GM, et al. Health care facility and community strategies for patient care surge capacity. Ann Emerg Med. 2004;44(3):253-61.
3. American Society of Health-System Pharmacists. ASHP statement on emergency preparedness. Am J Health Syst Pharm. 2003;60(24):2582-3.
4. Setlak P. Bioterrorism preparedness and response: emerging role for health-system pharmacists. Am J Health Syst Pharm. 2004;61(11):1167-75.
5. Bell C, Daniel S. Pharmacy leader's role in hospital emergency preparedness planning. Hosp Pharm. 2014;49(4):398-404.
6. Amaratunga CA, O'Sullivan TL, Phillips KP, Lemyre L, O'Connor E, Dow D, et al. Ready, aye ready? Support mechanisms for healthcare workers in emergency planning: a critical gap analysis of three hospital emergency plans. Am J Disaster Med. 2007;2(4):195-210.
7. Young D. Pharmacists play vital roles in Katrina response: more disaster-response participation urged. Am J Health Syst Pharm. 2005;62(21):2202-16.
8. Crane JS, McCluskey JD, Johnson GT, Harbison RD. Assessment of community healthcare providers ability and willingness to respond to emergencies resulting from bioterrorist attacks. J Emerg Trauma Shock. 2010;3(1):13-20.
9. U.S. Department of Health and Human Services. Strategic National Stockpile. Public Health Emergency. Washington, DC: HHS; 2019.
10. Hsu EB, Jenckes MW, Catlett CL, Robinson KA, Feuerstein C, Cosgrove SE, et al. Effectiveness of hospital staff mass-casualty incident training methods: a systematic literature review. Prehosp Disaster Med. 2004;19(3):191-9.

CHAPTER 14

CURRENT TRENDS IN MEDICATION SAFETY

Abstract

Current trends in medication safety reflect rapid innovation expanding capabilities while introducing novel considerations for implementation and oversight. Emerging technologies transforming medication management include advanced dispensing robotics reducing human manipulation errors, autonomous mobile robots providing reliable transportation, closed-loop administration systems creating comprehensive verification throughout medication processes, and Internet of Things applications connecting previously isolated systems into coordinated networks. Artificial intelligence applications create unprecedented capabilities through adverse event prediction models identifying patients at elevated risk, personalized dosing systems accounting for individual pharmacokinetic factors, adaptive alert systems reducing fatigue while maintaining critical warnings, and natural language interfaces enabling intuitive interaction with clinical systems, while raising important validation and regulatory considerations requiring new approaches to system verification. Global initiatives establish collaborative approaches transcending organizational and national boundaries through WHO programs including Medication Without Harm, international classification systems supporting consistent analysis, medication safety monitoring networks detecting patterns beyond individual country capabilities, and cross-border collaborations to overcome shared challenges across international boundaries.

Keywords: *Automation systems, artificial intelligence applications, predictive analytics, global collaboration, technological innovation*

Learning Objectives

After completion of the chapter, the learners should be able to:

- Remember main emerging technologies being applied to medication safety.
- Understand how artificial intelligence applications are transforming medication error prevention.
- Apply implementation science methodologies to support effective technology deployment.
- Analyze the potential benefits and limitations of advanced technologies in medication safety.
- Evaluate the impact of global initiatives on medication safety improvement.
- Create strategies for effectively implementing innovative approaches while addressing ethical considerations

EMERGING TECHNOLOGIES

Emerging technologies are rapidly transforming medication safety practices through innovative approaches that enhance detection, prevention, and management of medication-related risks. These technological advances create new capabilities that extend beyond traditional safety practices, offering unprecedented opportunities to address longstanding challenges while introducing novel considerations for implementation and oversight.

Automation and Robotics

Advanced dispensing robotics represents a significant evolution beyond first-generation automation, introducing sophisticated capabilities that reduce human manipulation while enhancing accuracy and efficiency. Contemporary systems employ computer vision for medication identification verification, precision robotics enabling exact measurement and preparation, gravimetric verification confirming dispensed quantities through weight comparison, and comprehensive transaction logging creating complete preparation documentation. Implementation in central pharmacy operations enables high-volume dispensing with minimal human intervention, while decentralized applications bring robotics to patient care areas through medication dispensing units with integrated automated selection. Specialized applications include chemotherapy robotics reducing staff exposure to hazardous agents, sterile product compounding systems minimizing contamination risk, and controlled substance automation enhancing security while maintaining accessibility for legitimate clinical needs. These advanced systems address the fundamental safety limitation of human manipulation errors while creating standardized processes with comprehensive documentation capabilities.

Autonomous mobile robots establish new medication delivery capabilities, creating reliable transport systems that operate independently throughout healthcare facilities. Contemporary implementations employ advanced navigation technologies including visual mapping, obstacle detection sensors, elevator interface capabilities, and secure access control for restricted areas. Medication-specific applications include scheduled medication delivery from pharmacy to patient care areas, specimen transport between clinical units and laboratories, supply distribution throughout healthcare facilities, and even direct patient room delivery in certain implementations. Safety features address both medication security through access-controlled compartments and environmental safety through sophisticated collision avoidance, emergency stopping capabilities, and pathway optimization preventing congestion in clinical areas. These automated delivery systems address transportation reliability challenges that frequently compromise medication availability, creating consistent delivery performance while freeing personnel for clinical activities requiring human judgment rather than simple transport functions.

Wearable robotics and augmentation technologies enhance human capabilities during medication preparation and administration, reducing physical limitations that can contribute to errors while maintaining human oversight for complex judgments. Applications include smart glasses displaying medication information during preparation and administration, wearable barcode scanners enhancing mobility during medication verification, exoskeleton devices reducing fatigue during extended medication preparation sessions, and voice-controlled documentation systems enabling simultaneous physical tasks and information recording. Advanced implementations integrate these wearable technologies with electronic health records and medication management systems, creating seamless information flow between facility systems and point-of-care wearable devices. These augmentation approaches address the complementary strengths of humans and machines, enhancing human capabilities where irreplaceable judgment proves valuable while supporting physical limitations that might otherwise compromise safety.

Intelligent automation systems incorporate adaptive

capabilities beyond simple programmed routines, creating responsive technologies that adjust operations based on changing conditions and learned patterns. Medication-specific implementations include inventory management systems that adjust stock levels based on observed usage trends, dispensing routines that adapt scheduling to patient administration patterns, preparation sequencing that optimizes workflow based on priority and resource availability, and quality control systems that intensify verification for error-prone situations identified through pattern analysis. The distinguishing characteristic of these intelligent systems involves closed-loop learning, where performance data continuously refines operational parameters without explicit reprogramming. This continuous adaptation addresses the limitations of static automation that maintains fixed operations regardless of changing circumstances, creating responsive systems matching actual operational conditions rather than predetermined assumptions that may poorly reflect reality.

Advanced Medication Administration Technologies

Smart infusion systems represent significant evolution beyond basic programmable pumps, incorporating sophisticated capabilities that prevent programming errors while providing comprehensive data for safety analysis. Contemporary systems implement dose error reduction software with customizable drug libraries establishing appropriate concentration, dosing, and rate parameters; interoperability with electronic health records enabling automatic programming based on verified orders; barcode verification ensuring proper medication selection before infusion initiation; and continuous monitoring with automated alerts for infusion abnormalities. Advanced capabilities include weight-based dosing calculators preventing mathematical errors, automated documentation creating complete infusion records, titration assistance supporting protocol-based adjustments, and integration with patient monitoring systems enabling physiological parameter correlation with medication administration. These sophisticated systems address the persistent safety challenges associated with high-risk intravenous medications, creating multiple layers of protection against programming errors while providing comprehensive data supporting both individual therapy optimization and system-level safety improvement.

Closed-loop medication administration technologies establish comprehensive verification throughout the medication use process, creating end-to-end confirmation from prescribing through administration. Fully implemented systems connect computerized provider order entry directly to dispensing automation, verify medication selection through barcode scanning, confirm patient identity before administration, document actual medication delivery including partial or refused doses, and record patient response completing the therapeutic cycle. Advanced implementations incorporate multiple technologies including barcode verification, RFID tracking, biometric patient identification, electronic medication administration records, and smart infusion systems into integrated verification networks rather than isolated technologies. This comprehensive approach addresses the traditional safety gaps between separate medication process stages, creating continuous verification throughout the medication use journey rather than isolated checks at discrete points with vulnerable transitions between systems.

Radio-frequency identification (RFID) medication tracking creates location awareness for medications throughout healthcare facilities, enabling physical tracking beyond the capabilities of traditional inventory and dispensing systems. Implementation approaches include RFID tagging of medication packages at distribution or preparation stages, strategic reader placement throughout facilities tracking movement between locations, integration with electronic health records connecting physical medication location with patient information, and alert capabilities identifying inappropriate medication movement or location. Advanced applications include expiration tracking with automatic alerts for soon-to-expire medications, temperature monitoring ensuring appropriate storage conditions throughout medication journeys, automatic inventory reconciliation without manual counting, and rapid recalls locating specific lots or products requiring removal. This location awareness addresses the persistent safety challenges of medication availability in appropriate locations, creating unprecedented visibility throughout complex healthcare environments with complete tracking from receipt through administration or disposal.

Advanced administration devices introduce novel delivery mechanisms beyond traditional approaches, creating new options for specialized medication delivery needs. Notable innovations include needle-free injection systems reducing sharps risks and improving medication absorption, implantable pumps providing continuous therapy for chronic conditions, smart inhalers confirming appropriate administration technique and documenting actual usage, and sensor-embedded pills verifying actual medication ingestion rather than assumed consumption based on dispensing alone. Safety features within these novel devices include precise dosing mechanisms preventing administration variability, confirmation systems documenting actual medication delivery, patient-specific calibration ensuring appropriate therapy matching individual needs, and communication capabilities sharing administration information with healthcare providers. These innovative approaches address the limitations of traditional administration routes and methods, creating new therapeutic options with enhanced safety features integrated directly into delivery mechanisms rather than relying solely on external verification systems.

Digital Health and Connected Systems

Internet of Things (IoT) applications in medication management create interconnected networks of devices sharing information and coordinating activities throughout the medication use process. Comprehensive implementations connect multiple systems including automated dispensing cabinets, refrigeration units, ambient storage conditions, preparation equipment, and administration devices into coordinated networks with centralized monitoring and management capabilities. Medication-specific applications include temperature monitoring systems ensuring appropriate storage conditions with automatic alerts for excursions, inventory tracking networks providing real-time availability information across multiple locations, preparation equipment sharing status information enabling workflow optimization, and administration devices communicating actual usage data to supply management systems. Security considerations include appropriate data protection preventing unauthorized access, authentication systems ensuring legitimate device connections, and resilience against connectivity disruptions maintaining critical functions despite network issues. These interconnected systems address the traditional isolation between separate medication technologies, creating cohesive information environments supporting comprehensive management rather than fragmented data trapped within individual system boundaries.

Table 14.1: Emerging Technologies in Medication Safety

Technology	Applications	Potential Impact
Closed-Loop Systems	Order to administration tracking Full process verification Complete documentation	50-80% error reduction Documentation improvement Workflow standardization
Smart Infusion Systems	Interoperability with EHR Auto-programming Comprehensive drug libraries	IV error reduction Programming time reduction Improved documentation
Medication Tracking	RFID medication tracking Real-time inventory Expiration management	Diversion reduction Inventory optimization Recall management
Telehealth Medication Management	Remote verification Virtual patient education Adherence monitoring	Access improvement Adherence enhancement Monitoring continuity

Mobile applications for medication management establish portable capabilities supporting medication safety throughout healthcare facilities and extending into patient homes. Clinical applications include mobile medication references providing instant information access at the point of care, barcode scanning applications enabling verification without fixed workstations, clinical decision support tools delivering personalized recommendations based on patient-specific factors, and documentation platforms capturing information during actual medication activities rather than requiring separate recording sessions. Patient-centered applications include medication reminder systems supporting adherence, educational tools explaining proper usage and potential effects, side effect tracking with appropriate escalation guidance, and secure communication channels connecting patients with healthcare providers for medication-related questions. These mobile capabilities address the limitations of stationary systems inadequately supporting dynamic healthcare workflows and patient self-management, creating accessible information and tools available whenever and wherever medication decisions occur.

Health information exchange specifically focused on medication information creates broader medication history accessibility beyond individual organizational boundaries, addressing the persistent safety challenge of fragmented information across multiple providers and pharmacies. Implementation approaches include shared medication history repositories accessible across healthcare organizations, community pharmacy networks contributing dispensing information to clinical care providers, prescription monitoring programs identifying concerning patterns across multiple prescribers, and standardized medication reconciliation platforms supporting information consistency during care transitions. Technical foundations include standardized terminology supporting consistent information interpretation, structured data formats enabling automated integration, appropriate privacy protections maintaining confidentiality while enabling necessary access, and identity management ensuring accurate patient matching across systems. This expanded information accessibility addresses the critical safety limitation of incomplete medication history during clinical decision-making, creating comprehensive medication visibility supporting appropriate therapeutic choices based on complete rather than partial information.

Patient engagement technologies establish direct connections between individuals and healthcare systems, creating new capabilities for medication self-management while generating valuable information supporting clinical care. Implementation approaches include patient portals providing access to medication lists with educational resources, secure messaging systems enabling medication questions without requiring appointments, remote monitoring platforms tracking therapy adherence and effects, and shared decision-making tools supporting collaborative medication choices based on individual preferences and clinical evidence. Advanced capabilities include personalized educational content matched to specific health literacy levels and language preferences, symptom tracking with algorithmic triage identifying concerning patterns requiring intervention, medication visualization tools illustrating proper administration techniques, and gamification elements encouraging consistent engagement with management activities. These engagement technologies address the traditional limitation of medication management confined within clinical encounters, extending support throughout daily life while creating continuous information flow between periodic healthcare visits.

Data and Analytics

Predictive analytics applications in medication safety utilize advanced statistical methods and machine learning to identify potential problems before actual harm occurs, shifting from reactive response to proactive prevention. Implementation approaches include risk prediction models identifying patients at elevated risk for adverse drug events based on demographic, clinical, and medication factors; early warning systems detecting subtle patterns suggesting developing complications before obvious symptoms appear; anomaly detection algorithms identifying unusual medication utilization patterns potentially indicating errors or quality issues; and workflow prediction forecasting resource needs and potential bottlenecks before operational problems develop. Technical foundations include large-scale data integration combining information across clinical, operational, and administrative systems; sophisticated model development using machine learning techniques with appropriate validation; and implementation systems delivering actionable insights to appropriate recipients capable of intervention. These predictive capabilities address the fundamental limitation of traditional safety systems that identify problems only after occurrence, creating anticipatory awareness supporting prevention rather than merely detecting adverse events after patients experience harm.

Real-time surveillance systems continuously monitor medication-related data streams, identifying potential safety issues requiring immediate attention through automated pattern recognition. Contemporary implementations analyze multiple data sources including electronic health record documentation, pharmacy dispensing records, medication administration data, laboratory results, and physiological monitoring parameters. Detection algorithms identify concerning patterns such as laboratory values suggesting medication toxicity, administration patterns indicating potential dosing errors, order combinations creating interaction risks, and physiological changes potentially representing adverse effects. Alerting systems deliver notifications to appropriate personnel through various modalities including electronic health record messaging, secure mobile communication, workstation alerts, and in highest-risk situations, automated paging or calling systems ensuring immediate awareness. These surveillance capabilities address the challenge of identifying safety concerns within massive data volumes exceeding human monitoring capacity, creating automated vigilance continuously evaluating information across entire patient populations rather than limited review possible through manual processes.

Natural language processing applications extract medication-relevant information from unstructured clinical documentation, transforming narrative text into structured data supporting safety applications. Implementation approaches include automated analysis of clinical notes identifying medication information not captured in structured fields; interpretation of patient-reported symptoms potentially representing adverse effects; extraction of medication instructions from discharge summaries supporting reconciliation; and identification of documented allergic reactions sometimes missing from formal allergy lists. Technical capabilities include named entity recognition identifying medication mentions within text; contextual analysis distinguishing between current, discontinued, and considered medications; semantic interpretation extracting dosing and timing information; and sentiment analysis identifying expressions of concern or uncertainty requiring additional attention. These capabilities address the significant safety limitation of critical medication information trapped within narrative documentation, creating structured data availability supporting automated analysis and clinical decision support beyond the limited information captured in dedicated medication fields.

Integrated analytics dashboards transform complex medication safety data into actionable intelligence supporting both operational management and strategic improvement. Implementation approaches include executive dashboards providing high-level safety metrics with drill-down capabilities revealing underlying factors; department-specific views presenting relevant information matched to specific roles and responsibilities; operational displays supporting daily management with real-time information; and analytical workbenches enabling interactive exploration for quality improvement activities. Visualization techniques include statistical process control charts distinguishing random variation from significant changes; comparative displays benchmarking performance against relevant standards; relationship diagrams illustrating connections between process factors and outcomes; and predictive visualizations showing projected trends supporting proactive intervention. These integrated perspectives address the challenge of extracting meaningful insights from increasingly complex and voluminous medication safety data, creating usable intelligence supporting both immediate operational decisions and strategic improvement initiatives rather than overwhelming information without practical application value.

ARTIFICIAL INTELLIGENCE

Artificial intelligence represents a transformative force in medication safety, introducing sophisticated capabilities that extend far beyond traditional rule-based systems to include advanced learning, reasoning, and adaptation addressing complex medication safety challenges. These technologies create unprecedented opportunities for safety enhancement while simultaneously introducing novel considerations for validation, implementation, and oversight.

Table 14.2: Artificial Intelligence Applications in Medication Safety

AI Application	Functionality	Challenges
Predictive Analytics	ADE risk prediction Intervention prioritization Resource allocation	Data quality requirements Algorithm validation Workflow integration
Clinical Decision Support	Intelligent alerting Context-aware recommendations Patient-specific dosing	Alert fatigue management Knowledge maintenance Clinical workflow integration
Error Detection	Pattern recognition Anomaly detection Near-miss identification	Data access requirements Validation processes Action protocols
Medication Management	Administration verification Patient identification Documentation assistance	Technology infrastructure Patient acceptance Staff adaptation

Machine Learning Applications

Adverse event prediction models employ sophisticated algorithms to identify patients at elevated risk for medication-related harm, enabling proactive intervention before adverse events occur. Contemporary implementations analyze multiple data elements including patient demographics, comorbidity profiles, laboratory values, medication regimens, prior adverse events, genetic information when available, and even social determinants of health influencing medication risks. Advanced models employ various techniques including supervised learning trained on historical adverse event data, deep learning identifying complex patterns beyond traditional statistical relationships, and reinforcement learning that continuously improves through outcome feedback. Clinical applications include risk stratification directing enhanced monitoring to highest-risk patients, intervention targeting focusing pharmacy review on vulnerable individuals, administration planning aligning observation intensity with predicted risk, and discharge preparation providing enhanced support for patients leaving with high-risk medication regimens. These predictive capabilities address the fundamental safety challenge of efficiently allocating limited resources, directing attention to patients most likely to benefit from intervention rather than applying uniform approaches regardless of individual risk profiles.

Medication error detection systems utilize artificial intelligence to identify potential mistakes throughout the medication use process, creating automated vigilance beyond human monitoring capabilities. Implementation approaches include pattern recognition identifying unusual medication orders requiring verification, image analysis detecting discrepancies during medication preparation, transaction review identifying potential dispensing errors, and documentation analysis revealing possible administration mistakes. Technical foundations include both supervised learning using known error patterns from historical data and anomaly detection identifying unusual patterns without specific pre-programming. Operational integration typically involves tiered alerting with different notification pathways based on error probability and potential severity, integration with existing workflow systems delivering alerts within normal processes rather than separate applications, and feedback mechanisms enabling continuous learning from alert outcomes. These automated detection capabilities address the inevitable limitations of human vigilance in complex, high-volume medication systems, creating continuous monitoring impossible through manual processes while reducing alert fatigue through sophisticated prioritization beyond simple rule-based warnings.

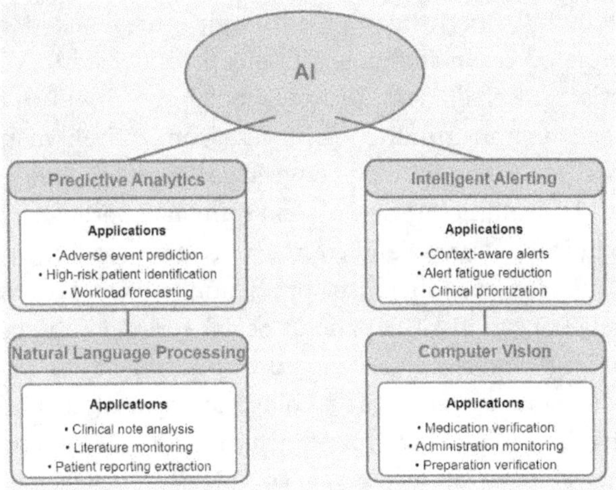

Figure 14.1 Artificial Intelligence Applications in Medication Safety

Medication reconciliation enhancement through artificial intelligence transforms this traditionally labor-intensive process through automated information processing capabilities. Advanced implementations employ natural language processing to extract medication information from various documents including admission notes, referral letters, and previous records; entity matching algorithms to identify the same medication across different terminology and naming conventions; intelligent form processing to extract information from scanned documents or external medication lists; and anomaly detection identifying potential discrepancies requiring human review. Workflow integration typically includes pre-processing systems preparing reconciliation information before clinician review, discrepancy highlighting focusing attention on potential issues rather than complete manual comparison, suggested resolution options based on common reconciliation patterns, and continuous learning improving performance through feedback from completed reconciliations. These capabilities address the persistent challenge of reconciliation quality and efficiency, transforming the process from entirely manual effort to collaboration between artificial intelligence handling routine processing and human experts focusing on clinical judgment and complex decision-making.

Medication adherence prediction utilizes artificial intelligence to identify patients at risk for non-adherence, enabling targeted interventions supporting appropriate medication use after prescribing. Sophisticated models analyze multiple factors including past adherence patterns, medication regimen complexity, socioeconomic factors, health beliefs and attitudes, side effect experiences, and practical barriers such as transportation or cost challenges. Technical approaches include supervised learning based on historical adherence data, temporal pattern analysis identifying changes potentially indicating declining adherence, and multimodal analysis integrating data across various sources including prescription fills, patient-reported information, and when available, direct medication consumption monitoring. Clinical applications include personalized intervention matching specific adherence barriers, resource allocation directing support services to highest-risk individuals, communication customization aligned with individual factors influencing adherence, and regimen simplification focusing on patients where complexity significantly impacts medication use. These predictive capabilities address the critical safety gap between prescribing and actual medication consumption, enabling proactive support rather than discovering adherence issues only after therapeutic failure or preventable complications.

Clinical Decision Support Evolution

Personalized dosing systems utilize artificial intelligence to recommend individualized medication regimens based on patient-specific factors beyond standard weight-based or population-derived dosing. Advanced implementations analyze multiple determinants including pharmacogenomic data affecting drug metabolism, organ function parameters influencing clearance, comorbidities altering medication response, concurrent medications creating interaction effects, age-related physiological changes, and when available, previous medication response patterns. Technical approaches include pharmacokinetic modeling predicting drug concentrations based on individual parameters, machine learning algorithms identifying optimal dosing from historical outcomes data, and reinforcement learning systems that continuously improve through outcome feedback. Clinical applications include initial dose selection matched to individual characteristics, adjustment recommendations based on monitoring results, adaptive titration guidance responding to observed effects, and therapeutic drug monitoring interpretation considering comprehensive individual contexts. These personalized approaches address the fundamental limitation of standard dosing recommendations based on population averages, creating individualized therapy matched to specific patient characteristics rather than generic regimens inadequately accounting for significant inter-individual variability.

Adaptive alert systems employ artificial intelligence to dynamically modify warning behavior based on context, user characteristics, and historical patterns, addressing the persistent challenge of alert fatigue compromising response to important warnings. Implementation approaches include user-specific adaptation adjusting alerting based on individual response patterns and expertise levels; contextual modification considering patient-specific factors affecting alert relevance; workload-sensitive timing presenting less critical alerts during lower-stress periods; and progressive disclosure providing basic information initially with additional detail available on demand. Technical foundations include reinforcement learning algorithms optimizing alerting based on response outcomes, pattern recognition identifying situations where alerts consistently provide value versus limited utility, and user modeling creating personalized alerting matched to individual work patterns and preferences. These adaptive capabilities address the fundamental limitation of static alerting treating all situations and users identically, creating dynamic warning systems matching information delivery to specific circumstances and recipients rather than one-size-fits-all approaches inevitably creating either excessive alerts or insufficient warnings for different users and situations.

Natural language interaction enables conversational engagement with clinical decision support systems, creating intuitive interfaces beyond traditional structured data entry and standardized display formats. Implementation approaches include voice-activated medication information retrieval providing hands-free access during clinical activities; conversational interfaces supporting natural questions about medication choices, dosing options, and potential interactions; contextual understanding maintaining conversation continuity across multiple exchanges; and multimodal interaction combining voice, text, and visual information based on clinical circumstances and user preferences. Technical foundations include natural language understanding interpreting clinical terminology and conversational language, contextual modeling maintaining awareness of previous interactions and current clinical situation, and response generation creating clinically appropriate answers matching user expertise level and information needs. These natural interfaces address the usability limitations of traditional decision support requiring structured interaction through rigid forms or specific query formats, creating accessible clinical intelligence available through intuitive communication rather than formal system interaction requiring specific technical knowledge.

Explainable AI for medication decisions establishes transparency in artificial intelligence recommendations, providing understandable rationales supporting clinical judgment rather than opaque "black box" guidance. Implementation approaches include decision path visualization showing logical progression from input data to recommendations; confidence indication communicating certainty levels with supporting evidence; counterfactual explanation demonstrating how different clinical circumstances would change recommendations; and comparative analysis showing alternative options with associated benefits and risks. Technical approaches include inherently interpretable models such as decision trees or rule lists providing directly understandable logic; post-hoc explanation methods generating interpretations of complex models; and hybrid systems combining transparent components for critical reasoning with higher-performance complex components for pattern recognition. These explainable capabilities address the fundamental tension between increasing model sophistication and clinical accountability, creating advanced systems that not only provide recommendations but also supply understandable reasoning supporting appropriate clinical assessment rather than requiring blind trust in algorithmic outputs without verification capability.

Validation Challenges

Validation methodologies for artificial intelligence in medication safety establish rigorous approaches to verifying performance and safety before clinical implementation, addressing the unique challenges of validating complex adaptive systems beyond traditional software verification methods. Comprehensive approaches include retrospective validation against historical data evaluating performance on known cases and outcomes; prospective evaluation running systems alongside standard practices without influencing decisions to compare recommendations; controlled clinical validation in limited environments before broader deployment; and continuous monitoring after implementation identifying any performance degradation or unexpected behaviors. Technical considerations include appropriate test dataset selection ensuring representative coverage across relevant clinical situations; bias assessment identifying potential unfairness across different patient populations; robustness testing evaluating performance with imperfect or missing data reflecting real-world conditions; and boundary testing examining behavior in unusual or extreme situations potentially revealing unsafe responses. These rigorous methodologies address the critical need for thorough validation before clinical deployment, establishing appropriate confidence in system performance while identifying limitations requiring mitigation or explicit acknowledgment during implementation.

Regulatory considerations for medication safety AI address the evolving oversight landscape for these novel technologies, navigating complex requirements while ensuring appropriate safety verification without unnecessarily impeding beneficial innovation. Current approaches navigate multiple systems including traditional medical device regulation when systems directly influence clinical care; software as a medical device (SaMD) classifications based on risk level and intended use; quality system requirements ensuring appropriate development, testing, and maintenance processes; and clinical evaluation expectations appropriate to potential patient impact. Implementation considerations include appropriate regulatory strategy development matching specific system characteristics and intended applications; documentation practices supporting regulatory review; postmarket surveillance planning detecting potential issues after deployment; and modification management ensuring appropriate revalidation after system changes. These regulatory navigation approaches address the challenge of ensuring appropriate oversight for patient safety while acknowledging the unique characteristics of artificial intelligence systems including continuous learning capabilities, complex performance characteristics, and potential for autonomous operation beyond traditional software limitations.

Ethical systems for AI in medication safety establish principled approaches to development and implementation, addressing the profound ethical questions raised by increasingly autonomous and influential technologies in safety-critical healthcare applications. Comprehensive systems address multiple dimensions including transparency regarding system capabilities and limitations; fairness ensuring equitable performance across diverse patient populations; privacy protection for sensitive data used in development and operation; autonomy preservation maintaining appropriate human oversight and decision authority; accountability establishing clear responsibility for system outcomes; and beneficence ensuring overall patient benefit as primary objective. Implementation considerations include ethical review processes during development, explicit consideration of potential unintended consequences, stakeholder engagement including patient perspectives, and governance structures providing ongoing ethical oversight throughout system lifecycle. These principled approaches address the fundamental need for ethical guidance beyond technical performance, ensuring that increasingly powerful artificial intelligence systems serve patient interests while respecting fundamental values and rights throughout their development and application.

Integration strategies for artificial intelligence in

clinical workflows establish practical approaches to incorporating advanced capabilities into actual care processes, addressing the critical gap between technical possibilities and operational reality that often limits real-world impact. Effective strategies include workflow analysis identifying appropriate integration points where AI can provide value without disruption; user-centered design creating interfaces matched to clinical needs and constraints; phased implementation beginning with limited applications before broader deployment; and collaborative development involving end users throughout the process rather than technical creation followed by attempted implementation. Organizational considerations include change management addressing transitional challenges; training programs developing appropriate user understanding without requiring technical expertise; feedback mechanisms capturing implementation experiences for continuous improvement; and support systems addressing inevitable questions and challenges during adoption. These practical approaches address the common failure point where technically impressive systems fail to achieve practical adoption due to workflow misalignment, creating implementations that effectively complement clinical processes rather than imposing technological solutions mismatched to operational realities.

Future Directions and Potential

Multimodal AI integrates diverse data types beyond traditional structured clinical information, creating comprehensive understanding supporting advanced medication safety applications. Implementation approaches include combined analysis of clinical documentation, medical imaging, physiological monitoring data, genomic information, social determinants of health, and even ambient intelligence from smart environments. Medication safety applications include comprehensive adverse effect detection through integrated analysis of documented symptoms, physiological changes, laboratory abnormalities, and patient-reported experiences; personalized risk assessment incorporating diverse factors beyond traditional clinical parameters; interaction detection considering broader influences beyond direct pharmacological effects; and therapeutic response prediction integrating multiple outcome indicators. Technical foundations include specialized processing for different data types, translation mechanisms creating comparable representations across modalities, fusion techniques integrating information at various processing levels, and advanced architectures handling fundamentally different data characteristics within unified systems. These integrative capabilities address the limitations of single-source analysis inadequately capturing complex medication effects manifesting across multiple clinical dimensions, creating comprehensive understanding supporting sophisticated safety applications beyond traditional compartmentalized approaches limited to isolated data categories.

Autonomous systems represent the frontier of artificial intelligence in medication safety, introducing capabilities for independent operation beyond traditional decision support requiring explicit human activation and oversight. Early implementations include autonomous monitoring systems continuously evaluating patient status and medication effects without requiring manual reviews; independent safety verification conducting automated checks without explicit human initiation; proactive intervention systems initiating safety measures based on detected risks; and self-optimizing processes that continuously improve based on operational experience and outcomes. Governance considerations include appropriate autonomy boundaries establishing clear limits on independent action; human oversight requirements specifying situations requiring expert intervention; transparency mechanisms ensuring visibility into autonomous operations; and accountability systems establishing clear responsibility for system actions and outcomes. These autonomous capabilities address the fundamental capacity limitations of human-centered safety systems, creating continuous vigilance impossible through manual processes while raising profound questions about appropriate balance between technological capability and human judgment in safety-critical healthcare contexts.

Federated learning enables artificial intelligence development across multiple organizations without sharing sensitive data, addressing the critical privacy and data ownership challenges limiting development of powerful medication safety models requiring diverse training information. Implementation approaches include distributed training where models learn from local data at multiple sites with only model parameters rather than actual data shared between organizations; secure computation techniques allowing collaborative analysis without exposing original information; privacy-preserving methods ensuring individual patient data remains protected while enabling population-level learning; and decentralized validation assessing performance across diverse environments. Medication safety applications include adverse event prediction models learning from wider patient populations than single organizations could provide; medication error detection systems incorporating patterns from diverse practice environments; drug interaction models integrating experience across varied patient cohorts; and personalized dosing systems learning from broader outcome data than available within individual institutions. These collaborative approaches address the fundamental tension between data privacy requirements and the need for diverse training information developing robust artificial intelligence systems, creating sophisticated models benefiting from broad experience while maintaining appropriate privacy protection and organizational data control.-AI collaboration models establish systems for effective partnership between clinicians and artificial intelligence systems, creating synergistic relationships leveraging the complementary strengths of human expertise and computational capability. Implementation approaches include mixed-initiative systems where either humans or AI can initiate interaction as appropriate; adaptive automation adjusting autonomy levels based on situation complexity and user preferences; transparent operation allowing human partners to understand AI reasoning and limitations; and calibrated trust supporting appropriate reliance without over-dependence or unwarranted skepticism. Medication safety applications include collaborative medication review where AI identifies potential issues for human evaluation; shared monitoring with AI conducting continuous surveillance while clinicians provide contextual interpretation; cooperative decision-making combining computational analysis with clinical judgment; and mutual learning where both human and artificial intelligence capabilities improve through collaboration. These partnership models address the limitations of both independent human judgment vulnerable to cognitive biases and information overload and autonomous artificial intelligence potentially lacking contextual understanding and moral reasoning, creating combined capabilities exceeding what either could achieve alone in ensuring medication safety.

GLOBAL INITIATIVES

Global initiatives in medication safety establish collaborative approaches transcending individual organizational and national boundaries, creating shared knowledge, standards, and practices that collectively advance safety across diverse healthcare environments worldwide. These international efforts acknowledge the universal nature of medication safety challenges while respecting contextual differences requiring adapted approaches in various settings.

World Health Organization Programs

The Global Patient Safety Challenge: Medication Without Harm represents a flagship World Health Organization initiative establishing medication safety as a worldwide priority through coordinated international action. This comprehensive program targets specific high-risk areas including transitions of care where information fragmentation creates vulnerability, polypharmacy situations creating complex interaction and adherence challenges, and high-risk medications with elevated harm potential when misused. Implementation focuses on four domains: patients and the public as active participants rather than passive recipients; medications themselves including naming, packaging, and labeling considerations; healthcare professionals and their education, training, and practice environments; and systems and practices of medication management across entire usage pathways. Country-level commitment involves specific action plans, measurement systems tracking progress, collaborative learning networks sharing effective practices, and alignment of national priorities with global objectives. This coordinated approach transforms medication safety from fragmented national or organizational efforts to synchronized global movement, establishing common direction while enabling context-appropriate implementation across diverse healthcare systems and resource environments.

International classification systems for medication errors create standardized taxonomies supporting consistent analysis and learning across organizational and national boundaries. WHO initiatives include the International Classification for Patient Safety establishing standardized terminology and relationships for safety events including medication errors; Minimal Information Model for Patient Safety providing core data elements for reporting and analysis; and International Classification of Diseases incorporating medication-related harm for systematic coding and tracking. Implementation includes translation into multiple languages ensuring global accessibility, mapping guidelines connecting local terminology to international standards, metadata repositories supporting consistent interpretation, and technical specifications enabling interoperable data exchange. These standardized approaches address the persistent challenge of inconsistent error classification preventing meaningful comparison and aggregation, creating common language and structure supporting collaborative learning and improvement across diverse settings rather than isolated understanding limited by incompatible categorization systems.

Table 14.3: Global Medication Safety Initiatives and Their Impact

Initiative	Sponsoring Organization	Focus Areas
Medication Without Harm	World Health Organization	High-risk situations Transitions of care Polypharmacy
Global Patient Safety Challenge	WHO/International Organizations	Standardized protocols Safety culture Patient engagement
ISMP International	International Medication Safety Network	Global medication alerts Best practice sharing Error reporting systems
International Pharmaceutical Federation	FIP	Pharmacist practice advancement Global standards Education systems

Medication safety monitoring networks establish international surveillance systems identifying emerging safety issues beyond the detection capabilities of individual countries or organizations. WHO programs include global pharmacovigilance networks connecting national reporting systems for broader pattern recognition; international alert mechanisms rapidly disseminating critical safety information across borders;

collaborative signal detection combining data from multiple sources for enhanced sensitivity; and coordinated investigation of significant safety concerns requiring multinational expertise. Technical infrastructure includes VigiBase maintaining the world's largest database of adverse drug reactions; VigiFlow supporting standardized case reporting across countries; VigiLyze providing analytical tools for signal detection; and VigiAccess offering public access to relevant safety information. These connected systems address the fundamental limitation of safety surveillance confined within national boundaries, creating comprehensive monitoring reflecting global medication usage patterns rather than fragmented oversight potentially missing important signals visible only through combined international data.

Capacity building programs develop medication safety capabilities in resource-limited settings, addressing the substantial global disparities in safety infrastructure and expertise. WHO approaches include technical guidance adapted for diverse resource environments; training programs developing core competencies among healthcare workers; mentorship initiatives pairing experienced organizations with developing programs; and appropriate technology solutions matched to local infrastructure and sustainability requirements. Implementation strategies emphasize contextually appropriate adaptation rather than direct transplantation of approaches from high-resource settings, capability development creating self-sustaining local expertise rather than perpetual dependence on external support, and phased implementation addressing highest-priority risks first within resource constraints. These development initiatives address the ethical imperative of equitable safety protection across global populations, creating appropriate safety capabilities throughout diverse healthcare environments rather than accepting persistent disparities as inevitable despite the universal nature of medication-related harm potential.

International Collaboration and Standards

International Society for Quality in Health Care (ISQua) initiatives establish global quality systems incorporating medication safety as essential component, creating standards and accreditation approaches supporting consistent improvement worldwide. Main programs include the International Accreditation Programme evaluating healthcare organizations against established safety standards; International Principles for Healthcare Standards providing fundamental guidelines for standards development organizations; and health service quality assessments supporting systematic improvement in diverse settings. Medication safety elements address comprehensive dimensions including governance structures, policy systems, professional practice expectations, technological infrastructure, patient engagement approaches, and outcome measurement methodologies. These international standards address the need for consistent safety expectations transcending national boundaries, establishing common quality systems supporting improvement across diverse healthcare systems while enabling appropriate contextual adaptation rather than rigid uniformity regardless of setting characteristics.

International Standards Organization (ISO) develops technical standards supporting medication safety through specifications for products, processes, and systems used in medication management worldwide. Relevant standards include ISO 9001 establishing quality management system requirements applicable to pharmaceutical operations; ISO 13485 specifying quality systems for medical devices including medication delivery systems; ISO 80369 preventing misconnections between medication delivery systems and other medical applications; and ISO IDMP (Identification of Medicinal Products) creating standardized identification supporting accurate information exchange. Development involves expert representation from multiple countries, consensus-building processes balancing diverse perspectives, systematic review maintaining relevance, and implementation support facilitating adoption. These technical standards address the essential need for consistent specifications supporting safe interchange of medication-related products and information across international boundaries, creating reliable interfaces between systems, products, and processes from different sources rather than hazardous incompatibilities potentially compromising safety.

International collaboration for medication naming standardization addresses the persistent safety challenges created by inconsistent nomenclature across global medication markets. Initiatives include the International Nonproprietary Name (INN) program establishing globally recognized generic medication names; tall man lettering standardization creating consistent approaches to distinguishing similar medication names; bar coding standards enabling reliable product identification across international boundaries; and global medication terminology systems supporting accurate information exchange despite language and naming differences. Implementation involves pharmaceutical manufacturer participation adopting standardized approaches, regulatory authority coordination enforcing consistent naming requirements, healthcare organization implementation incorporating standardized nomenclature into clinical systems, and technology vendor adherence ensuring software supports established standards. These harmonization efforts address the substantial safety risks created by nomenclature inconsistency in increasingly global pharmaceutical markets, establishing reliable identification despite diverse naming conventions and language differences rather than accepting perpetual confusion as inevitable aspect of international medication management.

Global health information exchange standards support medication information flow across organizational and national boundaries, creating interoperability supporting safe care transitions despite fragmented systems. Main standards include HL7 FHIR (Fast Healthcare Interoperability Resources) enabling structured data exchange; SNOMED CT providing clinical terminology for consistent concept representation; RxNorm establishing normalized naming for medications; and CDA (Clinical Document Architecture) supporting comprehensive clinical information exchange including medication data. Implementation approaches include standards development with international participation, harmonization between competing specifications, conformance testing ensuring reliable implementation, and certification programs validating standard adherence. These interoperability standards address the critical safety gaps created when medication information remains trapped within isolated systems, establishing reliable information flow supporting comprehensive medication management across care transitions and organizational boundaries despite diverse underlying technologies rather than perpetuating fragmentation compromising continuity and safety.

Table 14.4: Recent Trends in Medication Safety

Trend	Current Development Stage	Potential Benefits
Precision Medication Safety	Early adoption	Personalized risk profiles Targeted interventions Optimized therapy selection
Learning Health Systems	Pilot implementation	Real-time data utilization System adaptation Continuous improvement
Patient-Controlled Records	Early adoption	Improved information access Patient engagement Transition management
Blockchain Medication Tracking	Pilot testing	Supply chain integrity Complete traceability Counterfeit reduction

Cross-Border Initiatives

Multinational learning networks establish collaborative improvement communities transcending organizational and national boundaries, creating shared knowledge development accelerating safety advancement beyond individual capabilities. Implementation models include collaborative breakthrough initiatives addressing specific safety challenges through shared learning and coordinated implementation; communities of practice connecting professionals across diverse settings for knowledge exchange; virtual collaboration platforms supporting interaction despite geographic separation; and structured comparison methodologies identifying effective practices through systematic assessment across multiple organizations. Medication-specific networks focus on areas including high-alert medication management, medication reconciliation practices, technology implementation approaches, and safety culture development. These collaborative approaches address the inefficiency of isolated improvement reinventing solutions to common challenges, creating accelerated advancement through shared experience while enabling contextual adaptation rather than simplistic practice transplantation ignoring important setting differences.

Regional medication safety partnerships establish coordinated approaches across neighboring countries, addressing cross-border challenges while leveraging geographical proximity for collaborative activity. Notable examples include European Union medication safety initiatives coordinating regulatory approaches and surveillance systems across member states; Southeast Asian regional collaboration addressing cross-border medication supply chain security; Pan American Health Organization programs supporting medication safety development throughout the Americas; and African regional networks building medication safety capacity across neighboring countries with shared challenges and limited resources. Implementation approaches include harmonized regulatory systems supporting consistent safety standards, shared surveillance systems enabling broader pattern recognition, collaborative training developing regional expertise, and resource pooling creating capabilities beyond individual country capacity. These regional approaches address both cross-border medication movement creating safety implications transcending national oversight and the practical benefits of collaboration among countries with geographical proximity and often similar healthcare contexts, creating coordinated improvement leveraging shared characteristics while respecting necessary national adaptations.

Refugee and migrant population initiatives address the unique medication safety challenges faced by displaced populations crossing international boundaries, developing specialized approaches for these vulnerable groups with disrupted healthcare access and documentation. Implementation strategies include medication passport systems providing portable medication history documentation; translation tools supporting communication despite language barriers; cultural competency development among healthcare providers serving diverse populations; standardized approaches to medication reconciliation with limited historical information; and coordination mechanisms between non-governmental organizations, host country healthcare systems, and international agencies sharing responsibility for refugee healthcare. These specialized approaches address the particular vulnerability of populations receiving care across multiple countries with fragmented documentation and complex social determinants affecting medication management, creating appropriate safety protections for displaced individuals rather than accepting heightened risk as inevitable consequence of migration and displacement.

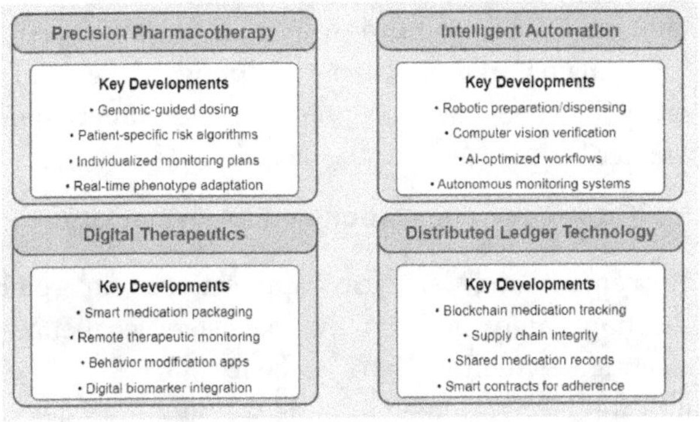

Figure 14.2 Recent Trends in Medication Safety

Global supply chain integrity initiatives establish international approaches to medication authenticity and quality, addressing the safety challenges created by increasingly complex multinational production and distribution networks. Implementation includes track-and-trace systems following medications from manufacture through distribution using standardized identification; international verification networks confirming product authenticity across borders; harmonized good manufacturing practice standards ensuring consistent production quality; coordinated inspection programs leveraging regulatory resources across countries; and rapid alert systems sharing information about identified counterfeit or substandard products. Technical foundations include serialization standards supporting unique product identification, blockchain implementations creating tamper-evident distribution records, data exchange protocols enabling information sharing between systems, and authentication technologies verifying product legitimacy at the point of dispensing. These international approaches address the fundamental safety threats created by globalized pharmaceutical production and distribution, establishing reliable quality assurance despite complex multinational supply chains rather than accepting compromised integrity as inevitable consequence of international commerce.

14.3.4 Knowledge Translation and Implementation

Implementation science applications in global medication safety address the persistent challenge of translating evidence into practice across diverse healthcare environments, developing systematic approaches to effective intervention deployment despite varying contexts. Methodologies include consolidated systems systematically assessing implementation factors including intervention characteristics, implementation setting, individual attributes, and process elements; determinant systems identifying factors influencing implementation success; implementation strategy taxonomies categorizing approaches supporting successful adoption; and evaluation models assessing both implementation processes and outcomes. Medication safety applications include structured assessment of contextual factors affecting technology implementation in different settings; tailored implementation strategies matched to specific organizational characteristics; barrier identification and mitigation planning before deployment; and appropriate adaptation preserving core safety elements while accommodating necessary contextual modifications. These scientific approaches address the frequent failure of demonstrably effective interventions during real-world implementation, creating systematic rather than haphazard approaches to successful deployment across diverse global healthcare environments.

Context-appropriate technology adaptation establishes principles for modifying technological approaches to medication safety based on setting characteristics, addressing the critical need for solutions matched to specific implementation environments rather than inappropriate technology transfer ignoring contextual realities. Main considerations include infrastructure requirements matching available resources, sustainability assessment ensuring ongoing operation capability, appropriate complexity aligned with local technical expertise, cultural factors affecting acceptance and utilization, and potential for incremental enhancement as capabilities develop. Implementation approaches include phased technology introduction beginning with fundamental capabilities before advanced features, hybrid systems combining technological and manual processes appropriate to transition stages, locally sustainable support models, and capability-building integrated with technology deployment. These adaptive approaches address the frequent failure of technology implementations misaligned with local contexts, creating appropriate solutions matched to actual implementation environments rather than imposing approaches developed for entirely different settings without necessary adaptation.

Knowledge mobilization strategies establish systematic approaches to sharing medication safety information across global contexts, addressing the persistent challenge of valuable knowledge remaining inaccessible where needed for improvement. Implementation approaches include multi-format dissemination creating accessibility regardless of technological limitations; translation services addressing language barriers; adaptation support modifying approaches for different contexts while maintaining core safety principles; and push-pull mechanisms combining proactive information distribution with user-initiated access based on specific needs. Technical foundations include open access publications removing financial barriers to information access; searchable repositories supporting efficient information location; metadata tagging enabling context-appropriate filtering; and rating systems identifying highest-value resources. These knowledge sharing approaches address the fundamental injustice of safety information inequity, creating appropriate accessibility throughout diverse global settings rather than confined availability in resource-rich environments despite universal relevance to medication safety improvement.

Sustainable capacity development establishes long-term capability building rather than temporary intervention, addressing the critical need for enduring medication safety improvement beyond short-term projects or external assistance. Implementation approaches include workforce development creating local expertise through structured training and mentorship; institutional capability building establishing organizational structures supporting ongoing improvement; leadership development ensuring appropriate governance and strategic direction; and resource mobilization developing sustainable funding supporting continued activities. Sustainability planning addresses critical elements including knowledge transfer creating local ownership; phased transition reducing external dependence; appropriate technology selection considering long-term maintenance capabilities; and integration with existing systems rather than parallel structures requiring separate support.

Things to Remember

- ☑ Emerging technologies include advanced dispensing robotics reducing human manipulation errors, autonomous mobile robots providing reliable transportation, closed-loop administration systems creating comprehensive verification, and Internet of Things applications connecting previously isolated systems.
- ☑ Artificial intelligence applications include adverse event prediction models identifying high-risk patients, personalized dosing systems accounting for individual factors, adaptive alert systems reducing fatigue, and natural language interfaces enabling intuitive interaction.
- ☑ Validation methodologies for AI must address the unique challenges of evaluating complex adaptive systems through rigorous testing across diverse clinical scenarios and continuous monitoring after implementation.
- ☑ Global initiatives establish collaborative approaches through WHO programs like Medication Without Harm, international classification systems, medication safety monitoring networks, and cross-border collaborations.
- ☑ Implementation science methodologies support effective technology and practice deployment across diverse healthcare settings through structured adaptation rather than simple adoption.
- ☑ Ethical rules addressing issues like transparency, equity, privacy, and autonomy must guide advanced technology implementation in safety-critical healthcare applications

Multiple Choice Questions

1. Emerging technologies transforming medication management include:
   a) Paper-based documentation systems
   b) Centralized medication distribution without automation
   c) Advanced dispensing robotics reducing human manipulation errors
   d) Manual verification processes without technological assistance
2. Artificial intelligence applications in medication safety include:
   a) Static alert systems without contextual adaptation
   b) Replacement of all human decision-making in medication processes
   c) Adverse event prediction models identifying patients at elevated risk
   d) Technology limited to data storage without analytical capabilities
3. Closed-loop medication administration systems create:
   a) Processes requiring minimal documentation
   b) Comprehensive verification throughout medication processes
   c) Systems focused exclusively on controlled substances
   d) Implementation without workflow consideration
4. Global initiatives establishing collaborative medication safety approaches include:
   a) Country-specific programs without international coordination

b) WHO programs including Medication Without Harm

c) Focus exclusively on high-income countries

d) Elimination of country-specific approaches in favor of standardization

5. Implementation science methodologies support effective technology deployment through:

   a) Rapid implementation without adaptation to local context

   b) Exclusive focus on technology without consideration of users

   c) Structured adaptation rather than simple adoption

   d) Identical approaches regardless of organizational characteristics

6. Ethical considerations in advanced technology implementation include:

   a) Focus exclusively on efficiency without safety consideration

   b) Addressing issues like transparency, equity, and privacy

   c) Implementation without regulatory oversight

   d) Prioritizing cost savings above patient outcomes

7. Internet of Things applications in medication safety involve:

   a) Isolated systems without connectivity between components

   b) Connecting previously isolated systems into coordinated networks

   c) Technology limited to pharmacy

environments without clinical areas

d) Focus exclusively on inventory management without safety applications

8. Adaptive alert systems in clinical decision support:

   a) Present identical alerts to all users regardless of context

   b) Reduce alert fatigue while maintaining critical warnings

   c) Function without integration with electronic health records

   d) Eliminate the need for clinical judgment in medication decisions

9. International classification systems supporting medication safety:

   a) Are relevant only for research without clinical application

   b) Ensure consistent categorization supporting cross-border learning

   c) Apply only to adverse events without near-miss situations

   d) Are limited to specific medication classes without comprehensive coverage

10. Natural language interfaces enabling intuitive interaction with clinical systems:

    a) Are primarily useful for non-clinical applications

    b) Require extensive technical training for effective use

    c) Support clinical workflows through simplified information access

    d) Function without integration with structured data systems

Self-Assessment Questions

1. Critically analyze how emerging technologies such as smart pumps, automated dispensing systems, and wearable monitoring devices are transforming medication safety practices.
2. Evaluate the current and potential applications of artificial intelligence in medication safety, including benefits, limitations, and ethical considerations.
3. Analyze global medication safety initiatives, comparing approaches between different regions and evaluating their effectiveness in improving patient outcomes.
4. Discuss how big data analytics is being applied to medication safety and its potential to transform adverse event detection and prevention strategies.
5. Evaluate the emerging role of patients as active participants in medication safety through technologies, engagement strategies, and shared decision-making models.
6. Analyze how telehealth and remote patient monitoring are changing medication safety practices and the unique challenges these modalities present.
7. Discuss the application of human factors engineering and design thinking to medication safety innovation, with examples of successful implementations.
8. Evaluate how precision medicine and pharmacogenomics are influencing medication

safety considerations and personalized risk mitigation strategies.

9. Analyze emerging approaches to medication safety education for healthcare professionals, including simulation, interprofessional learning, and continuous professional development.
10. Discuss how social, economic, and political factors are influencing the future direction of medication safety research, policy, and practice globally.

Bibliography

1. Bates DW, Saria S, Ohno-Machado L, Shah A, Escobar G. Big data in health care: using analytics to identify and manage high-risk and high-cost patients. Health Aff (Millwood). 2014;33(7):1123-31.
2. Bates DW, Gawande AA. Improving safety with information technology. N Engl J Med. 2003;348(25):2526-34.
3. Obermeyer Z, Emanuel EJ. Predicting the future - big data, machine learning, and clinical medicine. N Engl J Med. 2016;375(13):1216-9.
4. Shortliffe EH, Sepúlveda MJ. Clinical decision support in the era of artificial intelligence. JAMA. 2018;320(21):2199-200.
5. Beam AL, Kohane IS. Big data and machine learning in health care. JAMA. 2018;319(13):1317-8.
6. Rajkomar A, Dean J, Kohane I. Machine learning in medicine. N Engl J Med. 2019;380(14):1347-58.
7. Saria S, Butte A, Sheikh A. Better medicine through machine learning: what's real, and what's artificial? PLoS Med. 2018;15(12):e1002721.
8. Doan S, Maehara CK, Chaparro JD, Lu S, Liu R, Graham A, et al. Building a natural language processing tool to identify patients with high clinical suspicion for Kawasaki disease from emergency department notes. Acad Emerg Med. 2016;23(5):628-36.
9. Agrawal A. Medication errors: prevention using information technology systems. Br J Clin Pharmacol. 2009;67(6):681-6.
10. World Health Organization. Medication Without Harm - Global Patient Safety Challenge on Medication Safety. Geneva: World Health Organization; 2017

ANSWERS TO THE MCQS

Chapter 1
1. b
2. a
3. b
4. c
5. c
6. b
7. c
8. a
9. c
10. c

Chapter 2
1. b
2. b
3. c
4. b
5. b
6. c
7. c
8. c
9. b
10. c

Chapter 3
1. c
2. c
3. c
4. c
5. b
6. c
7. c
8. c
9. b
10. b

Chapter 4
1. b
2. d
3. c
4. b
5. c
6. a
7. b
8. c
9. c
10. b

Chapter 5
1. c
2. b
3. c
4. b
5. b
6. c
7. b
8. c
9. b
10. b

Chapter 6
1. b
2. b
3. b
4. b
5. c
6. c
7. c
8. b
9. c
10. c

Chapter 7
1. c
2. d
3. b
4. c
5. b
6. b
7. c
8. b
9. c
10. b

Chapter 8
1. b
2. c
3. b
4. c
5. b
6. b
7. c
8. b
9. b
10. c

Chapter 9
1. b
2. c
3. c
4. c
5. c
6. b
7. c
8. c
9. b
10. c

Chapter 10

1. b
2. c
3. c
4. c
5. b
6. b
7. c
8. c
9. c
10. b

Chapter 11

1. b
2. c
3. b
4. b
5. d
6. c
7. b
8. d
9. c
10. c

Chapter 12

1. b
2. b
3. c
4. c
5. b
6. c
7. b
8. c
9. b
10. c

Chapter 13

1. b
2. b
3. b
4. c
5. b
6. b
7. c
8. c
9. b
10. c

Chapter 14

1. c
2. c
3. b
4. b
5. c
6. b
7. b
8. b
9. b
10. c

ABOUT THE AUTHORS

Dr. RAJKIRAN KOLAKOTA

Dr. Rajkiran Kolakota serves as Principal and Professor of Pharmacology at Sri Sivani College of Pharmacy, Srikakulam. He earned his postgraduate and doctoral degrees from Andhra University, Visakhapatnam. With 18 years of experience in pharmaceutical research, teaching, and administration, he has authored over 50 publications in reputed journals and holds four patents. His work focuses on advancing pharmacological education and innovation.

Mr. SRI VENKATESH URITI

Mr. U. Sri Venkatesh is an Associate Professor in the Department of Pharmacology at Sri Sivani College of Pharmacy, Srikakulam, Andhra Pradesh. With over eight years of experience in academia, he has published 30 research articles, secured four patents, and contributed to two book chapters. He actively participates in faculty development programs, ATAL workshops, and UGC-MMTC short-term courses. He holds lifetime memberships in professional organizations including APTI, IPA, OPF, and SPER. In 2024, he received the "Outstanding Liaison in Community Engagement Award" from the Council for Skills and Competencies.

Mr. MANOJ KUMAR GEMBALI

Mr. Manoj Kumar Gembali is an Associate Professor at Sri Sivani College of Pharmacy. He holds a Master's degree in Pharmacy and brings more than 12 years of teaching experience. He has guided over 20 M.Pharm and 60 B.Pharm students in their research projects throughout his academic career.

Mrs. MANJULATHA KORNU

Mrs. Manjulatha Kornu is an Assistant Professor in the Department of Regulatory Affairs at Sri Sivani College of Pharmacy, Srikakulam, Andhra Pradesh. She brings over four years of combined experience from industry and academia, and has secured three patents. She actively participates in professional development through ATAL workshops, UGC-MMTC courses, and FDPs. She is a lifetime member of the Association of Pharmaceutical Teachers of India (APTI).

www.ingramcontent.com/pod-product-compliance
Lightning Source LLC
Chambersburg PA
CBHW062132160726
48282CB00027B/797
* 9 7 8 8 1 9 7 9 7 3 1 4 7 *